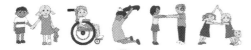

Models of Child Health Appraised
(A Study of Primary Healthcare in 30 European countries)

ISSUES AND OPPORTUNITIES IN PRIMARY HEALTH CARE FOR CHILDREN IN EUROPE

ISSUES AND OPPORTUNITIES IN PRIMARY HEALTH CARE FOR CHILDREN IN EUROPE

The Final Summarised Results of the Models of Child Health Appraised (MOCHA) Project

EDITED BY

MITCH BLAIR, MICHAEL RIGBY, DENISE ALEXANDER

Imperial College London, UK

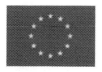

The project was funded by the European Commission through the Horizon 2020 Framework under the grant agreement number: 634201. The sole responsibility for the content of this work lies with the authors. It does not necessarily reflect the opinion of the European Union. The European Commission is not responsible for any use that may be made of the information contained therein

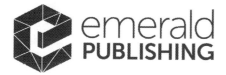

United Kingdom – North America – Japan – India – Malaysia – China

Emerald Publishing Limited
Howard House, Wagon Lane, Bingley BD16 1WA, UK

First edition 2019

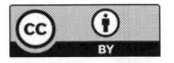
British Library Cataloguing in Publication Data
A catalogue record for this book is available from the British Library

ISBN: 978-1-78973-354-9 (Print)
ISBN: 978-1-78973-351-8 (Online)
ISBN: 978-1-78973-353-2 (Epub)

The ebook edition of this title is Open Access and is freely available to read
online.

Open Access

ISOQAR certified
Management System,
awarded to Emerald
for adherence to
Environmental
standard
ISO 14001:2004.

ISOQAR
REGISTERED

Certificate Number 1985
ISO 14001

INVESTOR IN PEOPLE

Contents

List of Figures

List of Tables

List of Contributors

Denise Alexander	Imperial College London, UK
Manna Alma	University Medical Center Groningen, Netherlands
Amina Al-Yassin	Imperial College London, UK
Jay Berry	Boston Children's Hospital, USA
Mitch Blair	Imperial College London, UK
Magda Boere-Boonekamp	University of Twente, Netherlands
Maria Brenner	Trinity College Dublin, Ireland
Anne Clancy	University of Tromsø, Norway
Barbara Corso	CNR Neuroscience Institute (IN), Padova, Italy
Shalmali Deshpande	Imperial College London, UK
Filipa Ferreira	University of Surrey, UK
Heather Gage	University of Surrey, UK
Karin Groothuis-Oudshoorn	University of Twente, Netherlands
Carol Hilliard	Our Lady's Children's Hospital, Crumlin, Dublin
Eleanor Hollywood	Trinity College Dublin, Ireland
Uy Hoang	University of Surrey, UK
Danielle Jansen	University Medical Center Groningen, Netherlands
Stine Lundstroem Kamionka	University of Southern Denmark, Denmark
Nicole van Kesteren	TNO (Netherlands Organisation for Applied Scientific Research), Netherlands
Paul Kocken	TNO (Netherlands Organisation for Applied Scientific Research), Netherlands
Grit Kühne	Imperial College London, UK
Uttara Kurup	Imperial College London, UK
Philip Larkin	Université de Lausanne, Switzerland, *previously*
Sapfo Lignou	King's College London, UK
Gaby de Lijster	TNO (Netherlands Organisation for Applied Scientific Research), Netherlands
Harshana Liyanage	University of Surrey, UK
Simon de Lusignan	University of Surrey, UK

Daniela Luzi	CNR Institute for Research on Population and Social Policies (IRPPS), Rome, Italy
Ekelechi MacPepple	University of Surrey, UK
Michael Mahgerefteh	Imperial College London, UK
Arjun Menon	Imperial College London, UK
Pierre-André Michaud	University Hospital of Lausanne, Switzerland
Nadia Minicuci	CNR Neuroscience Institute (IN), Padova, Italy
Elena Montañana Olaso	Trinity College Dublin, Ireland
Miriam O'Shea	Trinity College Dublin, Ireland
Catharina Nitsche	Imperial College London, UK
Colman Noctor	Trinity College Dublin, Ireland
Fabrizio Pecoraro	CNR Institute for Research on Population and Social Policies (IRPPS), Rome, Italy
Sijmen A. Reijneveld	University Medical Center Groningen, Netherlands
Michael Rigby	Imperial College London, UK
Ilaria Rocco	CNR Neuroscience Institute (IN), Padova, Italy
Mariana Miranda Autran Sampaio	Imperial College London, UK
Rose Satherley	King's College London, UK
Tamara Schloemer	Maastricht University, Netherlands
Peter Schröder-Bäck	Maastricht University, Netherlands
Oscar Tamburis	CNR Institute for Research on Population and Social Policies (IRPPS), Rome, Italy
Keishia Taylor	Trinity College Dublin, Ireland
Janine van Til	University of Twente, Netherlands
Johanna P. M. Vervoort	University Medical Center Groningen, Netherlands
Annemieke Visser	University Medical Center Groningen, Netherlands
Eline Vlasblom	TNO (Netherlands Organisation for Applied Scientific Research), Netherlands
Austin Warters	Trinity College Dublin, Ireland
Helen Wells	Keele University, UK
Ingrid Wolfe	King's College London, UK
Kinga Zdunek	Medical University of Lublin, Poland
Renate van Zoonen	TNO (Netherlands Organisation for Applied Scientific Research), Netherlands

Foreword

When I reflect back on the last 35 years of clinical practice as a paediatrician, I am very aware of the considerable changes to children's health which have occurred in my country and in Europe. Many diseases I saw as a student and young trainee have all but disappeared through the development and administration of new vaccines or the introduction of novel technological discoveries such as artificial surfactant, home ventilation and new drugs for cancer treatment. These have resulted in improved survival of so many children and young people who would have otherwise suffered premature death from the myriad of different congenital or acquired conditions. At the same time, I am all too cognisant of the effects of the degree of social change both in terms of the changing nature of family structure and stability, of unacceptable levels of poverty and inequity, environmental challenges such as nutrition, housing and pollution, the effects of national and international conflict leading to unprecedented movement of families between continents and of the huge changes in the speed and breadth of communication and social media. In parallel, there are increased levels of mental health disorder, obesity, neurodevelopmental issues such as specific learning difficulties, ADHD and autism and the sheer complexity of multimorbidity of twenty-first-century children and young people.

How do we ensure that we keep up to date and that clinical care remains relevant and effective in such circumstances? Clearly, clinical practice not only depends on the capacity and competence of well-trained practitioners but also depends on the context of a country or region's health care system and this, in turn, has its own historical, cultural, political and economic origins. And in any country, primary care is the first port of call, where the great majority of prevention, diagnosis and treatment are carried out.

It is the attention to both the clinical and the wider aspects of primary child health care which was the focus and purpose of the Models of Child Health Appraised (MOCHA) project, funded by the European Union's Horizon 2020 programme from 2015 to 2018. MOCHA set out to describe the organisation of primary care for children and young people in all 28 EU and two EEA countries in Europe. We originally set out to answer which systems work best and how might we use such knowledge to improve the delivery of primary care for this population; it also allowed us a unique view of the current situation in Europe and how we might shape the next era. As a multidisciplinary international research team of over 80 individuals, we wanted to explore this from multiple perspectives and this is reflected in the fact that we drew expertise from many different professional and scientific disciplines: paediatrics, school and adolescent specialists, public health and family practice, nursing, social science and care, political science, economics, health management, informatics, epidemiology, statistics and even criminology.

Michael, Denise and I have worked with each other for at least two decades on a number of European projects and for MOCHA – this itself is a story, to be told elsewhere, of the slow evolution of European child public health projects. In MOCHA, we were most ably supported by our project manager, Christine Chow. My respect for and gratitude to them all is immeasurable. This core team, along with the committed group of co-worker scientists slowly growing in number and influence over this period, very much bonded as a 'family' over the last four years, and together we have been on a fascinating voyage of discovery, challenge and mutual learning. In another aspect of development, eight babies were born to members of the MOCHA family over that time!

It has been an extraordinarily rich experience for me personally and I am sure this is the same for many of those involved. We have had many challenges. It was frustrating and disappointing that we were unable to find robust and readily available routine data to inform so many of our appraisal processes, an important discovery in itself. However, we gained enormously from the insights of children in a number of countries who told us what they thought about the services offered, and especially and uniquely, from the detailed answers from the country agents in each country and from the extensive literature and other reviews carried out by the MOCHA scientists. This book is the culmination of that joint learning which I know will help us all to take the next steps in further improving the outcomes for millions of children and young people in Europe.

Professor Mitch Blair – Principle Investigator, MOCHA.
Imperial College, London, UK

Chapter 1

The MOCHA Project: Origins, Approach and Methods

Mitch Blair, Denise Alexander and Michael Rigby

Abstract

Primary care (PC) is a strong determinant of overall health care. Children make up around a fifth of the population of the European Union and European Economic Area and have their own needs and uptake of PC. However, there is little research into how well PC services address their needs. There are large differences in childhood mortality and morbidity patterns in the EU and EEA countries, and there has been a major epidemiological shift in the past half century from predominantly communicable disease, to non-communicable diseases presenting and increasingly managed in PC. This increase in multifactorial morbidities, such as obesity and learning disability, has led to the need for PC systems to adapt to accommodate these changes. Europe presents a challenging picture of unexplained variation in health care delivery and style and of children's different health experiences and health-related behaviour. The Models of Child Health Appraised (MOCHA) project aimed to describe the PC systems in detail, analyse their components and appraise them from a number of different viewpoints, including professional, public, political and economic lenses. It did this through nine work packages supported by a core management team, and a network of national agents, individuals in each MOCHA country who had the expertise in research and knowledge of their national health care system to answer a wide range of questions posed by the MOCHA scientific teams.

Keywords: Child health; primary care; scientific appraisal; research; child morbidity; child

Background and Origins

Primary care (PC) is the first point of contact with the health services for most people. Almost all health care, except for major trauma, starts in PC.[1] PC, therefore, strongly determines the overall pattern of health care, and also to a great extent, it influences the pattern of health of the population. Children are a fifth of the population and have their own needs for and patterns of uptake of PC. Despite this, there is little research into the use of PC by children and young people and into how well PC services address the needs of children and young people.

Children's health affects the future of Europe. Children are citizens, future workers, future parents and carers and the future elderly population. Ensuring an optimum healthy start to each child's life is the basis for later active and healthy ageing. Children may only make up to a fifth of the population of each country, but they are 100% of our future.

A child's health is determined by many factors over the life course, including the influence of the family, peers, culture, beliefs, education, physical environment and of course health services (World Health Organization, 2008). These elements can either protect and promote health, or restrict the family's choices about health. A child changes considerably at different ages and at developmental stages. At the beginning of life, he or she is entirely dependent on others and highly influenced by the family, social, educational and natural environment. In the teenage years, there is a shift to increasing independence and autonomy, requiring a different health service response.

PC health services are influenced by many determinants, such as the history, culture, politics and economics of a country (see Chapter 17; Blair, Stewart-Brown, Waterson, & Crowther, 2010). The child and family, also, exert a powerful influence in shaping health services through co-creation with health professionals (Ferrer, 2015). It is this dynamic interaction between the developing child and family and the health services that is a core aspect of the Models of Child Health Appraised (MOCHA) project, funded by the European Commission's Horizon 2020 research programme (European Commission, 2018).

Society has a duty to provide health care. Though much reliance is placed, rightly, on the family, it has to be recognised that for some children, this support is missing or compromised. In addition, a child's health is strongly affected by the immediate physical, economic and cultural environment; this can take the form of, among other factors, the relationship between pollution and respiratory health; the availability of toys or books in the house and cognitive and language development; or the impact of social media on self-image, peer relationships and well-being. The health services play an important role in safeguarding children from such threats to their health. Essentially, not only is a child's good health

---

[1]According to the UK Royal College of General Practitioners in evidence to the UK Parliamentary Select Committee on Health, primary care accounts for 90% of patient contacts with the English NHS, but the source is not cited, and no equivalent figure is available from WHO, OECD or Eurostat.

desirable, but it is a fundamental right, as set out by the UN Convention on the Rights of the Child in Article 24 (United Nations, 1989; Chapter 4).

Children's Health in Europe

The variations in child and adolescent health status in Europe are well described in the latest Report from the World Health Organization (World Health Organization Regional Office for Europe, 2018b). In the past decade there have been considerable improvements in overall childhood mortality with major reductions being seen in all countries over time. Seventeen of the 30 MOCHA countries have adopted the WHO Child and Adolescent Health Regional Strategy 2015–2020 (Regional Committee for Europe, 2015) which was designed to help member states develop:

> evidence-based frameworks for review and improvement of child and adolescent health and development policies, programmes and action plans from a life-course perspective; promote multisectoral action; and identify the health sectors role in developing and coordinating policy and delivering services that meet children's and adolescent's health needs.
>
> (World Health Organization Regional Office for Europe, 2018b, p. 3)

Twelve of the 17 countries adopting the Strategy have reported that they specifically allocated budgets and have monitoring systems in place (World Health Organization Regional Office for Europe, 2018b).

Despite this, there are large differences between Member States in both mortality and morbidity patterns, risk-taking and exploratory behaviours, mental health and well-being, infectious diseases and environmental health, nutrition and physical activity levels and the degree to which rights and participation of children and young people are exercised. For example, the difference in recently reported hospitalisation rates of 0- to 14-year-olds varies fivefold between Spain and Bulgaria (52/1,000 and 256/1,000, respectively). About 90% of Lithuanian 15-year-old boys report "high life satisfaction levels" compared to 84% in the UK. Variations in PC family practitioner service provision indicate that Greece has almost nine times fewer general practitioners (GPs) per 100,000 population than Portugal (World Health Organization Regional Office for Europe, 2018b).

Thus, Europe presents a challenging picture of unexplained variation in health care delivery and style and of children's different health experiences and health-related behaviour. This also means that Europe provides a unique laboratory to examine different health systems in depth and, in particular, the PC system contribution to health and well-being and its contribution to the health of Europe's children. There is little knowledge relevant to twenty-first-century Europe of the effects on child health of publically funded health systems versus insurance based, and the relative access and provision of services (especially preventive services) to children within these, together with regulatory and governance issues; the benefits or otherwise of some direct personal service provision (such as immunisation and screening) by dedicated public sector child health services; the role of and provision of different models of school health services; models of the availability and adequacy of direct access for adolescents to mental health and reproductive health services in particular, to avoid unnecessary morbidity and mortality; and models of care for children and their families at the acute—community interface and at health—social care interface for children at risk or in receipt of social care.

Changing Epidemiology

The last 50 years has seen a major shift in disease patterns in many countries from a predominance of communicable disease to one of the non-communicable morbidities, such as mental health, long-standing illness and injury (Haggerty, 1995; Wolfe, Thompson, et al., 2013). This epidemiological shift from single agent causes, such as infectious disease, to multifactorial morbidities such as obesity or learning disability requires a change in emphasis in PC practice. Specific professional skills are necessary to tackle these issues, while ensuring that the key attributes of PC — access, coordination, continuity and equitable service provision — are maintained (Starfield, Shi, & Macinko, 2005).

Defining Primary Care and Its Scope

The MOCHA project has worked to certain definitions of functions and features of PC:

- *Primary health care (PHC)* refers to the concept elaborated in the 1978 Declaration of Alma-Ata (World Health Organization, 1978), which is based on the principles of equity, participation, inter-sectoral action, appropriate technology and a central role played by the health system.
- *PC* is first-contact, accessible, continued, comprehensive and coordinated care. Ideally, first-contact care is accessible at the time of need, ongoing care focuses on the long-term health of a person rather than the short duration of a specific disease, comprehensive care is a range of services appropriate to the common problems in the respective members of the population, and coordination is the role by which PC acts to coordinate other specialists that the patient may need (World Health Organization, 2018a).
- *General practice* is a term now often used loosely to cover the general practitioner and other personnel and is therefore synonymous with PC and family medicine (FM). Originally, it was meant to describe the concept and model around the most significant single player in PC: the general practitioner or PC physician, while FM originally encompassed the notion of a team approach as well as recognition of the patient's family own setting. The general practitioner is the only physician who operates at the nine levels of care: prevention, screening, early diagnosis, diagnosis of established disease, management of disease, management of disease complications, rehabilitation, palliative care and counselling (World Health Organization, 2018a).

- *FM or PC teams* can vary between countries and in size: the core team usually is the general practitioner and a nurse, but can comprise a multidisciplinary team of up to 30 professionals including community nurses, midwives, feldshers,[2] dentists, physiotherapists, social workers, psychiatrists, speech and language therapists, dietitians, pharmacists, administrative staff and managers. PC/FM teams should be patient-centred, so their composition and organisational model can change over time (World Health Organization, 2018a).
- *PC paediatricians* deal comprehensively with the health and well-being of infants, children and adolescents within the context of their families, communities and cultures. PC paediatrics sees infants, children and adolescents as its main subject of care, respecting their autonomy and involving parents, guardians and/or custodians as integral part of the 'unit of care'. They may or may not work with multidisciplinary teams (ECPCP, 2018).
- *Nursing* encompasses autonomous and collaborative care of individuals of all ages, families, groups and communities, sick or well and in all settings. Nursing includes the promotion of health, prevention of illness and the care of ill, disabled and dying people. Advocacy, promotion of a safe environment, research, participation in shaping health policy and in patient and health systems management, and education are also key nursing roles. Nurses include professional nurses, enrolled nurses, auxiliary nurses and other nurses such as dental or PC nurses (International Council of Nurses, 2015).

Scope of Primary Child Health Care in MOCHA

The principles of PC can be described by their functioning; however, the pattern of provision of each can vary according to regulation and governance, funding mechanism, access rules and distribution within a community. Thus, there are many forms of PC for children across Europe which are taken as being within the scope of the MOCHA project. They are as follows:

- physician care for acute (in and out of office hours) and chronic illness;
- nursing care including home visiting (especially where the nurse acts autonomously or with only very broad supervision);
- school health (school is frequently considered as 'outside' the usual model of PC services – but is often the primary access point for health care for this cohort of children)
- direct access services, particularly for adolescents (also often considered outside PC, but a vital first contact point);
- community pharmacy;
- community dental services;
- health promotion services; and
- society-facing e-health (telephone hotlines, websites and apps).

---

[2]A health care professional who provides various medical services limited to emergency treatment and ambulance practice.

Despite PC being an important aspect of health care for children, it is at the same time a relatively under-addressed area of health systems research. This is despite the importance and potential for massive health gains that focusing on the child population of Europe can provide both for children and young people themselves (well-being) and for future adults (well becoming). On this background, a number of publications have described the previous provision of paediatric services in PC in Europe and have demonstrated a pattern of decreasing numbers of PC paediatric providers and an increase in GP led and mixed medical and nursing systems (Ehrich et al., 2015; van Esso et al., 2010; Katz, Rubino, Coller, Rosen, & Ehrich, 2002). However, evidence of differences in outcomes attributable to different systems is somewhat scant (Wolfe, Thompson, et al., 2013) and certainly there has to date been no systematic research of all 30 EU and EEA countries carried out prior to the MOCHA project.

The EC Horizon 2020 call in the area of public health care research in 2014 (*H2020-PHC-23-2014, Developing and comparing new models for safe and efficient, prevention oriented health and care systems*) gave an opportunity for us to bid successfully for a €6.8m grant to enable the Imperial College-led team to research the primary child health care provision in 28 EU and two EEA countries with the objective of describing and appraising this diversity of health care systems in relation to child health and with the advantage of a number of different and complementary scientific disciplines. We were keen to build on the knowledge and experience gained on previous European projects on which many of the scientists had worked together. These included CHILD (on indicators), PHASE (on public health actions for a safer Europe), EUGLOREH (on state of health), RICHE (on child health research gaps) and TRANSFoRm (on linking health databases), as well as the WHO European Region Child and Adolescent Health and Development Strategy 2005 and its monitoring subproject.

A strong feature of MOCHA, as was also the case in the aforementioned projects, has been the assembly of a very broad multidisciplinary research team of selected scientists from across Europe, together with focussed American and Australian input. The team consisted of 19 institutional partners in 11 countries with expert scientists in the fields of paediatric, adolescent and family practice medicine, child public health, nursing, psychology, policy and health management, political science, sociology, statistics, informatics, epidemiology and health economics. Like a kaleidoscope, we were able to shine many different lights on the issue and look at PC in its many forms. The following sections describe the overall aims and how the project was structured to meet these.

MOCHA Project Aims

A key objective for MOCHA was firstly to describe the PC systems in detail and their components and to appraise them from a number of different viewpoints, professional, public (including parents, children and wider community), political and economic lenses.

More specifically, we wished:

- to describe the various models of PC that exist in the 28 EU countries and two EEA countries;
- to describe the full scope of PC that exists for young people including school and adolescent health services, helplines, community pharmacy and dental services;
- to research existing theoretical appraisal frameworks for PC systems and their use;
- to source measures of health systems outcomes and PC quality including national and regional databases;
- to describe the workforce structure in each country and economic aspects of health-care funding and spend and their relationship;
- to analyse equity of provision of the various models;
- to describe the types and use of health records systems as an integral part of a modern effective system;
- to explore child centred socio-political and cultural context and obtain patient and stakeholder views of the system;
- to identify optimal models of patient-centred, prevention-oriented, efficient, resilient, safe and sustainable child health system provision; and
- to raise awareness of the issues and assess transferability between settings.

MOCHA Project Structure and Operation

The project was designed around a number of discrete Scientific Work Packages (WPs) with their own leads and focusing on specific interrelated themes listed below:

- WP1: Identification of the various models of children's PHC;
- WP2: Safe and efficient interfaces of models of children's PHC;
- WP3: Effective models of school and adolescent health services;
- WP4: Identification and application of innovative measures of quality and outcomes of models;
- WP5: Identification and use of derivatives of large data sets and systems to measure quality;
- WP6: Economic and skill set evaluation and analysis of models;
- WP7: Ensuring equity for all children in all models;
- WP8: Use of electronic records to enable safe and efficient models; and
- WP9: Validated optimal models of children's prevention-oriented PHC.

The various scientific WPs were supported by a core project management team also responsible for dissemination strategy for the outputs. An external advisory board (EAB) was assembled to give further scientific and contextual support to the core team and WP leads throughout the project period. This consisted of individuals drawn from international scientists, non-government organisations and European specialist associations, with its own chairperson.

A full list of the scientists in each WP and the leads and EAB members is given in Appendix 1.

Country Agents

Another principle feature has been the extensive use of country agents as informants with local knowledge of the national situation, who have responded to the survey questions set by the scientist teams.

Identifying the Country Agents

Each of the 11 EU/EEA Scientific Partner countries nominated one individual who could act as country agent for their country. In the remaining 19 countries where there was no research partner, the MOCHA country agents were identified through a combination of previous European Union research projects, word of mouth, contacts and requests. This group of individuals were required to undertake specific information gathering tasks to defined instructions and supply academically robust material (see Appendix 2 for a list of Country Agents). The MOCHA project used a mixed-methods approach, reflecting the many influences and components of PC. The agents were expected to have a good knowledge of children's health issues and the national health system and health determinant issues in their country. In addition, they needed to recognise the importance of complete and accurate data being obtained for research and to work with high integrity and have the ability to deal with vernacular material. High levels of trustworthiness and confidence were necessary prerequisites for the scientific team.

We knew that The MOCHA question topics were likely to be diverse, ranging from the care in the community of children with complex care needs, to national data surveillance of child PC tracer conditions, to qualitative research into cultural influences on child health policy-making. Thus, there was a clear expectation that they were also expected to have access to an adequate network to enable the collection of material on aspects on which they themselves were not necessarily always expert.

Developing the Country Agent Working Process and Project Timetable

The Country Agent process was based on 'rounds' of questioning; which began in October 2015 and ended in March 2018. Each round took approximately eight weeks to complete, and each stage within the process was timetabled so that everyone in the project knew when to expect questions and resulting data. In total, 15 rounds of questions were completed during the project.

Broadly, a round consisted of between two and four sets of questions from one or more of the MOCHA WPs. Within the overall scientific plan of the project, each WP team set out its own data requirements strategy, and this was shared at project level to maximise corporate ownership and depth of use. Each WP research team booked a question for a particular round via the project's Research Coordinator, depending on when the relevant deliverable was due, and the logistics of analysis and reporting.

Each WP devised a question set relevant to their research topic, which was then sent to the research coordinator. The objective, rationale and content of each question set were discussed in depth by the MOCHA management team to ensure scientific validity, linguistic clarity and relevance to the overall aims of the MOCHA project. Once agreement at this stage was reached, the questions were then sent to a technical subgroup of the project's EAB for further feedback and revision if necessary, in conjunction with the question authors and research coordinator. The technical subgroup comprised four EAB members who expressed an interest in reviewing the country agent questions. They were sent the questions and given approximately two weeks to give feedback via the research coordinator who discussed suggestions with the relevant WP research team.

The questions were then finalised by the research coordinator and then sent to the country agents who were given approximately four weeks to return the data. This was sent to the research coordinator, who then passed the answers to the research teams for analysis. Any late answers were chased up by the research coordinator, who kept constant communication with each country agent throughout the project. The question process methods are summarised in Figure 1.1.

Data Collection by the Country Agents

The country agents had to fulfil a number of tasks in the project: to gather data for each country, identify expert informants, collate and synthesise data, seek clarification of the data and review project reports. Over the course of the project, they had to answer 15 rounds of questions, which totalled over 900 individual questions and, throughout the life of the project, contact over 100 expert informants. Identifying and contacting the relevant experts in each country was

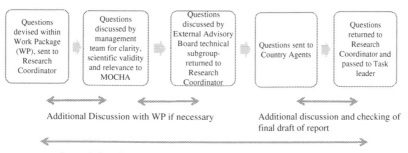

Figure 1.1.   The Country Agent process.

a key skill of the country agent, requiring tenacity and perseverance throughout. The country agents were professional and skilled in research, able to assess and collate data, avoiding artificially showing their country in a falsely positive (or negative) light, as well as adhering to the schedule of the rounds of questions as far as possible.

Data Analyses

Each WP was responsible for the collation of data passed on by the Research Coordinator, and these first-level analyses were made available to other WP teams via the MOCHA project web portal. A number of different techniques were used by the WP scientists in analysing the data from multiple sources. Some of these are listed below and included the following:

- systematic and narrative review and meta-analysis of key functions in relation to life course related tracer conditions;
- the use of case studies and clinical scenarios to reveal the underlying structural and process mechanisms in each country;
- use of standardised survey tools, for example, Standards for Systems of Care for Children and Youth with Special Health Care Needs (WP2) applied to an EU setting;
- structural equation modelling (SEM) and unified business modelling techniques (UML) were applied for a number of tracer conditions or programmes of care; respectively;
- public preference studies were used to ascertain multiple stakeholder perspectives on scenarios of optimal care; and
- qualitative research using thematic analysis of CA text responses and child and parent interviews.

Coordination and WP Interaction

A key aspect of the project management has been the cross fertilisation of individual WPs by regular half-yearly face-to-face meetings and monthly Skype conferencing which facilitated joint learning, supplemented on occasions by specific topic-based workshops. This was a very formative process over the duration of the project, allowing the development of a number of core themes to emerge. Figure 1.2 indicates how this was facilitated.

Throughout the project period, dissemination at a variety of different discipline national and international conferences has allowed us to test some of our emerging ideas with wider scientific and policy audiences. The MOCHA website www.childhealthservicemodels.eu contains a full list of dissemination activities.

There is no doubt that we set itself a challenging remit with a responsibility to the 100 million children living in Europe today. The remainder of this publication details the journey we have taken over the last 42 months and the key items of what our extended team has discovered.

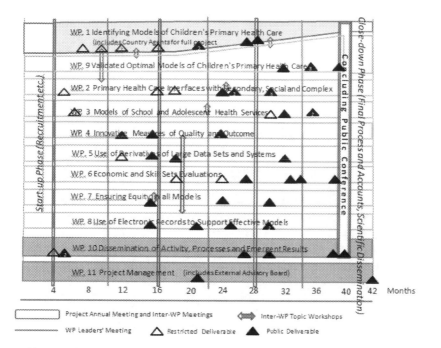

Figure 1.2.   Integration of MOCHA project activities over 42 months.

References

Blair, M., Stewart-Brown, S., Waterson, T., & Crowther, R. (2010). *Child public health*. Oxford: Oxford University Press. Retrieved from http://www.oxfordscholarship.com/view/10.1093/acprof:oso/9780199547500.001.0001/acprof-9780199547500

Ehrich, J. H. H., Tenore, A., del Torso, S., Pettoello-Mantovani, M., Lenton, S., & Grossman, Z. (2015). Diversity of pediatric workforce and education in 2012 in Europe: A need for unifying concepts or accepting enjoyable differences? *Journal of Pediatrics, 167*(2), 471−476.e4. doi:10.1016/jpeds.2015.03.031

van Esso, D., del Torso, S., Hadjipanayis, A., Biver, A., Jaeger-Roman, E., Wettergren, B., ... Primary Secondary Working Group (PSWG) European Academy of Paediatrics. (2010). Paediatric primary care in Europe: Variation between countries. *Archives of Disease in Childhood, 95*(10), 791−795. doi:10.1136/adc.2009.178459

European Commission. (2018). *Horizon 2020*. Retrieved from https://ec.europa.eu/programmes/horizon2020/

European Confederation of Primary Care Paediatrics (ECPCP). (2018). *About us*. Retrieved from https://www.ecpcp.eu/about-us/primary-care-paediatrics/

Ferrer, L. (2015). *Engaging patients, carers and communities for the provision of coordinated/integrated health services: Strategies and tools*. Copenhagen, Denmark: World Health Organization. Retrieved from: http://www.euro.who.int/__data/

assets/pdf_file/0004/290443/Engaging-patients-carers-communities-provision-coor-dinated-integrated-health-services.pdf?ua=1

Haggerty, R. J. (1995). Child health 2000: New pediatrics in the changing environment of children's needs in the 21st century. *Pediatrics, 96*(4), 804−812. Retrieved from http://pediatrics.aappublications.org/content/96/4/804

International council of nurses. (2015). *Nursing definitions*. Retrieved from https://www.icn.ch/nursing-policy/nursing-definitions

Katz, M., Rubino, A., Coller, J., Rosen, J., Ehrich, J. H. (2002). Demography of pediatric primary care in Europe: Delivery of care and training. *Pediatrics, 109*(5), 788−796.

Regional Committee for Europe. (2015). *64th Session regional committee for Europe: Investing in children: The European child and adolescent health strategy 2015−2020*. Retrieved from http://www.euro.who.int/__data/assets/pdf_file/0010/253729/64wd12e_InvestCAHstrategy_140440.pdf?ua=1

Starfield, B., Shi, L., & Macinko, J. (2005). Contribution of primary care to health systems and health. *The Milbank quarterly, 83*(3), 457−502. doi:10.1111/j.1468-0009.2005.00409.x

United Nations. (1989). *Convention on the rights of the child, New York*. London UK: UNICEF UK. Retrieved from https://downloads.unicef.org.uk/wp-content/uploads/2010/05/UNCRC_united_nations_convention_on_the_rights_of_the_child.pdf?_ga=2.209651665.27443 7633.1540996300-199092997.1540996300

Wolfe, I., Thompson, M., Gill, P., Tamburlini, G., Blair, M., van den Bruel, A., Ehrich, J., ... McKee, M. (2013). Health services for children in Western Europe. *The Lancet, 381*(9873), 1224−1234. doi:10.1016/S0140-6736(12)62085-6

World Health Organization. (1978). *Declaration of Alma-ata international conference on primary health care*. Alma-Ata, USSR, September 6−12, 1978. Retrieved from http://www.who.int/publications/almaata_declaration_en.pdf

World Health Organization. (2008). *Commission on social determinants of Health: Closing the gap in a generation* (p. 247). Retrieved from https://www.who.int/social_determinants/thecommission/finalreport/en/

World Health Organization Regional Office for Europe. (2018a). *Primary health care main terminology*. Retrieved from http://www.euro.who.int/en/health-topics/Health-systems/primary-health-care/main-terminology

World Health Organization Regional Office for Europe. (2018b). *Situation of child and adolescent health in Europe*. Retrieved from http://www.euro.who.int/__data/assets/pdf_file/0007/381139/situation-child-adolescent-health-eng.pdf?ua=1

Chapter 2

Models of Primary Care and Appraisal Frameworks

*Mitch Blair, Mariana Miranda Autran Sampaio,
Michael Rigby and Denise Alexander*

Abstract

The Models of Child Health Appraised (MOCHA) project identified the
different models of primary care that exist for children, examined the particular attributes that might be different from those directed at adults and
considered how these models might be appraised. The project took the multiple and interrelated dimensions of primary care and simplified them into a
conceptual framework for appraisal. A general description of the models in
existence in all 30 countries of the EU and EEA countries, focusing on lead
practitioner, financial and regulatory and service provision classifications,
was created. We then used the WHO 'building blocks' for high-performing
health systems as a starting point for identifying a good system for children.
The building blocks encompass safe and good quality services from an educated and empowered workforce, providing good data systems, access to
all necessary medical products, prevention and treatments, and a service
that is adequately financed and well led. An extensive search of the literature failed to identify a suitable appraisal framework for MOCHA, because
none of the frameworks focused on child primary care in its own right.
This led the research team to devise an alternative conceptualisation, at the
heart of which is the core theme of child centricity and ecology, and the
need to focus on delivery to the child through the life course. The MOCHA
model also focuses on the primary care team and the societal and environmental context of the primary care system.

Keywords: Child; primary care; appraisal framework; conceptual
framework; health system; models of care

Introduction

> The primary care values to achieve health, for all require health
> systems that 'Put people at the centre of health care'. (World
> Health Organization, 2008a)

Thirty years after the Alma Ata Declaration (World Health Organization, 1978), the World Health Organization Report: Primary Care More than Ever (2008) highlights the increasing emphasis on person-centred care, as health systems adapt to rapidly changing social circumstances and increasing public expectations. It is in this context, and a decade later, that the Models of Child Health Appraised (MOCHA) project has attempted to appraise the current primary care systems for children and placing them very much at the centre of health care (see Chapter 3).

Children are not mini adults. Their needs for primary care services are specific in a number of ways: from clinical knowledge and skills required to treat them to means of access and types of advocacy. The MOCHA project set out to identify which models of primary care exist for children, whether there are particular attributes which might be different from those directed at adults and how might these models be appraised. To achieve this, it is essential to first be clear about what is meant by a 'model'. In the MOCHA project, we have defined a model as a simplified description of the primary care system, but one that is comprehensive enough to describe the complexity and coordination of its components. Pragmatically, the model allows an overall view of a system, and enables comparison between systems. Thus we have taken the multiple and interrelated dimensions of primary care and attempted to simplify them into a conceptual framework for appraisal in a number of attributes. Ultimately, in the same way as a model farm operates, in which exemplars are produced to maximise crop or animal yields, we set out to identify a validated effective and efficient model or model components which can be assembled in such a way as to lead to optimum health outcomes (Wade-Martins, 2002).

With this meaning in mind, a summary of the findings of an extensive review of the literature on primary care models with particular focus on the child and family led to building on the work of researchers such as Starfield, who was among the first pioneers to research what constitutes a 'good' primary care system (Starfield, Shi, & Macinko, 2005). Thus, we describe the model types and apply this to practical application of appraisal methodologies in the MOCHA project.

Model Types

The many different forms of primary child health care provision are described in Chapter 1.

Given the finite project resources and the greatest and most strategic foci of primary care activity for children, the MOCHA project has concentrated primarily on the general practice or family practice (seeing all ages but optionally with specialisation), primary care paediatricians (seeing only child patients), community nursing with their own child caseload, practice-based nurses working in tandem with a primary care and school health services. The other contributors to primary care received some attention in our scientific survey questionnaires analysing service patterns.

A MOCHA literature review (Alexander & Blair, 2016) identified a number of models used to classify primary care systems. In summary, these included one or more axes: European paediatric professional associations and country agent classifications of lead practitioner in terms of general practitioner (GP), primary care paediatrician or mixed systems (Ehrich, Namazova-Baranova, & Pettoello-Mantovani, 2016; Katz, Rubino, Collier, Rosen, & Ehrich, 2002; van Esso et al., 2010); the system of regulation, financing and service provision; and separately State, health insurance or private provider as 'actors' (Böhm, Schmid, Götze, Landwehr, & Rothgang, 2013), or a combination of state or professional control (hierarchy) and gatekeeping (Bourgueil, Marek, & Mousques, 2009).

Lead Practitioner Classifications

The lead clinician has often been the key focal point of a model and the classification by which it has been defined. The clinician is the point of entry into the primary care system in most, but not all, models. The clinician acts as a medical advocate for the patient and may coordinate further care (Kringos, Boerma, Hutchinson, & Saltman, 2015a, 2015b). This is a somewhat simplistic, but pragmatic means of describing a model of primary care. The MOCHA project has echoed previous research by describing models by means of three types of lead clinician (see Chapter 13):

(1) a paediatrician-led model;
(2) a GP/Family doctor-led model; and
(3) a mixed model.

Within a country, there may be transition from one type to another, for example from paediatrician-led services to a GP-led service at a certain point in childhood (Alexander & Blair, 2016), and there is very little evidence to show outcomes related to the type of model or variation in outcomes within a country's model (Ehrich et al., 2016; Katz et al., 2002; van Esso et al., 2010).

Financial Classifications

In Europe, countries are generally divided into tax-based national health systems and social insurance systems (Saltman, Rico, & Boerma, 2006), but the manifestations of each funding system by societal and political decisions leads to a diversity in models. Funding is a very important factor in shaping a health care system, but it is unable to explain the diversity in Europe on its own (see Chapters 8 and 9). The Expert Panel on Effective Ways of Investing in Health (European Commission, 2018) recommends that all EU Member States have adequate financing for primary care, to guarantee a certain level of population health and well-being. Any system must have a degree of financial stability to function properly and to remain accessible and effective (European Commission, 2018). In most countries, there is free or almost free access to primary care for children, but there are also hidden costs that can result in inequity of provision (see Chapters 9 and 15), which is perhaps exacerbated by the recent financial crises in Europe.

Regulatory, Financial and Service Provision Classifications

Another means of classifying the diversity of models of primary health care is on the type of service offered and how it is organised. These have been described by Kringos et al. (2015a, 2015b) among others in three model subtypes:

(1) The public hierarchical normative model − this is where primary care is central to the health system and is run by the state rather than by health professionals. In these systems, health care facilities provide voluntary coverage and are governed by decentralised authorities or regions, and GPs or primary care paediatricians are usually salaried. Examples of countries with this type of system are Finland, Lithuania, Portugal, Spain and Sweden.
(2) The professional hierarchical gatekeeper model − in these systems, GPs are the cornerstone of primary care and usually hold a gatekeeper role to other services. The primary care professionals are accountable for the management of resources used for health care. Remuneration of professionals is mixed between fee-for-service, self-employed and salaried. Examples of this system are Denmark, Estonia, Poland, the Netherlands, Slovenia and the United Kingdom.
(3) The free professional non-hierarchical model − health professionals organise care independently, without strong regulation from the state or insurance funding. This model emphasises patient and professional freedom. There is an absence of a list system or a gatekeeping role. Primary care professionals work alongside each other, but not necessarily in collaborative teams. Countries with this system include Austria, Belgium, France, Germany and Switzerland (see Chapter 9). Not all countries fit neatly into these classification systems, however. For example, Italy has a combination of a public hierarchical normative model and a professional hierarchical gatekeeper model. Other research has extended these classifications further, based on contextual factors including funding, clinic types and community settings. These are discussed in detail in Alexander and Blair (2016).

In the MOCHA project, a combination of our own country-based studies with reference sources and literature, we were able to map the different models in the EU and EEA countries. Table 2.1 was used to highlight the different classification types described above and to support the Work Package scientists in their task of appraising the model characteristics against a variety of outcomes.

A number of additions were made to the Table 2.1 as the project progressed; including workforce training, presence of multidisciplinary teams, school and adolescent health services, amount of funding, background factors such as GDP and PPP and types of record systems.

Table 2.1. Mapping of models of provision in MOCHA countries.

	Practitioner at First Point of Contact*	Lead Practitioner – Clinical Responsibility				Financial Organisation		Referral/Access System to Secondary Care
	From CA Questions and Bourgueil et al. (2009)	From: WP1 CA Questions	From van Esso et al. (2010)	From Ehrich et al. (2016)	MOCHA Agreed Primary Care Lead Practitioner	From Relevant HIT Documents (European Observatory on Health Systems & Policies, 2018)	OECD Classification From Böhm et al. (2013)	From Relevant HIT Documents/Country Agent Comments
Austria	GP or paediatrician	GP and paediatrician	Combined – Both	'Pediatric primary health care in Austria involves the services of general pediatricians and general practitioners' http://www.jpeds.com/article/S0022-3476(16)30142-1/fulltext	Both (GP/ paediatrician)	Compulsory health insurance, children up to age 18, or 21 if unemployed, 26 if in full-time education are insured with close relatives (e.g. parent)	Social health insurance	Open access
Belgium	Family doctor or first line paediatrician	Family doctor or first line paediatrician	Combined		Combined (GP/ paediatrician)	Mixture of state social security and private health insurance. Fee for service	Etatist social health insurance	Open access
Bulgaria	GP or paediatrician	GP for those with health insurance. Pre-2000 was mandatory for community paed for children up to 18; younger GPs only have nine weeks paeds training.	GP Led		GP	State health insurance and voluntary health insurance		Primary care is gatekeeper to other health services GP has a limited number of referrals per year. 70% use primary care as entry point to system

Table 2.1. (*Continued*)

	Practitioner at First Point of Contact*	Lead Practitioner – Clinical Responsibility				Financial Organisation		Referral/Access System to Secondary Care
	From CA Questions and Bourgueil et al. (2009)	From: WP1 CA Questions	From van Esso et al. (2010)	From Ehrich et al. (2016)	MOCHA Agreed Primary Care Lead Practitioner	From Relevant HIT Documents (European Observatory on Health Systems & Policies, 2018)	OECD Classification From Böhm et al. (2013)	From Relevant HIT Documents/Country Agent Comments
Croatia	GP or paediatrician	Primary care paediatrician or GP		'Paediatricians and school medicine specialists provide comprehensive preventive health care for both preschool and school-aged children' http://www.jpeds.com/article/S0022-3476(16)30143-3/fulltext	Primary care paediatrician	Mandatory health insurance fund and private insurance for additional services. Children are free	Etatist social health system	Primary care is mainly gatekeeper to other health services
Cyprus	Paediatrician	Private paediatrician or public hospital paed	Paediatrician led		Primary care paediatrician	Two parallel systems, the state and private sector. Since the economic crisis more uptake of public sector. 5–10% have private health insurance	Government and private health system	Open access
Czech Republic	Paediatrician	'Registering paediatrician' Accessed via triage nurse	Paediatrician led However, this may be misleading. The Czech Republic has a 'specialty' called PLDD 'praktický lékar pro deti a	'Does not involve general practitioners (GPs) in primary child health care. Indeed, all parents in the Czech Republic can choose their own pediatrician at the	Primary care paediatrician	90% have health insurance via public health insurance companies 'so-called sickness funds': For people who are not employed (including children, pensioned,	Etatist social health insurance	Access to secondary care is open but at the same time a referral system is functional

Denmark	dorost' 'General Practitioner for Children and Adolescents' who, when selected by parents becomes the 'Registering pediatrician' for the child	GP	level of primary care'. www.jpeds.com/article/S0022-3476(16)30144-5/fulltext	'child primary care is taken care of by general practitioners who have six months of pediatric training as part of their specialty training and, therefore, are qualified to work as gatekeepers for the secondary health care at the hospitals' http://www.jpeds.com/article/S0022-3476(16)30145-7/fulltext	Combined GP/health nurse	job-less), the fund receives monthly payments form the state	State funded, but voluntary health insurance as well Overall tax financed – voluntary health insurance exist but is very seldom relevant in this situation because the access to health nurse/GP is not a problem	National health service	Primary care is gatekeeper to other health services. For school children, the health nurse attached to the school or the school dentist service (which is more constant present) may be the primary contact and may, in many cases, solve the minor problems
Estonia	GP	GP	'For the last 20 years, family doctors have been responsible for the primary care of children. Paeciatric subspecialists work mainly in 2 children's hospitals' http://www.jpeds.com/article/S0022-3476(16)30146-9/fulltext	GP	Estonian health insurance fund (mandatory) covers 95% of population	Etatist social health insurance	Primary care is *partial* gatekeeper to other health services Some can be contacted directly

Table 2.1. (*Continued*)

	Practitioner at First Point of Contact*		Lead Practitioner – Clinical Responsibility			Financial Organisation		Referral/Access System to Secondary Care
	From CA Questions and Bourgueil et al. (2009)	From: WP1 CA Questions	From van Esso et al. (2010)	From Ehrich et al. (2016)	MOCHA Agreed Primary Care Lead Practitioner	From Relevant HIT Documents (European Observatory on Health Systems & Policies, 2018)	OECD Classification From Böhm et al. (2013)	From Relevant HIT Documents/Country Agent Comments
Finland	Nurse in health centres (public health nurses, nurses and midwives have a limited right to prescribe, for children less than 12 years only)	GP	GP		Combined other (nurse/GP/paed)	Municipality financed	National health service	Primary care is gatekeeper to other health services. Nurse acts as gatekeeper to GP
France	GP or paediatrician. The direct access to a specialist usually involves an extra cost for the patients, except for paediatricians (along with gynaecologist ophthalmologist, psychiatrist)	Family physician who is either a paediatrician or a GP	Combined		Combined other (nurse/GP/paed). Nurses are generally supervised by doctors, except in a few institutions (PMI- Maternal and Infant Protection, 'crèches', school) where they can have a role of screening and orientation	Social insurance, but strong state influence on health	Etatist social health insurance	PC has a *Semi-gatekeeping* functioning. There are incentives to use primary care as gatekeeper. But the scarcity of liberal doctors, especially in large cities, makes direct use of hospital emergencies specifically paediatric very frequent, and without financial consequences

Country	Paediatrician or GP	Paediatrician	Combined	Primary care paediatrician	Mandatory health insurance	Social health insurance	Open access
Germany							
Greece		GP or paediatrician chosen from insurance co. list. Usually paediatrician up to 18 years old	Paediatrician led	Primary care paediatrician	Economic crisis severe in Greece. NHS and social insurance systems co-exist		Primary care is gatekeeper to other health services
Hungary	GP or paediatrician		Combined	Combined (GP/paediatrician)	Health insurance fund	Etatist social health insurance	Primary care is partial (but more or less acts as the) gatekeeper to other health services. Partial gatekeeping
Iceland	GP or paediatrician	One family doctor from a health care centre or private paediatrician	Combined	GP	Health insurance covers all who have lived in Iceland for six months or more	National health service	Open access so far, no user charges for children in PHC but minor costs with private consultations. After 1 February 2017, it is to become a referral system with the GP as lead practitioner and continued low cost for specialist consultation; if not GP referral to specialist, increased costs for families
Ireland	GP	GP	GP	GP	Tax funded state health system with extra health insurance funding. Policy is currently changing, with phased introduction of free GP care for children based on	National health insurance	Primary care is gatekeeper to other health services

'There is free access to acute hospital care, but not for primary care, for all children. About 40% of the

Table 2.1. (*Continued*)

	Practitioner at First Point of Contact*	Lead Practitioner – Clinical Responsibility				Financial Organisation		Referral/Access System to Secondary Care
	From CA Questions and Bourgueil et al. (2009)	From: WP1 CA Questions	From van Esso et al. (2010)	From Ehrich et al. (2016)	MOCHA Agreed Primary Care Lead Practitioner	From Relevant HIT Documents (European Observatory on Health Systems & Policies, 2018)	OECD Classification From Böhm et al. (2013)	From Relevant HIT Documents/Country Agent Comments
Italy	Paediatrician or GP	<6 have paediatrician (or GP, only if no paed locally available)	Combined	'Italian pediatricians related to the Public Health Care System work in their own private offices, providing primary care of patients from birth to 14 years of age (to 16 for some population have free access to primary care. Universal preventive public health services, including vaccination and immunisation, newborn blood spot screening, and universal neonatal hearing screening are free'. http://www.jpeds.com/article/S0022-3476(16)30149-4/fulltext	Combined (GP/ paediatrician)	government reimbursement of general practitioners. From 2015, all children under six years receive free primary health care if their parents register with a GP participating in the national scheme. Also free GP care for children whose families do not meet an income threshold or children with certain long-term conditions	National health insurance	Primary care is gatekeeper to other health services

Latvia	GP	GP/family doctor or a paediatrician	Max 800 children per paediatrician (in several areas, 1,000–1,200)	6–14 have paediatrician or GP	cases of chronic diseases) [...] parents can choose between a paediatrician and a GP for their children who are between 6 and 14 years of age'. http://www.jpeds.com/article/S0022-3476(16)30151-2/fulltext6	GP	The financial system the same in 2016. Resources mainly come through general taxation, but out of pocket payment (OOP) are as well, like private voluntary insurance or for services with a long waiting time or services not covered by state budget and provided by private doctors. National Health service (HHS) under the Ministry of Health acts a pooler of health funds and the purchaser of service. Service providers may be public or private. In primary care, predominantly all GP are private, but secondary care providers predominantly are public	Between national health service and national health insurance system. The Latvian HC system is between – in inpatient care for children, state gives money and majority of providers are state hospitals, but in outpatient care (primary care), money comes from state, but providers (GP) are private	Primary care is gatekeeper to other health services. But once referred can choose specialist

Table 2.1. (*Continued*)

	Practitioner at First Point of Contact*		Lead Practitioner – Clinical Responsibility			Financial Organisation		Referral/Access System to Secondary Care
	From CA Questions and Bourgueil et al. (2009)	From: WP1 CA Questions	From van Esso et al. (2010)	From Ehrich et al. (2016)	MOCHA Agreed Primary Care Lead Practitioner	From Relevant HIT Documents (European Observatory on Health Systems & Policies, 2018)	OECD Classification From Böhm et al. (2013)	From Relevant HIT Documents/Country Agent Comments
Lithuania	GP or paediatrician	Family doctor/GP or paediatrician	Combined		Combined (GP/paed)	National health insurance fund	National health service	Primary care is gatekeeper to other health services (developing)
Luxembourg	Paediatrician or GP	Family doctor or paediatrician	Combined		Combined (GP/paed)	Three company insurance schemes	Social health insurance	Open access
Malta	GP	Family doctor (private) or walk in community health centre			GP	Public – free; private care accounts for two-thirds of primary care workload		Open access
Netherlands	GP	GP (triaged by nurse)	GP	'The GPs treat almost all uncomplicated health problems; as a consequence, Dutch paediatricians see few common child health problems'. http://www.jpeds.com/article/S0022-3476(16)30153-6/fulltext	GP Footnote: preventive care in children has a separate lead; the preventive child physician		Etatist social health insurance	Primary care is gatekeeper to other health services
Norway	GP	GP	GP		Combined (GP/paed) Paediatrician or GP at the municipal health care centres / clinics see children at regular periods, have	Taxes and grants Primary care is financed from municipal taxes, block grants from the central government	National health service	Primary care is gatekeeper to other health services

		an important public health role (and screening vaccination), but GP are most important with acute illness or concerns			and earmarked grants for specific purposes. A major source of financing of primary care is also the NIS (through fee-for-service payments and reimbursement of user fees). Reference: Health in Transition: Norway 2013	Primary care is gatekeeper to other health services
Poland	GP/ paediatrician	A new law from 27 October 2017 states that the Primary health physician has to be: (1) specialist in the field of family medicine or (2) during the specialised training in the field of family medicine or (3) specialist in the field of general medicine or (4) specialist in paediatrics or (5) physician with specialist title in the field of internal medicine (has no right to take care of children) In Poland, there is no longer training in general medicine; this has been replaced by family medicine specialisation This change is in transition and is the consequence of the newly adopted (November 2017) Primary Health Care Act. Law: http://www. dziennikustaw.gov.pl/ DU/2017/2217	Combined (GP/paed) This is in accordance with the currently binding legislation the primary health care might be provided by both (1) the medical doctor specialised in family medicine or general medicine and (2) medical doctor specialised in paediatrics	The vast majority is from public universal health insurance; voluntary health insurance limited role	Etatist social health insurance	
Portugal	GP				GP	

Table 2.1. (*Continued*)

Practitioner at First Point of Contact*	Lead Practitioner – Clinical Responsibility				Financial Organisation		Referral/Access System to Secondary Care
From CA Questions and Bourgueil et al. (2009)	From: WP1 CA Questions	From van Esso et al. (2010)	From Ehrich et al. (2016)	MOCHA Agreed Primary Care Lead Practitioner	From Relevant HIT Documents (European Observatory on Health Systems & Policies, 2018)	OECD Classification From Böhm et al. (2013)	From Relevant HIT Documents/Country Agent Comments
GP (80%) or private paediatrician			Mixed (GP and paediatrician) mostly offered by general practitioners (GPs) (approximately 70% of patients) or by paediatricians (caring for approximately 30% of children). There are an estimated number of children that are followed by both GPs and paediatricians. http://www.jpeds.com/article/S0022-3476(16)30154-8/fulltext	Combined (GP/paediatrician)		National health service	Primary care is gatekeeper to other health services
Romania Family doctor (the function is called family doctor, and the training is general practitioner)	Family doctor			GP	State health insurance system, based on individual contribution of insured adults. Primary care is a mix of funded and fee-for-service care. All children have free	Etatist social health insurance (the state holds the regulatory power, grants privileges for the financing and provision of health services and allows private health services at all levels)	Mixed access. As there are many private health services for adults and children where anybody has access if they pay, we can call it open access; however, the primary health care (family health care (family

Slovenia	Paediatrician (family doctor if paediatrician is not available locally)	Paediatrician	Primary care paediatrician	health care at all levels	Etatist social health system	doctors) acts as gate keeper for all free health care services and even some of the specialised treatments
		'Physicians working with children and adolescents in primary level have a 5-year specialisation in paediatrics'.		Mandatory health insurance, private insurance becoming more common	However: Slovenia stands out as a special case. Slovenia is characterised by universal coverage, financing through earmarked taxes, a purchaser–provider split, public hospitals, and private or mixed delivery in the outpatient sector	Primary care is gatekeeper to other health services
		General practitioners (GPs) and family doctors provide care for 1.5% of children of 0–6 years of age and 7.7% of children of 7–18 years of age		Children under 18 years of age, students under 26 years of age are entitled to the health benefits covered under compulsory insurance scheme		Primary paediatricians are holders of lists of patients as patients (parents for their children) are entitled to select their own/ their child's personal physician
		http://www.jreds.com/article/S0022-3476(16)30161-3/fulltext		Children under 18 years of age, students under 26 years of age are exempt from co-payments and therefore do not need to pay voluntary health insurance	The state still provides most of the health care services with own facilities while funding is delegated to a social health insurance scheme	Primary paediatricians have the role of gatekeepers to secondary and tertiary health care level
					Social-based mixed type	But patient can choose specialist once referred
					Slovenia challenges theoretical assumptions about the specifications of dimensions in health	

Table 2.1. (*Continued*)

	Practitioner at First Point of Contact*		Lead Practitioner – Clinical Responsibility			Financial Organisation		Referral/Access System to Secondary Care
	From CA Questions and Bourgueil et al. (2009)	From: WP1 CA Questions	From van Esso et al. (2010)	From Ehrich et al. (2016)	MOCHA Agreed Primary Care Lead Practitioner	From Relevant HIT Documents (European Observatory on Health Systems & Policies, 2018)	OECD Classification From Böhm et al. (2013)	From Relevant HIT Documents/Country Agent Comments
							care through the combination of state-led provision with societal financing and regulation. http://edoc.vifapol.de/opus/volltexte/2012/4221/pdf/AP_165_2012.pdf	
Spain	Paediatrician	Primary care paediatrician	Paediatrics-based system	Primary care paediatrician Primary paediatric care is provided by employed paediatricians in the primary care centres public network	Primary care paediatrician	National health service/Primary care services funded through general taxation	National health service (NHS)	Primary health care is gatekeeper to other NHS services/health care levels
Sweden	Nurse or doctor in health centres (nurses can prescribe)	Primary care for children in Sweden is divided in two parts: nurse-led preventive services and GP-led curative services Nurse-led preventive services are based in child health centres – nurses consult a team of consultants (e.g. GPs or paediatricians) as necessary	GP	Within the primary care sector, most children receive care from family physicians Irrespective of registration, however, primary care rarely has a formal gatekeeping role and, thus, patients are free to contact specialists directly	GP	Health services in Sweden are run by 21 county councils using funds from national taxation	National health service	Open access (PC has guiding role) The positioning of the paediatricians vary somewhat between counties. In Stockholm county (about 30% of the Swedish population), a referral is not needed to see a paediatrician in outpatient clinics, but in most counties, a referral from a GP is

	Curative primary care is built around GPs in primary care health centres, supported by nursing staff			http://www.jpeds.com/article/S0022-3476(16)30161-5/fulltext	needed to see a paediatrician and he/she only work in hospitals. GP referral is necessary for most secondary care, but child psychiatric services is quite often, but not always open access
				National Health Service	Primary care is gatekeeper to other health services
				Tax-based national health system. Some differences in funding arrangements in the four devolved countries such as England/Wales/Scotland and Northern Ireland	
		GP	GPs are the usual first port of call if a child is unwell, acting as gatekeepers for further referrals to other specialists. Children are immunised either in primary care or in school. http://www.jpeds.com/article/S0022-3476(16)30164-0/fulltext		
	GP as a named accountable professional	GP			
United Kingdom	Nurse or doctor in PC group practice (nurses can prescribe)				

Source: Blair, Rigby, & Alexander (2017).

Identifying Appraisal Frameworks

Having described the model components and their variations across the 30 countries, the next and central MOCHA project challenge was how to appraise the various combinations. We used the World Health Organization 'building blocks' (World Health Organization, 2010) for high-performing health systems which might act as useful starting point when looking at primary care for children to try to establish what makes a good system and from which perspective. The building blocks are as follows:

- Good health services are those which deliver effective, safe, quality personal and non-personal health interventions to those that need them, when and where needed, with minimum waste of resources.
- A well-performing health workforce is one that works in ways that are responsive, fair and efficient to achieve the best health outcomes possible, given available resources and circumstances (i.e. there are sufficient staff, fairly distributed; they are competent, responsive and productive).
- A well-functioning health information system is one that ensures the production, analysis, dissemination and use of reliable and timely information on health determinants, health system performance and health status.
- A well-functioning health system ensures equitable access to essential medical products, vaccines and technologies of assured quality, safety, efficacy and cost-effectiveness and their scientifically sound and cost-effective use.
- A good health financing system raises adequate funds for health, in ways that ensure people can use needed services and are protected from financial catastrophe or impoverishment associated with having to pay for them. It provides incentives for providers and users to be efficient.
- Leadership and governance involve ensuring strategic policy frameworks exist and are combined with effective oversight, coalition-building, regulation, attention to system design and accountability.

Specifically for primary care, Starfield et al. (2005) identified six mechanisms, alone and in combination which may account for the beneficial impact of primary care on population health:

(1) greater access to needed services;
(2) better quality of care;
(3) a greater focus on prevention;
(4) early management of health problems;
(5) the cumulative effect of the main primary care delivery characteristics (first-contact access for each new need, long-term person (not disease)-focused care, comprehensive care for most health needs and coordinated care); and
(6) the role of primary care in reducing unnecessary and potentially harmful specialist care.

Appraisal of the models of primary care for children and young people is considered through a number of different lenses. These include effectiveness or health gain, acceptability against child, family and societal expectations and economic efficiency.

To identify a suitable appraisal framework for MOCHA, we carried out a detailed literature review of the conceptual frameworks that could be applied. This work identified 13 specific frameworks that focused on the overall health system and eight specifically on primary care (Sampaio & Blair, 2018). No published literature was found to specifically focus on primary child health care in its own right. This reinforces our overall finding that despite the importance of child health, it is an inadequately studied field of health care (see Chapters 6 and 7). The 13 frameworks have been used at national, international and regional levels and are summarised in Table 2.2. Table 2.3 is a summary of the dimensions of the eight conceptual frameworks applied to primary health systems across different countries.

Tables 2.2 and 2.3 do not show the relationship between the dimensions, but they demonstrate that improved health status (or health outcomes/effectiveness) appear in all frameworks, while access, efficiency, equitable outcomes, responsiveness, human resources, physical resources, financial resources, political and socio-economic factors are present in most of them, both in general and in primary health frameworks. Although general and primary health frameworks have a similar pattern, it is possible to highlight some differences between their dimensions. Quality appears in most general health frameworks but in only two primary health ones. Health system use, governance, continuity and health system management appear in most primary health frameworks but are infrequent in general health frameworks.

Health outcome (or effectiveness) is always a goal of the system and eventually may also compose the performance dimension. Efficiency, however, is present as an outcome or system goal (Aday et al., 1999; Handler et al., 2001; Kringos, Boerma, Bourgueil et al., 2010; Starfield, 2001; Veillard et al., 2017; Watson et al., 2004; Wong et al., 2010; World Health Organization, 2007), performance measurement (Hsiao, Heller, & Reisman, 2008; Sibthorpe & Gardner, 2007; World Health Organization, 2007) or both. The same is the case of responsiveness that can figure as an outcome (Hsiao et al., 2008; Murray & Frenk, 2000; World Health Organization, 2007), performance dimension (Aday et al., 1999; Arah et al., 2006; Starfield, 1998; Tham et al., 2010; Watson et al., 2004) or both (Canadian Institute for Health Information CIHI, 2012; van Olmen et al., 2010; Wong et al., 2010; World Health Organization, 2009).

Equity appears in many frameworks, but in different places, nevertheless highlighting equitable access to health services (procedural equity) as a cause of equitable outcomes (substantive equity). The World Health Organization (2008b) stated that health inequities (inequities in outcomes) are caused by unequal access to health care and many other visible or invisible circumstances, such as unequal distribution of power, income and goods. Nevertheless, no framework considered equity at a structural or contextual level.

Table 2.2. Dimensions of the conceptual general health frameworks.

	Aday et al. (1999)	Murray and Frenk (2000)	Starfield (2001)	Handler, Issel, and Turnock (2001)	Watson, Broemeling, Reid, and Black (2004)	Arah, Westert, Hurst, and Klazinga (2006)	WHO (2007)	Hsiao et al., (2008)	WHO (2009)	CIHI (2012)	European Commission Health (2015)	Total
Improved health status, wellness, functioning/effectiveness	X	X	X	X	X	X	X	X	X	X	X	11
Equitable outcomes (equity)	X	X	X	X	X	X	X		X	X	X	9
Efficiency/value for money	X			X	X	X	X	X	X	X		8
Responsiveness/public satisfaction	X	X			X	X	X	X	X	X		8
Access/accessibility[a]	X				X	X	X	X	X	X	X	8
Quality					X	X	X	X	X	X	X	7
Political and socio-economic factors[d]	X		X	X	X	X				X	X	7
Financial resources/expenditure/cost	X			X	X	X				X	X	6
Human resources[c]		X		X	X				X	X	X	6
Physical resources (facilities, medical products, vaccines and equipment)	X			X	X				X	X	X	6
Financing process (collecting, pooling and purchasing)	X			X	X	X					X	5

Behavioural and cultural factors	X							5
Physical environment		X	X		X	X	X	4
Equitable access to health services (equity)					X	X	X	4
Safety			X	X		X	4
Governance/stewardship/policy development	X		X	X		X	4
Health system's use/service delivery/clinical activities[b]	X		X	X	X	4
Informational resources		X		X	X	X	4
Genetic endowment	X		X	X		4
Social/financial risk protection			X	X	X	3
Innovation	X		X		X	3
Organisation	X		X	X	3
Sustainability			X	X	2
Risk factors and behaviours	X		X	X	2
Appropriateness		X	X		2
Comprehensiveness		X	X	2
Coverage		X	X	2
Continuity		X	X	2
Regulation		X	X	X	2
Health system characteristics/processes non-specified		X		2

Table 2.2. (*Continued*)

	Aday et al. (1999)	Murray and Frenk (2000)	Starfield (2001)	Handler, Issel, and Turnock (2001)	Watson, Broemeling, Reid, and Black (2004)	Arah, Westert, Hurst, and Klazinga (2006)	WHO (2007)	Hsiao et al., (2008)	WHO (2009)	CIHI (2012)	European Commission Health (2015)	Total
Demographic characteristics										X	X	2
Coordination										X		1
Health system management					X							1
Demand/need				X								1
Network/linkages												0
Service availability/range of services												0

Notes: [a] Geographical, financial, administrative, cultural and timeliness.
[b] Volume, distribution, type and qualities.
[c] Workforce availability, competence, motivation and development.
[d] Socioeconomic position, life conditions and political context.
(See Sampaio and Blair (2018) for further information)

Table 2.3. Dimensions of the primary health care conceptual frameworks.

	Starfield (1998)	Sibthorpe and Gardner (2007)	Kringos, Boerma, Hutchinson, van der Zee, and Groenewegen (2010)	van Olmen et al. (2010)	Wong et al. (2010)	Tham et al. (2010)	Jahanmehr et al. (2015)	Veillard et al. (2017)	Total
Improved health status, wellness, functioning/effectiveness	X	X	X	X	X	X	X	X	8
Access/accessibility[a]	X	X	X	X	X	X	X	X	8
Health system's use/service delivery/clinical activities[b]	X	X	X	X	X	X	X	X	8
Human resorces[c]	X	X	X	X	X	X	X	X	8
Governance/stewardship/policy development	X	X	X	X	X	X		X	7
Physical resources (facilities, medical products, vaccines and equipment)	X	X		X	X	X	X	X	7
Efficiency/value for money		X	X		X	X	X	X	6
Responsiveness/public satisfaction	X	X		X	X	X		X	6
Continuity	X	X	X		X	X		X	6
Health system management	X	X		X	X	X		X	6

Table 2.3. (Continued)

	Starfield (1998)	Sibthorpe and Gardner (2007)	Kringos, Boerma, Hutchinson, van der Zee, and Groenewegen (2010)	van Olmen et al. (2010)	Wong et al. (2010)	Tham et al. (2010)	Jahanmehr et al. (2015)	Veillard et al. (2017)	Total
Financial resources/expenditure/cost	X		X		X	X	X	X	6
Equitable outcomes (equity)		X	X		X		X	X	5
Political and socio-economic factors[d]	X			X	X		X	X	5
Appropriateness		X			X	X			3
Comprehensiveness			X		X			X	3
Coordination			X		X			X	3
Equitable access to health services (equity)		X	X				X		3
Financing process (collecting, pooling, purchasing)		X		X				X	3
Network/linkages		X	X			X			3
Innovation		X	X					X	3
Informational resources		X		X				X	3
Service availability/range of services	X		X					X	3

							Total
Demand/need	X				X		X	3
Sustainability			X				X	2
Risk factors and behaviours		X					X	2
Coverage	X				X			2
Quality	X					X		2
Safety						X	X	2
Organisation						X	X	2
Genetic endowment	X						X	2
Behavioural and cultural factors					X		X	2
Physical environment				X			X	2
Social/financial risk protection					X			1
Regulation					X			1
Demographic characteristics		X						1
Health system characteristics/processes								0
non-specified								0

Notes: [a]Geographical, financial, administrative, cultural and timeliness.
[b]Volume, distribution, type and qualities.
[c]Workforce availability, competence, motivation and development.
[d]Socio-economic position, life conditions and political context (see Sampaio and Blair (2018) for further information).

Notwithstanding the importance social determinants of health, contextual dimensions were not included in seven frameworks (Hsiao et al., 2008; Kringos, Boerma, Hutchinson et al., 2010; Murray & Frenk, 2000; Sibthorpe & Gardner, 2007; Tham et al., 2010; World Health Organization, 2007, 2009). Even when the objective is to appraise the primary child health system, which may not be responsible for changing variables out of its domain, health determinants were not present in any framework. Contextual factors allow a broader understanding of the system (see Chapter 17), and it has been shown that health determinants can have a higher impact on health outcomes than health care (Donkin, Goldblatt, Allen, Nathanson, & Marmot, 2017).

Obviously, 'it is hard to isolate the impact of health care from the impact of other determinants of health status' (Hurst & Jee-Hughes, 2001). However, a conceptual framework ideally will contribute to operationalise statistical models to measure the impact of each variable. Sometimes, a concept is not easily identified in the framework figure. Yet, it is implicit in the description of another concept. This is described in Kringos, Boerma, and Hutchinson et al. (2010), which included effectiveness as a feature of quality dimension. A different situation occurred in Starfield's, 1998 framework (Starfield, 1998), where the author acknowledges equity's importance as a system goal, but did not include it explicitly in her framework, not even in its description. Additionally, the frameworks vary in focus, being broader or more specific. For example, Starfield produced two separate frameworks with differing emphasis of the health system within the wider context of health (Starfield, 1998, 2001).

Moreover, as already mentioned, there is variation in the definitions of the concepts, when available. Responsiveness, for example, varies between patient 'satisfaction and acceptability', which depend on expectations, and 'experience', which 'seeks to describe objective characteristics of health service delivery, such as whether patients were (factually) given a choice of treatment' (Hurst & Jee-Hughes, 2001).

Adapting Frameworks for MOCHA

A major concern for the MOCHA project is that none of the identified frameworks are child specific (see Chapter 6), which is important because of the specific needs of children from primary care (see Chapter 1).

Many of the appraisal frameworks are constructed on a structure-process-outcome theme; describe capacity-performance-health status; or are focused on input/output and outcomes. Thus, all attempt to relate the various components in a linear framework, rather than either looking at a dynamic interactive system or focussing on the individual child as the reactive and proactive subject of care. Nearly all of the frameworks recognise that health status of a population cannot solely be attributable to the health system but must be analysed in the context of broader environmental, economic and social situations. This raises the conundrum of how to estimate the balance between primary care combatting the adverse effects of external determinants of health as they adversely affect individual child, as opposed to the effort that can be invested in preventively addressing the deterents such as by combating household smoking or advocating for better housing for families with small children. Overall, however, the utility of having such appraisal frameworks does allow a conceptual framework to be developed, which can contribute to seeking to operationalise statistical models to measure the impact of each variable.

The Primary Health Care Activity Monitor for Europe (PHAMEU) is a significant research group that has attempted to develop a scoring system following a structure−process−outcome framework. This project concluded that a generic all-ages primary care system can be defined and approached as:

> a multidimensional system structured by primary care governance, economic conditions and primary care workforce development, facilitating access to a wide range of primary care services in a coordinated way, and on a continuous basis, by applying resources efficiently to provide high quality care, contributing to the distribution of health in the population. Primary care contributes through its dimensions to overall health system performance and health. (Kringos, Boerma, Hutchinson et al., 2010)

This European primary care monitor was subsequently tested to rate the strength of primary care systems across Europe (Schäfer et al., 2011). While this work did not consider the specific needs of children (such as different types of access), we have included this in our table of components as a variable that may be used to analyse the primary care systems for children.

Recognising the value of a conceptual framework, but the failings of the existing published ones to meet the specific needs of children, and in a primary care setting, the MOCHA research team devised an alternative conceptualisation. At the heart of this has been our core theme of child centricity (see Chapter 4) and the need to focus on delivery to the child through the development of the life course. The MOCHA working model focuses on the child, the life course, the primary care team and the societal and environmental context (see Figure 2.1).

The MOCHA model is based on three theoretical frameworks, Bronfenbrenner's ecological model of determinants of health (Bronfenbrenner, 1986), a modified PHAMEU; model of determinants of quality of primary care (Kringos, Boerma, Hutchinson et al., 2010); and a life course epidemiological framework for childhood health and disease (Kuh, Ben-Schlomo, Lynch, Hallqvist, & Power, 2003). The left-hand circle was inspired by the visualisation of positive and negative health determinant forces developed by the Child Health Indicators of Life and Development (CHILD) (Rigby & Köhler, 2002) project and describes influences on health and health policy decisions. Within the community setting, a family makes choices and decisions about health based on what is available, knowledge and cultural influences, and finally − potentially influenced by all of these practices − the child. Alternatively, viewed from the inside out, it can be seen as the child in the centre, able to influence and make

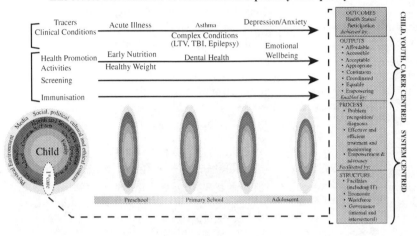

Figure 2.1.   The MOCHA working model.

decisions about what is available to him or her in terms of health in the context of the family, and with appropriate support the child can further exert some influence on the wider determinants. In practice, both situations occur in a dynamic process which is constantly in flux.

The variation in the respective widths of the coloured elements of the diagram as the child moves from one age range to another indicates how the various determinants are weighted for a typical child over time. For example, there is a relatively large influence from parents and family in the early years, and great influence of school, peer groups and external influences such as the media, as children grows older.

A combination of preventive care, physical and mental health and short-term and long-term conditions has been selected as tracer conditions, examples of which appear in the diagram above the circles. Project scientists have surveyed the country agents concerning various different aspects of the MOCHA Working Model so that there is a balance of acute conditions, long-term conditions, mental health and the well child. The primary care system is closely related, in the left-hand circle, to secondary and tertiary care, in other words, vertical, aspects and to social care education and justice as a horizontal axis of interaction.

Practical Application of Appraisal Methodologies

Identification of models to form a visualisation is one part of the appraisal process in the MOCHA project. A second necessary part has been empirical analysis, though as will emerge this has been severely hampered by the lack of accessible data (see Chapter 7).

To seek to achieve meaningful appraisal, the project's scientists looked in particular at the following aspects: health status of children and clinical outcomes which are theoretically attributable to the primary care system, patient perspectives of the primary care system derived from interviews with children in five countries, an economic appraisal in relation to infant mortality rates and the influence of incentives and penalty systems, the ability of the system to provide equitable provision (preventive care, immunisation, diagnosis of development disorders, diagnosis of congenital anomalies, ambulatory sensitive conditions) and appraisal in terms of children's rights (consent and participation).

A number of tracer conditions have been identified to allow us to assay the different structures and processes that exist in the 30 countries in relation to the key functions of primary child health care. Clinical scenarios were developed to illustrate how these functions operated in each country. These were first access care in acute illness, chronic management of disease and its impact, prevention of disease through screening and immunisation, early detection of developmental or congenital disorders, support in coordinating care for children with complex physical and mental health care needs. We also attempted to harvest data at national and regional level using the MIROI tool (see Chapter 7) and worked with a selected number of countries who had sufficiently granular data on different socio-economic dimensions to allow us to appraise the ability of the primary care system to provide equitable service provision/health outcome (see Chapter 7). The MOCHA approach to the model structures is summarised in Table 2.4. The appraisal process and the use of case studies to develop these in the different countries are described in Table 2.5. Table 2.6 describes the approach to the life course of the child. Each table represents a different appraisal lens whether from a pure health care system perspective, a child and family-centric perspective or using a developmental time basis. The following chapters describe in more detail how this was achieved and the results from the country agent's responses and scientific reviews of the literature.

Summary

In order to successfully appraise the models of primary care for children, the MOCHA project has systematically identified the different types of models that exist, acknowledging the complexity of doing this, particularly with respect to the lack of child focus in more previous researches. An analysis of the existing appraisal frameworks also highlighted the lack of a child-centric perspective, leading to the creation of the MOCHA working model. The project has addressed this appraisal in a number of ways, not least because of the range of expertise and subject focus on the different elements of primary care as they relate to children. The results are shown in the subsequent chapters of this report.

Table 2.4. Structure of a model in terms of the MOCHA project.

	Structure	Process	Outputs	Outcomes
	Facilities (inc IT), Economic, Workforce, Governance	**Problem Recognition, Diagnosis, Treatment, Monitoring**	**Affordable, Accessible, Acceptable, Appropriate, Continuous, Confidential, Equitable, Empowering**	**Health Status, Participation**
Identification of models (WP1)	Existing model concepts	Existing model concepts	Existing model concepts	Conceptual framework
Interface with secondary care for children needing complex care (WP2)	Mechanisms for coordination and communication of care such as IT facilities and communication pathways	Monitoring and communication between primary and secondary care. Communication between services (e.g. health, social care, education, leisure, etc)	Continuous care, dignity of care	Optimum health for the child
School and adolescent health (WP3)	Structure of school health services	Monitoring of conditions in schools, treatment, handling of medicines in schools, preventive medicine in schools, health education	Accessibility for adolescents	Conditions, indicators of outcomes
		Transition of care for adolescents into adult care	School health contributing to health education, health promotion	
Quality measures and outcomes (WP4)	System based on evidence, data available to assess quality and evaluate	Evaluation of quality of care	Reliable, valid, relevant and useable performance information for policy-makers, patients, providers and citizens	Optimum care and efficient health service

Use of large datasets (WP5)	Access to data	Use of databases to appraise and evaluate care	Child-specific data	Identification of innovative outcome measures
		Use of large data sets to devise innovative quality measures	Appropriate data	Identifying unifying common clinical concepts relevant to children
Economic and skill set evaluation and analysis (WP6)	Economic structure of health systems	Training of health workforce		Effect of different systems on health outcomes to children
	Workforce capacity of health systems, including planning and incentives	Analysis of health needs to inform workforce		
Equity (WP7)	Health system accessible to all	Capacity in the system to ensure equity	Accessible service for all	Optimum health for disadvantaged population groups
		Methods to encourage hard-to-reach populations to make use of health service	Adaptable service for all types of user	
Electronic records (WP8)	eHealth system in place	Continuity of care (affecting also quality of care); for older children balancing holistic record keeping with confidentiality; effective monitoring of individual and	Confidential and secure records	Population confidence in confidentiality and security
			Accessible to the correct health personnel	Improved communication

Table 2.4. (*Continued*)

Structure	Process	Outputs	Outcomes
Facilities (inc IT), Economic, Workforce, Governance	**Problem Recognition, Diagnosis, Treatment, Monitoring**	**Affordable, Accessible, Acceptable, Appropriate, Continuous, Confidential, Equitable, Empowering**	**Health Status, Participation**
	population health, across health models (primary, secondary, tertiary) and across national boundaries		and collaboration between disciplines
		Aids efficiency of care across disciplinary boundaries and national boundaries in the EU	Improved efficiency of care
Optimal models (WP9)	MOCHA recommendations for structural elements of health service		

Table 2.5. Primary care in a child centred ecological model and MOCHA.

	Child	Family	School/Community/Peers/Extended Family/Carers	Health and Social Care Services, Secondary Care, Tertiary Care, Social Care	Social and Political Context, Media
Identification of models (WP1)	Case study focus	Case study focus	Case study focus – overlaps with WP3	Case study focus – overlaps with WP2	Workstream on social and political context
Interface with secondary care for children needing complex care (WP2)	Uses case studies – child focus (overlap with WP1)	Case study focus complex care and family; social care perspective; child protection (connects to WP1)	Case study focus – extended family and external carers; social care context, education (Connects to WP1)	Focus on interaction between primary and secondary/tertiary care; interaction with social care services	
School and adolescent health (WP3)	Adolescent care – focus on empowerment of child; accessibility; autonomy in decision-making	Family relationship with school? Family relationships (problematic?) in terms of well-being in adolescence?	School health focus; peer influence on health, autonomy in adolescence and greater influence of friends.	Structure and function of school health services Alternative focus of services for appropriate and accessible adolescent health care	Social media Social acceptance of school health services Encouragement for adolescents to use outreach/other adolescent-specific services

Table 2.5. (*Continued*)

	Child	Family	School/Community/Peers/Extended Family/Carers	Health and Social Care Services, Secondary Care, Tertiary Care, Social Care	Social and Political Context, Media
Quality measures and outcomes (WP4)	Child vaccinations, conditions	Family involved in service, engaged in service	Health system appropriate for community needs/setting	Good communication and coordination between different services and models	Social acceptance of quality Good understanding of quality evidence base Social agreement on what is a good outcome
Use of large datasets (WP5)	Consent for data to be collected and used	Acceptance of need for data, consent for child and family data to be collected and used	Data availability and use in community services.	Data availability Use of data to inform service structure and communication needs	Social acceptance of data collection and use
Economic and skill set evaluation and analysis (WP6)	Appropriate workforce for child's needs (skilled)	Communication between family and health workforce to	Accessible and appropriate workforce in community settings	Motivated and skilled workforce in health system	(Earned) Respect for health workforce

	Accessible (friendly, knowledgeable) workforce	common aim (good outcome)		Workforce communication between primary, secondary, tertiary care etc.	Social context taken into account to adapt health service so that all populations can access if needed
Equity (WP7)	Child is able and willing to access and engage with health service	Family is able and willing to access and engage with health service	Community access equitable to all	Equity of access to health service (based on clinical/social need?)	
Electronic records (WP8)			Sharing of eHealth records across disciplines and services (when appropriate)	Sharing of eHealth records across disciplines and services (when appropriate)	
Optimal models (WP9)	Child centredness taken into account in optimum model recommendations; positioning of the health system in wider ecological model				

Table 2.6. Life stage of a child and the MOCHA project (Broadly illustrated by school ages, which may have different parameters in different countries).

	Preschool	School	Adolescent	Adult
Identification of models (WP1)	Case study of young child in particular health service model	Case study using school-aged child	Case study of adolescent (in conjunction with WP3?)	Case study – transition to adulthood
Interface with secondary care for children needing complex care (WP2)	Infant acquired/congenital conditions managed in primary and secondary care	Acquired/congenital conditions managed at school. Challenges of child with chronic condition	Effects of puberty/development on child with chronic condition (e.g. mental health, brain injury)	Transition to adult services
	Growth and development of a child with chronic condition		Ability of services to coordinate care to a child preparing for adulthood	Developmental age (learning disability) not related to chronological age
School and adolescent health (WP3)		School health services (SHS)	Specific adolescent health services	
Quality measures and outcomes (WP4)	Measures of quality of care for young children;	Measures of quality of care for school-aged children	Measures of quality of care for adolescents	
	Appropriate care built into model	Appropriate care built into model	Appropriate care built into model	
Use of large datasets (WP5)	Age group data	Age group data	Age group data	

Economic and skill set evaluation and analysis (WP6)	Workforce specific for early years (training, capacity)	Appropriate workforce for school-aged children (inc. school health services in conjunction with WP3)	Appropriate workforce for adolescents (with WP3) — Transition to adult services (financial aspects)
Equity (WP7)	Equity for young children, child rights, advocacy for young children / Accessibility for all population groups	Child rights, advocacy, accessibility and equality for all population groups	Child rights, dignity, respect for young person / Accessibility for all population groups
Electronic records (WP8)	Electronic records from birth	Electronic records encompassing different services (education, SHS, social, etc.)	Electronic records encompassing different services (education, SHS, social, etc.)
Optimal models (WP9)	Age and developmental stage of child taken into account in optimum model		

References

Aday, L. A., Begley, C. E., Lairson, D. R., Slater, C. H., Richard, A. J., & Montoya, I. D. (1999). A framework for assessing the effectiveness, efficiency, and equity of behavioral healthcare. *American Journal of Managed Care.* 5 Spec No, SP25-44. Retrieved from https://www.ajmc.com/journals/issue/1999/1999-06-vol5-n1sp/jun99-899psp025-sp04

Alexander, D., & Blair, M. (2016). *Current models of child primary health care.* Retrieved from http://www.childhealthservicemodels.eu/publications/technical-reports/

Arah, O. A., Westert, G. P., Hurst, J., & Klazinga, N. S. (2006). A conceptual framework for the OECD health care quality indicators project. *International Journal for Quality in Health Care, 18*(Suppl 1), 5–13. Retrieved from http://www.ncbi.nlm.nih.gov/pubmed/16954510%5Cnhttp://intqhc.oxfordjournals.org/cgi/doi/10.1093/intqhc/mzl024

Blair, M., Rigby, M., & Alexander, D. (2017). *Final report on current models of primary care for children.* Retrieved from www.childhealthservicemodels.eu/wp-content/uploads/2017/07/MOCHA-WP1-Deliverable-WP1-D6-Feb-2017-1.pdf

Böhm, K., Schmid, A., Götze, R., Landwehr, C., & Rothgang, H. (2013). Five types of OECD healthcare systems: Empirical results of a deductive classification. *Health Policy, 113*(3), 258–269. doi:10.1016/j.healthpol.2013.09.003

Bourgueil, Y., Marek, A., & Mousques, J. (2009). Three models of primary care organisation in Europe, Canada, Australia and New Zealand. *Questions d'economie de la Sante, 141*, 1–4.

Bronfenbrenner, U. (1986). Ecology of the family as a context for human development: Research perspectives. *Developmental Psychology, 22*(6), 723–742.

Canadian Institute for Health Information (CIHI). (2012). *A performance measurement framework for the Canadian Health System.* Retrieved from https://secure.cihi.ca/free_products/HSP-Framework-ENweb.pdf

Donkin, A., Goldblatt, P., Allen, J., Nathanson, V., & Marmot, M. (2017). Global action on the social determinants of health. *BMJ Global Health, 2*(4), e000603. Retrieved from http://gh.bmj.com/lookup/doi/10.1136/bmjgh-2017-000603

Ehrich, J., Namazova-Baranova, L., & Pettoello-Mantovani, M. (2016). Introduction to diversity of child health care in Europe: A study of the European Paediatric Association/Union of National European Paediatric Societies and Associations. *Journal of Pediatrics, 177*, S1–S10. doi:10.1016/j.jpeds.2016.04.036

European Commission. (2015). *Towards a joint assessment framework in the area of health work in progress: 2015 update.* Retrieved from ec.europa.eu/social/BlobServlet?docId=17033&langId=en

European Commission. (2018). *Report of the expert panel on effective ways of investing in Health (EXPH). Expert panel on tools and methodologies for assessing the performance of primary care.* Retrieved from https://ec.europa.eu/health/expert_panel/sites/expertpanel/files/docsdir/opinion_primarycare_performance_en.pdf

European Observatory on Health Systems and Policies. (2018). *Health system reviews (HiT series).* Retrieved from http://www.euro.who.int/en/about-us/partners/observatory/publications/health-system-reviews-hits

Handler, A., Issel, M., & Turnock, B. (2001). A conceptual framework to measure performance of the public health system. *American Public Health Association.*, *91*(8), 1235–1239.

Hsiao, W. C., Heller, P. S., & Reisman, D. (2008). What macroeconomists should know about health care policy. *Singapore Economic Review*, *53*(2), 341–344.

Hurst, J., & Jee-Hughes, M. (2001). Performance measurement and performance management in OECD health systems. *OECD Labour Market and Social Policy Occasional Papers*, 1–69. doi:10.1787/788224073713

Jahanmehr, N., Rashidian, A., Khosravi, A., Farzadfar, F., Shariati, M., Majdzadeh, R., … Mesdaghinia, A.(2015). A conceptual framework for evaluation of public health and primary care system performance in Iran. *Global Journal of Health Science*, *7*(4), 341–357. doi:10.5539/gjhs.v74p341

Katz, M., Rubino, A., Collier, J., Rosen, J., & Ehrich, J. H. (2002). Demography of pediatric primary care in Europe: Delivery of care and training. *Pediatrics*, *109*(5), 788–796.

Kringos, D., Boerma, W., Hutchinson, A., & Saltman, R. B. (2015a). *Building primary care in a changing Europe: European observatory on health systems and policies.* Retrieved from http://www.euro.who.int/__data/assets/pdf_file/0018/271170/BuildingPrimaryCareChangingEurope.pdf

Kringos, D. S., Boerma, W. G., Bourgueil, Y., Cartier, T., Hasvold, T., Hutchinson, A., … Wilm, S. (2010). The European primary care monitor: Structure, process and outcome indicators. *BMC Family Practice*, *11*(1), 81. doi:10.1186/1471-2296-11-81

Kringos, D. S., Boerma, W. G. W., Hutchinson, A. L., & Saltman, R. B. (2015b). *Building primary care in a changing Europe – Case studies.* Retrieved from http://www.euro.who.int/__data/assets/pdf_file/0018/271170/BuildingPrimaryCareChangingEurope.pdf

Kringos, D. S., Boerma, W. G. W., Hutchinson, Al., van der Zee, J., & Groenewegen, P. P. (2010). The breadth of primary care: A systematic literature review of its core dimensions. *BMC Health Services Research*, *10*(65). doi:10.1186/1472-6963-10-65

Kuh, D., Ben-Schlomo, Y., Lynch, J., Hallqvist, J., & Power, C. (2003). Life course epidemiology. *Journal of Epidemiology and Community Health*, *57*, 778–783. doi:10.1136/jech.57.10.778

Murray, C. J., & Frenk, J. (2000). A framework for assessing the performance of health systems. *Bulletin of the World Health Organization*, *78*(6), 717–731.

Rigby, M., & Köhler, L. (2002). *Child health indicators of life and development (CHILD): Report to the European Commission.* European Commission Health Monitoring Programme. Retrieved from https://ec.europa.eu/health/ph_projects/2000/monitoring/fp_monitoring_2000_frep_08_en.pdf

Saltman, R., Rico, A., & Boerma, W. (2006). Primary care in the driver's seat? *Organizational Reform in European Primary Care.* Oxford: Oxford University Press.

Sampaio, M. M. A., & Blair, M. (2018). *Literature review of conceptual frameworks that could be applied to appraise primary child health systems across different countries.* Retrieved from http://www.childhealthservicemodels.eu/publications/technical-reports/

Schäfer, W. L. A., Boerma, W. G. W., Kringos, D. S., de Maeseneer, J., Gress, S., Heinemann, S., ... Groenewegen, P. P. (2011). QUALICOPC, a multi-country study evaluating quality, costs and equity in primary care. *BMC Family Practice*, *12*(1), p. 115. Retrieved from http://bmcfampract.biomedcentral.com/articles/10.1186/1471-2296-12-115

Sibthorpe, B., & Gardner, K. (2007). A conceptual framework for performance assessment in primary health care. *Australian Journal of Primary Health*, *13*(2), 96–103.

Starfield, B. (1998). *Primary care: Balancing health needs, services, and technology.* New York, NY: Oxford University Press.

Starfield, B. (2001). Improving equity in health: A research agenda. *International Journal of Health Services*, *31*(3), 545–566. Retrieved from https://doi.org/10.2190/DGJ8-4MQW-UP9J-LQC1

Starfield, B., Shi, L., & Macinko, J. (2005). Contribution of primary care to health systems and health. *The Milbank Quarterly*, *83*(3). Retrieved from https://www.ncbi.nlm.nih.gov/pmc/articles/PMC2690145/pdf/milq0083-0457.pdf

Tham, R., Humphreys, J., Kinsman, L., Buykx, P., Asaid, A., Tuohey, K., & Riley, K. (2010). Evaluating the impact of sustainable comprehensive primary health care on rural health. *Australian Journal of Primary Health*, *18*(4), 166–172. doi:10.1111/j.1440-1584.2010.01145.x

van Esso, D., del Torso, S., Hadjipanayis, A., Biver, A., Jaeger-Roman, E., Wettergren, B., ... Primary Secondary Working Group (PSWG) European Academy of Paediatrics. (2010). Paediatric primary care in Europe: Variation between countries. *Archives of Disease in Childhood*, *95*(10), 791–795. doi:10.1136/adc.2009.178459

van Olmen, J., Criel, B., Van Damme, W., Marchal, B., Van Belle, S., Van Dormael, M., ... Kegels, G. (2010). *Analysing health systems to make them stronger.* Vol. 16, Studies in health services organisation & policy. Retrieved from http://www.strengtheninghealthsystems.be/doc/SHSO&P27_HS.ANALYSIS_FINAL.pdf

Veillard, J., Cowling, K., Bitton, A., Ratcliffe, H., Kimball, M., Barkley, S., ... Wang, H. (2017). Better measurement for performance improvement in low- and middle-income countries: The primary health care performance initiative (PHCPI) experience of conceptual framework development and indicator selection. *Milbank Q*, *95*(4), 836–883. doi:10.1111/1468-0009.12301

Wade-Martins, S. (2002). *The English model farm – Building the agricultural ideal, 1700–1914.* Oxford: English Heritage/Windgather Press.

Watson, D. E., Broemeling, A.-M., Reid, R. J., & Black, C. (2004). A Results-based logic model for primary health care: Laying and evidence-based foundation to guide performance measurement, monitoring and evaluation. *Central Health Services Policy Research*, *34*. Retrieved from https://open.library.ubc.ca/cIRcle/collections/facultyresearchandpublications/52383/items/1.0048322

Wong, S. T., Yin, D., Bhattacharyya, O., Wang, B., Liu, L., & Chen, B. (2010). Developing a performance measurement framework and indicators for community health service facilities in urban China. *BMC Family Practice*, *11*(1), 91. Retrieved from http://www.biomedcentral.com/1471-2296/11/91

World Health Organization. (1978). *Declaration of Alma-Ata international conference on primary health care.* Alma-Ata, USSR, 6-12 September 1978. Retrieved from http://www.who.int/publications/almaata_declaration_en.pdf

World Health Organization. (2007). *Everybody's business: Strengthening health systems to improve health outcomes: WHO's framework for action.* Retrieved from http://www.who.int/healthsystems/strategy/everybodys_business.pdf

World Health Organization. (2008a). *The world health report 2008: Primary health care: Now more than ever.* Retrieved from http://www.who.int/whr/2008/whr08_en.pdf

World Health Organization. (2008b). *Commission on social determinants of health: Closing the gap in a generation.* Retrieved from https://www.who.int/healthinfo/HSS_MandE_framework_Nov_2009.pdf

World Health Organization. (2009). *Monitoring and evaluation of health systems strengthening: An operational framework.* World Health Organization. 2009. Retrieved from http://www.who.int/healthinfo/HSS_MandE_framework_Nov_2009.pdf

World Health Organization. (2010). *Monitoring the building blocks of health systems: A handbook of indicators and their measurement strategies.* Geneva: World Health Organization. Retrieved from https://www.who.int/healthinfo/systems/WHO_MBHSS_2010_full_web.pdf

Chapter 3

Listening to Young People

Kinga Zdunek, Manna Alma, Janine van Til,
Karin Groothuis-Oudshoorn, Magda Boere-Boonekamp and
Denise Alexander

Abstract

Children's voices are seldom heard directly. Most often, children, particularly young children, are represented by adults acting on their behalf who may or may not best represent the child's views or best interests. This can be beneficial or problematic, if the child's needs are not appreciated or recognised. This chapter looks at the changing attitudes to listening to young people, and the growing recognition of the value of children's needs, as well as the growing voices of the children themselves, who make their needs increasingly clear. The results of our Models of Child Health Appraised (MOCHA) interviews with children and young people via the DIPEx International organisation give us clear direction as to the importance children using primary care services place on being taken seriously, being listened to and being able to make their own decisions. Other researchers asked input from primary care professionals on children's autonomy and how the current and future primary care systems can best address the needs of young people, as well as the placing of these issues in a wider cultural context, and how this influences and is influenced by children's choices. Finally, we look at how the MOCHA country agents have reported the assessment of the importance and function of listening to young people in our research.

Keywords: Child; children; patient participation; autonomy; primary care; listening; interviews

Introduction

Listening to users, and adjusting services to make them relevant, attractive and accessible, is important in any dimension of health care. With children, this is equally important, as in this life period, health issues are best detected and addressed early, and salutogenic behaviour established, but of course listening to children does have practical and ethic challenges (Roth-Cline & Nelson, 2013). However, as demonstrated by the various approaches developed during the Models of Child Health Appraised (MOCHA) project, these challenges can be overcome successfully and fruitfully.

In this chapter, we look at the importance of listening to children and young people. Child centricity is an important tenet of the MOCHA project (see Chapter 4), and as part of this, we have tried to ensure that we not only have explored how children's experiences, views and needs are taken into account of in the appraisal of primary care services for them in Europe, but also investigated how children's experiences are taken into account, or influence the way primary care policy and services evolve in European Union (EU) and European Economic Area (EEA) countries. Sometimes, this is problematic, for example, children from marginalised populations (see Chapter 5) are poorly listened to or represented. The MOCHA project has investigated how the changing attitudes to children and young people have (or haven't) shaped primary care services, what young people are saying about their care and the service primary care provides, what the public believe to be the case about care for children and societal reactions to child-centred issues that influence or change policy-making. Finally, in an exploration of the MOCHA results, we identify where there is disconnect between what children need and what is in place in the primary care systems of the EU and the EEA countries (see also Chapters 19 and 20).

Changing Attitudes to Listening to Young People

A fundamental premise of the MOCHA project is that of respecting the needs and rights of children as a unique population group (see Chapter 4). We committed to being child-focussed and child-centric, with services being designed to meet need. In this context, we sought to identify what constitutes optimal care for children in primary care services and to find means by which this can be achieved by the different primary care services in Europe. This cannot be achieved without seeking the views of young people themselves.

Children are far more than 'adults in waiting', but have specific health needs and requirements of the primary care health services. We have seen, in the process of the MOCHA project, that children are often required to mould their needs of health care into a structure that is exclusively adult-focused and adult-designed. In addition, research into children's health and health services is more often than not an exercise in navigating systems and structures that are not designed with children in mind, and even basic statistics on services for children and their outcomes are hard to obtain (see Chapters 6 and 7).

As described in Chapter 4, the perception of 'what is a child' has changed, resulting in today's concept of child empowerment, not as a mini adult, but as a distinct individual with specific needs. This has resulted in the recognition that there is a need to define and respect a child's health and role in the health services (Rosa & Matysiuk, 2013). Current thinking on child rights acknowledges that children's views and rights are recognised by the United Nations (UN) and almost all UN member states including all EU and EEA nations (UNHCR, 2018) and by the World Health Organization as a fundamental tenet of health, ensuring their healthy growth and development ought to be a prime concern of all societies (Chapters 2 and 4; WHO, 2018).

Such a change can be seen as a shift in socio-cultural perceptions of the child as having intrinsic, rather than extrinsic value, and this is explored in more detail in Chapters 4 and 17 of this report. Culture in this sense can be defined as the results of material and ideas-based concepts. Values and accepted ways of doing things are adopted and objectified by groups of individuals, transferred to other groups and to the next generations (Szczepański, 1963). It is this process that creates societal attitudes towards children and the value that we place on them. This was reflected in health policy analysis, which has developed to seek to understand the actors involved, including children (see Chapter 1). This approach to policy-making and enabling children via their agents (see Chapter 4), to contribute to policies that affect them can be seen as a cultural change. It is one that allows deep insight into the analysis of primary care for children and is one that MOCHA has adopted.

In the MOCHA project, through analysis of national information received from the MOCHA country agents (see Chapter 1) and from other research activity, increasing focus on the child as a central actor in policy-making has been identified. We found that children are often the main object (directly and indirectly) of debates and discussions related to child primary health care across most of the European countries (Blair, Rigby, & Alexander, 2017; Zdunek, Schröder-Bäck, Blair, Rigby, 2017). This focus can take many forms, such as the child as an object of policy decisions:

- as a well-child embedded in a family context and a broadly understood social environment or preventive care context; and
- the child with long-term illnesses and/or complex health care needs at the centre of the debate.

Although the child is not usually an active participant in policy creation or shaping, he or she becomes a causative actor in the process, because they are the subject of the policy. As described in Chapter 4, the child is surrounded by a range of representatives – who either have a direct influence on the child (as part of the family or immediate social environment – including teachers, neighbours, family physicians and nurses), or an indirect and more distant involvement (including professional groups, health care practitioners representing the health care system, government representatives and the media). At present, changing attitudes to the child have resulted in a number of influences on child health policy, including the child and proximal and distal agents of representation.

Incorporating Young People's Views and Experiences

It is particularly important, when thinking about a child's experience of primary health care, to listen to what children need and understand what they expect and experience from primary care services. Children's lack of autonomy and power means they have very little opportunity to effect change or influence how care is delivered to them. By assessing a child's experience of the health care service, this provides important evidence about the best way to run and provide services.

Including the views of children, young people and their parents are essential components in the appraisal of primary health care for children in Europe. This needs to be proactive and planned, since children do not complete surveys, fill out comments cards or make complaints. Parents, particularly of younger children, or parents faced with newly arising health problems in their child, may not want to antagonise the health professionals and system with which they are dealing and may not know what service norm to expect. It is necessary to actively seek such views.

DIPEx: Qualitative Inquiry into Children's Experiences

Qualitative inquiry into children's and parent's experiences of primary health care for children provided valuable triangulation of results and identification of areas of concern for children, young people and their families. Qualitative researchers from institutions in five different countries that are part of the DIPEx International network (www.dipexinternational.org) worked collaboratively to explore children's experiences of primary care in their respective countries across Europe: Czech Republic, Germany, The Netherlands, Spain and the United Kingdom. These were the only EU/EEA countries with a DIPEx member, but this list included a representative sample of different types of primary care system. The specific objective of this task was to provide insights into the experiences of children and parents in terms of primary health care for children.

Data Collection

The qualitative research methodology used by the MOCHA project was developed by the Health Experiences Research Group (HERG) University of Oxford (Ziebland & Herxheimer, 2008). This methodology includes narrative and semi-structured interviews. The relatively unstructured, open-ended nature of the interview method helps to identify participants' own concerns, meanings and priorities rather than being led by a highly focused research interest (Riessman, 2008). We focused on the experiences of children as well as their parents. Participants were recruited using maximum variation sampling, which involves including a broad range of experiences and demographic characteristics (Coyne, 1997; Marshall, 1996). We aimed to identify and include the widest range of experiences of children and parents in terms of primary care services for children, rather than to identify the numerical distribution that exists in the wider population. We focused on the experiences of 'healthy' children, children with

Table 3.1. Overview of number of children and number and type of interviews in each country.

	Total	Czech Republic	Germany	Netherlands	Spain	UK
# in-depth interviews	38	13	1	7	6	11
# focus group interviews[a]	5 (26)	1 (5)	2 (14)	–	1 (3)	1 (4)
# secondary analysis interviews	20	–	14	–	–	6

Note: [a]In brackets number of participants of the focus group interview.

(complex) mental health conditions and children with (complex) physical health conditions and their parents. In total, 84 children participated in the study.

Data collection consisted of in-depth interviews, focus group interviews and a secondary analysis of interviews conducted in earlier studies in one of the five countries. Interviews and focus group discussions were analysed for themes that structured participants' experiences using a thematic analysis combined with constant comparison. Table 3.1 gives an overview of the number of children that participated in the study per country.

Communication and Relationships with Health Care Professionals

The complete findings of this research can be found in Alma, Mahtani, Palant, Klůzová Kráčmarová, and Prinjha (2017) which discusses in detail the issues that are important to children, young people and their families. Examples of these issues are described here, including communication and relationships with primary care and the importance of involvement and participation in care. Communication and relationships with health care professionals play pivotal role for children in terms of what is good about primary care and what they felt needs to be improved. Communication and relationships were reported as a key quality component. Issues about communication skills, positive attitude towards the child and parents, a trustful relationship and professionalism were the main aspects valued by the participants. Openness to discussion, communication and taking into account the child's opinions about treatment were seen as a sign the child is respected by the health care professional. Other communications skills that were valued were being empathetic, easy to talk to and really listening to what the child or parent is saying.

> What I think they should do – they should, they should be relaxed. I know being a doctor's really stressful and it's very [...] well I don't know that, I don't know why I'm saying that. But I know it can be stressful because of having a job like that is stressful. But I feel like they should be [...] they should relax

themselves, should be relaxed. They should interact, they should
[...] because if you, if you just [...] if you tone it down [...] if you
tone down your, if you tone down the professionalism to some
extent and to more of a social [...] to more of a [...] to more of
an informal sort of stance, then it would definitely have [...] it
will definitely [...] you'll definitely engage with teenagers that
way. Because teenagers don't like formality, and I feel like it's
important to engage with teenagers and so it'll be a bit more [...]
to be a bit more chilled. (UK, M, child)

Children stressed also the importance of building a trusting relationship with
their health care professional. In order to be able to build such a relationship,
children stressed the importance of seeing the same professional every time.
Meeting with the same health care professional helps young people to have
relaxed conversations, feel at ease and build a relationship.

I think it is better to see the same doctor every time, especially
the same GP. Because I know, the doctors ask you about your
medical history every time. And then you do not have to tell
them the same things all over again. (G, F, child)

Although seeing the same doctor every time was important to almost all participants, many recalled seeing different professionals every time they visited the
doctor. Many children perceived a lack of continuity of care. This resulted in
distress, as children met new people each time and had to repeat their story to
different health care professionals as a result. A lack of coordination in primary
care systems was perceived by several participants. This can have serious consequences for children, particularly for a child with complex long-term conditions.

Involvement and Participation in Care
Children and young people felt that they should be involved in managing their
own care. They varied in how much parental involvement they desired and if
they prefer to visit a primary health care professional alone or with their parents.
Many children we interviewed said they visited primary health care services with
their parents. Factors influencing the decision to visit the general practitioner
alone or with someone else included: age, the reason for the visit, level of control
by the parents, accessibility and transport. The disadvantages of visiting health
care professionals with parents were discussed.

Another key point identified was that of being part of the conversation.
Several children recalled that the doctor often spoke to the adult rather than to
the child, which they found annoying.

I can remember thinking I hope this goes away but also that
I was slightly annoyed that they had not paid any attention on
mine to what I'd been saying. (UK, M, child)

> So I think the GP, or the health professional in general, should really just ask the young people what they feel like they need. (UK, F, child)

For successful participation of children in health care, it is important that children's contributions are taken into account and acted upon (Schalkers, Dedding, & Bunders, 2014). However, decisions are often made in cooperation with parents.

> I think the doctors should speak more with the child. [...] I don't know why they cannot ask the child directly. When I am ill and I go to the doctor, I lie down, the doctor examine me, leave me lying there and then he speaks with my father about everything. 'Since when does she feel sick?' and I could be sick earlier, I just didn't say that at home, right? And I think it is wrong, they should talk to the child who is sick [...]. (CZ, F, child)

A number of other issues that are important to children and young people were identified in this qualitative study: accessing primary care services, physical environment of the primary care facility, role of schools, financial issues and medical records. These are fully discussed in Alma et al. (2017).

Parent's Opinions and Experiences on Children's Autonomy

In addition to gathering the views of a group of children, the MOCHA project also sought public views on primary care services and how they address the needs of children. This gave us the views of adults on behalf of children they represent. The report: *Public Priorities for Primary Care for Children. A report on public preferences for patient-centred and prevention oriented primary child health care models for children* (van Til, Groothuis-Oudshoorn, & Boere-Boonekamp, 2018) aimed to elicit formative values from the general public in five European countries and determine public priorities in the assessment of the quality of a child-oriented primary care system. This was a descriptive, cross-sectional, quantitative study of a representative sample of the general public in five European countries (Germany, the Netherlands, Poland, Spain and the United Kingdom). We sought the public's experiences and perceptions of the quality of the currently provided primary care for children, particularly with respect to the children's primary care. We developed the Preferences for Child Health Care Assessed (POCHA) questionnaire as a research instrument, which was translated into Dutch, German, Polish and Spanish (van Til et al., 2018).

In accordance with the children's need for good communication, good access and the need for trust and respect from their primary care providers, one of the foci of the POCHA questionnaire was autonomy of children. This relates in particular to the attributes of quality of care in terms of accessibility, confidentiality and empowerment.

In total, 2,403 adult respondents filled out the POCHA questionnaire. To be able to analyse specifically the opinions and experiences of parents about child autonomy, the respondents who are parents of a child or children aged under 18 years (N = 872) were selected. This resulted in 143 respondents from Germany (DE), 148 from the Netherlands (NL), 173 from Poland (PL), 235 from Spain (ES) and 173 from the United Kingdom (UK).

The results presented in this chapter are based on the topics of what parents consider to be desirable with respect to children's autonomy (10 questions) and what parents have experienced with respect to children's autonomy (nine statements).

Opinions

In the beginning of the POCHA questionnaire, we asked respondents with children aged under 18 years: 'Can you tell us at what age you think a child should be able to do the following?' for ten items related to autonomy.

The overall opinion of respondents of the five countries on the age a child 'should be able to do' the items is presented in Figure 3.1. For all ten autonomy items, the age of 16 years seems to be an important marker to respondents. The figure also shows that respondents think differently about the different items, for example they feel that a child should know about the range of services at a much younger age (89% said at least at the age of 16 years) than that a child should be able to limit access to his or her medical records from his or her parents, in order to protect privacy (43% said at least at the age of 16 years).

In order to study how the five countries relate to each other in terms of the overall opinion on autonomy of children, the respondents' answers on the ten questions were averaged. Figure 3.2 shows that respondents from the Netherlands and Germany assign autonomy to children at a younger age than, for example, respondents from Spain or Poland.

As the age of 16 years seems to be an important marker to respondents, we analysed whether countries differ in opinion on what a child should be able to do first. The five countries' respondents agreed that knowing about the range of services available in health care and how to access them is the item a child should be able to do first. They also agreed on the item that a child should be able to do the latest: namely limiting access to his medical records from his parents. However, agreement on this item ranges a lot; 23.7% of respondents in Poland agree that a child should be able to do this at age 16 compared to 62.4% in the United Kingdom.

Experiences

In the POCHA questionnaire, we also asked respondents with children under 18 years of age about the experiences they have had with primary care for children in their country. Each participant was presented with statements about potential quality of primary care for children and was asked to indicate to what extent he/she agreed or disagreed. We used a scale of 'strongly disagree' to 'strongly agree'. Again, this exercise was designed to measure the experiences of parents

Autonomy per item

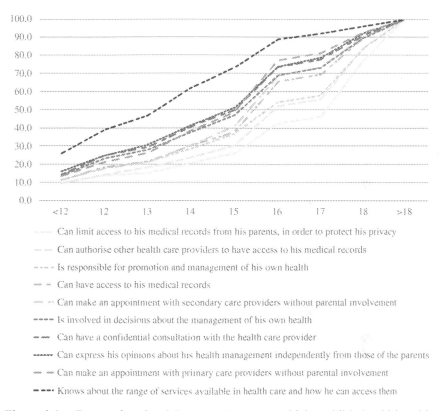

<12   12   13   14   15   16   17   18   >18

------ Can limit access to his medical records from his parents, in order to protect his privacy

—— Can authorise other health care providers to have access to his medical records

~~~~ Is responsible for promotion and management of his own health

—— Can have access to his medical records

—— Can make an appointment with secondary care providers without parental involvement

━━━ Is involved in decisions about the management of his own health

—— Can have a confidential consultation with the health care provider

~~~~~ Can express his opinions about his health management independently from those of the parents

—— Can make an appointment with primary care providers without parental involvement

■━━■ Knows about the range of services available in health care and how he can access them

Figure 3.1.   Respondents' opinions on the age at which a child should be able to do the activities mentioned in the 10 Questions, presented as cumulative percentages of respondents of the five countries together.

about child autonomy. Therefore, we selected the nine items related to accessibility, confidentiality and empowerment to illustrate this.

The results are presented in Table 3.2 and visualised in Figure 3.3.

Accessibility

Respondents' experiences show that improvements with regard to accessibility are achievable. More than half of respondents (53.8%; range 36.1% for Poland to 69% for Germany) agree that children and/or their parents can make an appointment with other primary care providers without a referral from the main primary care provider; percentages are slightly higher for making an appointment with secondary or other health care providers (59.0%; range 40.5% for the UK to 69% for the Netherlands). Almost three-quarters of respondents agree that children and/or their parents (73.1%; range 52.9% for Germany to 84.4% for the UK) are well

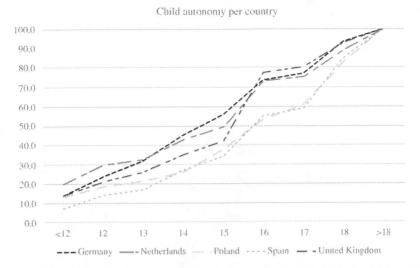

Child autonomy per country

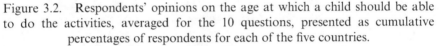

--- Germany ----- Netherlands ------ Poland ---- Spain --- United Kingdom

Figure 3.2.   Respondents' opinions on the age at which a child should be able to do the activities, averaged for the 10 questions, presented as cumulative percentages of respondents for each of the five countries.

informed about the range of services available in primary care and how they can access them. More than two-thirds of respondents (70.8%; range 59.7% for Spain to 88.0% for the Netherlands) have the experience that their child and/or they themselves have access to the child's medical record.

Confidentiality
With respect to confidentiality items, 60.8% (range 37.8% for Poland to 80% for Germany) confirms that a child has the right to a confidential consultation with his primary care provider. Only 32.7% (range 11.6% for Poland to 48.7% for Germany) of respondents agree that in primary care a child can limit parental access to the child's medical records in order to protect his privacy. About two-thirds (66.0%; range 47.4% for Spain to 86.1% for Poland) confirm that the child and/or the parents have to authorise other health care providers accessing the record.

Empowerment
Respondents' experiences related to empowerment items are diverse. More than half of respondents (52.5%; range 40.5% for Poland to 63.9% for the Netherlands) answer that a child can express his opinions about his health management independently from those of the parents. almost three-quarters (74%; range 61.4% for Spain to 93.6% for the UK) agree that in primary care, children and/or their parents are involved in decisions about the management of the child's health.

Societal Reactions

The context of child primary care is not just placed with the users and providers, but is inextricably linked with the wider cultural context (see also Chapters 4 and 17).

Table 3.2. Percentage of agreement (summed percentage of respondents that agree and strongly agree) with the statements on autonomy-related attribute items, indicated by the respondents of the five countries.

Statements	% Agreement with Statement, Per Country*						Pearson χ^2	p-value
	DE	NL	PL	ES	UK	Average		
Children and/or their parents can make an appointment with other primary care providers without a referral from the main primary care provider (accessibility)	69.0	56.4	36.1	50.9	58.8	53.8	30.6	0.015
Children and/or their parents can make an appointment with secondary or other health care providers without a referral from a primary care provider (accessibility)	64.9	69.0	65.2	57.4	40.5	59.0	19.0	0.268
Children and/or their parents know about the range of services available in primary care and how they can access them (accessibility)	52.9	72.7	74.4	64.2	84.4	73.1	22.7	0.119
A child and/or his parents have access to a child's medical records (accessibility)	65.4	88.0	80.5	59.7	75.9	70.8	32.1	0.010
A child has the right to a confidential consultation with the primary care provider (confidentiality)	80.0	75.0	37.8	52.4	66.7	60.8	39.1	0.001
In primary care, a child can limit their parents' access to the child's medical records in order to protect his privacy (confidentiality)	29.4	48.7	11.6	33.3	41.5	32.7	30.7	0.014

Table 3.2. *(Continued)*

Statements	% Agreement with Statement, Per Country*						Pearson χ^2	*p*-value
	DE	NL	PL	ES	UK	Average		
In primary care, the child and/or the parents have to authorise other health care providers accessing the child's medical records (confidentiality)	68.1	64.1	86.1	47.4	49.0	66.0	12.5	0.706
In primary care, a child can express his opinions about his health management independently from his parents (empowerment)	60.7	63.9	40.5	41.4	63.4	52.5	28.2	0.030
In primary care, children and/or their parents are involved in decisions about the management of the child's health (empowerment)	85.2	68.6	67.9	61.4	93.6	74.0	35.8	0.003

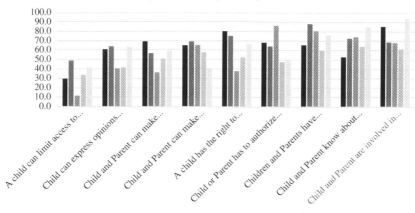

Figure 3.3. Percentage of agreement (summed percentage of respondents that agree and strongly agree) with the statements on autonomy-related attribute-items, indicated by the respondents of the five countries, based on their experiences.

As part of the MOCHA project, we investigated the effect of societal reactions to issues that affect children. We looked at particularly sensitive national concerns and how they affected popular perceptions of what child primary care should be for and how it is run in countries (Zdunek, Schröder-Bäck, Blair, Rigby, 2017). The MOCHA country agents identified two or three recent societal debates in their country, which involved children's health and well-being. They described wide variety of cases, demonstrating the broad perspectives of children's health and health services. Many of the issues described were very different, but all had certain elements in common. Essentially, the concerns in Europe about children's health are twofold. On the one hand, attention was given to issues relating to organisational factors of the care of children, involving those indirectly concerned with children as patients; on the other hand, some issues directly involved children themselves, such as cases of child abuse, care of children in hospital, childhood obesity, homelessness or poverty (Zdunek, Schröder-Bäck, Blair, Rigby, 2017). Children are seen in two broad domains – either that of the generally healthy child embedded in a family context, where attention is focused on preventive actions, or as a sick child, or a child with a long-term condition, who has need of specific attention from the health services.

Child health issues can be particularly sensitive and thus can provoke strong societal reactions that may eventually shape national health policy. Public voices can stimulate policy change, when a government is reluctant or unable to deliver because of lack of political interest, inflexible public administrations, resource constraints or lack of trust in certain populations (Greer, Kosińska, & Wismar, 2017). Civic society, in the form of informal movements or public discussions, brings expertise, ideas and diverse perspectives to the field of health policy-making, particularly child health policy-making. Indeed, the effectiveness of child health policy initiatives increases the more there is involvement of relevant actors.

The means by which the public express their dismay or support of an initiative or system change can also support or hinder the process of policy development (see also Chapter 17). In addition, public expression can also stimulate change without appropriately informed debate as to the intended or unintended consequences of the resulting action. In MOCHA, we investigated the vehicles of public expression, to characterise how the public sentiment was raised and continued.

In the research process, we were able to identify four distinct areas of public expression: actors, actions, communication and information. *Actors* who were directly involved in the process of children's health care, such as parents and individuals, politicians and academics, experts and stakeholders and non-governmental organisations (NGOs), expressed opinions through *actions* such as protests and strikes, campaigns, debates and petitions, social media activity or emotional reactions. Additionally, they were often supported by philanthropic and political initiatives. Public attention was maintained through various *communication channels*, most commonly social media, traditional media and the internet. *Information* is becoming more readily available, via official government internet websites, social media or other channels, such as articles in the press, documentaries and educational films, as well as publications of reports, which help to keep the issue in the public eye. Those elements supplement each other and therefore they cannot be analysed separately

Actors

Expression of the process of policy change or the desire for change is manifested by certain actors, including those representing children in the proximal and distal sense (see Chapter 4). These could be individuals such as children, parents or journalists, or organisations such as political parties or NGOs. For instance, childhood obesity in Malta was highlighted as an issue and an object of policy campaigning by politicians and academics in the country, and political debates in Finland and the United Kingdom were held about the services and treatment given to unaccompanied child asylum-seekers.

In Ireland, objections to changes in the Discretionary Medical Card (which enables health care free of charge) were voiced by a range of actors who inspired much public support. These actors organised a strong social media campaign and online petition to the government and were supported by public support foundations and NGOs. These actors aimed to reverse a decision that many felt resulted in inequity of (lack of) provision to vulnerable children. In Romania, the inappropriate treatment and overmedication of children in residential children's home was exposed by journalists as actors representing the rights and needs of the children.

A private foundation (Paracelsus NGO) advocated 'freedom of choice' by publicising an anti-vaccination rhetoric in the media in the Czech Republic, against the mandatory vaccination policy of that country. There has also been much debate in Italy, where compulsory vaccination has recently been revoked due to the influence of anti-vaccination sentiments.

Public expression can take place by the actors directly involved, or opinions are expressed through actions, such as a strike (as was the case in Poland), or a vigil (such as that held by parents protesting at changes to eligibility for Discretionary Medical cards).

Actions

Actions such as public protests, strikes, campaigns, debates and petitions are common societal reactions to issues that are perceived to affect children unjustly. Examples of this have been reported in relation to issues pertinent to children in Greece, Italy, Ireland Lithuania and Norway (Blair et al., 2017) among other countries. In Croatia, there were public protests related to mandatory vaccination, disabled children's rights and child abuse. In Poland, the nurses went on strike in protest at poor remuneration and stressful working conditions, which were supported by patients and nurses from health centres other than the hospital where the protest initiated. The nurses' strike was also met by protests by groups of parents who argued that they should find another means of expressing their discontent, as their actions risked harming children further in their eyes.

Another form of action is the creation of a petition, which is a demonstration of the depth of support for an issue. In France, there was a public protest against the DTP vaccination, an action that began with a petition which eventually collected over one million signatures. In the Czech Republic in 2010, a group of parents presented a petition against mandatory vaccination. A petition was also created in the Czech Republic to express disquiet about the need to unify services, despite the fact that concern had been previously raised about the fragmentation of services and the complex system. In Ireland, a petition was organised by those objecting to the decision to build a national children's hospital in the centre of Dublin. Social media and Web-based campaigns resulted in over 60,000 signatures.

Media campaigns are another common action that has been used to increase public awareness about an issue. In Ireland, the issue of homelessness was discussed nationally after being highlighted in a television programme, and within the UK, and in Northern Ireland, child sexual exploitation was exposed in this way.

Philanthropic actions can also be seen as a form of societal reaction to national situations. The presence of food banks in Spain is one such example as a reaction to the hardship felt by many families. In Norway, the scandal of a young boy who was a victim of child abuse led to members of the public leaving flowers at the entrance to the hospital where he was treated. Emotional actions, similarly, are often used to support and stimulate the retention of an issue in the public psyche. In Poland, for example, support for and resistance to the nurses' strike was maintained by stressing the emotional aspects of events that led to the strike. This was characterised by presenting the children as innocent victims of a 'heartless system', 'insensitivity of officials', 'nurses concerned only with money', and 'political manipulation'. Politicians were also seen to use emotional pressure on the striking nurses, and the opposition politicians accused the government of disinterest in the fate of nurses and their patients.

Communication

For any protest or reaction to be successful, communication is essential. The means of this is changing, relying increasingly on social media rather than official methods such as printed media or television. Social media, in particular, is increasingly powerful as it functions to support campaigns. Electronic communication played a crucial role in almost all cases described by the MOCHA country agents.

Shocking events were almost always reported in the media – such as news, newspapers, online and so on, and these provoked a national discussion. This allowed the actors, such as parents and other stakeholders, to speak publicly about their issues.

For example, in Croatia, a parent witnessed child abuse by an employee at the Croatian 'Special Hospital for Protection of Children with Neurodevelopmental and Motor Disorders'. This was shared through social media, which caused a scandal and resulting heavy coverage by the national media. An explanation and disciplinary action were demanded by the public as a result. In the United Kingdom, the news and social media were instrumental in raising concerns about immigration and facilitating actions. Images and stories were shared regularly and societal actions resulted. These ranged from a public march to welcome refugees, which saw thousands congregate to support asylum-seekers and refugees in September 2016, to petitions that oppose refugees and asylum-seekers entering the United Kingdom.

New regulations on nutrition for young people sparked social media protests in Poland. High school students claimed that they wanted to decide on their own diet, resulting in a petition and discussion among young people, parents, politicians and businesses.

Traditional media, such as newspapers, television and radio remain a key aspect of societal reactions to policy changes. Public debates are sustained through Web-based initiatives and traditional press. Awareness of childhood obesity was raised in Austria through daily newspapers, televisions and other campaigns. They often used attention-grabbing headlines such as 'Each fifth child is overweight' or 'the fight against obesity', 'Our children grow ever fatter'.

Information

Without information, societal reactions do not happen. What is an issue is whether the information is reliable and truthful. Information is shared by active actors, through various communication channels. National and local news reports are instrumental in raising many types of concerns, and as a result, public opinion and trends can have a significant impact on decisions about health systems. For example, an Irish television documentary called 'My Homeless Family' about the experiences of homeless families and those living in emergency accommodation was televised a month before a general election. This, combined with wider debate and emerging statistics about the increase in homelessness in Ireland, turned it into an election issue. This was also informed by a report entitled Homeless Truths (Ombudsman for Children's Office, 2012), which described children's experiences of homelessness; simultaneously, the Ombudsman for Children also launched a series of recordings of the young people's interviews that were used in the study. In Latvia, educational films about bullying in schools and cyberbullying were created from national reports and research, to respond to increasing concerns about bullying. The goal of these films was to provide information to empower pupils and teachers to understand and deal with bullying, its nature and consequences. The Association of Hungarian primary care paediatricians produced publications outlining the issue of unclear health certificates for children attending summer camps in Hungary; in the United Kingdom, charities and other organisations produced reports on the challenges faced by unaccompanied asylum-seeking children and called upon the government to do more to help them.

The childhood obesity debate in the United Kingdom, particularly in Scotland, was fuelled by a number of reports published by the Scottish Government on the health and economic burden of obesity in Scotland in 2015. Targets were subsequently set to reduce the prevalence of obesity, and a ban on advertising junk food was extended in the country.

Environmental pollution was a topic of discussion in Italy, after a number of press articles and the Higher Institute of Health report known as the ISTISAN Report. The data in this report were published on the website of the Higher Institute of Health and refer to a study commissioned by the Ministry of Health to implement prevention strategies after increased mortality and hospitalisation had occurred in an area where considerable amount of waste was incinerated (Blair et al., 2017)

MOCHA Country Agent Questions about Children

In addition to independent research in MOCHA to listen to children and young people, or to gain the views of their representatives, we also asked the country agents to identify policies and practices in their countries that facilitated or restricted children from giving their views or influenced health services for young people. The country agents were not able to obtain views of children themselves, because of ethical permissions, nor were they able to give opinions about their country. However, they were able to provide examples and instances of where each country was particularly child-friendly, or which countries made it more difficult for children to participate and collaborate in their own primary care.

Within 40 sets of questions to the country agents, all of which were child-focused in some way; 15 directly investigated children's experiences. Subjects that were subject to MOCHA's attention were migrant and refugee children, long-term complex conditions, chronic physical and mental conditions; vulnerable children (e.g. those in the care system); children's corporate autonomy and how well this is catered for in each country; the use and regulation of health apps and helplines; and home-based records where parents and children can have access and input.

Equity of Provision for Young People

MOCHA country agents answered questions about equity of provision for two particularly vulnerable groups of individuals, refugee and asylum-seeking children and children living in out of home societal care (foster or residential care). These child populations can be seen as representative of the equity of provision in primary health care in their countries, more about which is discussed in Chapter 7. The country agents were asked to provide policy references, about whether these children received the same health care as other children in their country and whether they received less care or par-ticularly targeted care − which may or may not result in intended or unin-tended consequences.

Children with Complex Care Needs in the Community

Country agents identified particular points of care for children living with com-plex care needs. Tracer conditions chosen to represent this group of vulnerable individuals were those on long-term ventilation, those with traumatic brain injury and those with intractable epilepsy. In order to establish the primary care and community support that children and families had in their countries, country agents identified the different agencies involved in every day care, the extent to which families and children are consulted and input into their care plans, and the ease at which good quality and relevant support could be obtained and sustained.

Children with Long-term Mental Health Needs in the Community

Country agents were tasked with identifying the level of support and care children with long-term mental health needs experience in primary care and the community. Tracer conditions of Autism and ADHD were used to represent all children with complex needs, as the management and treatment of these are typical of many other forms of mental health care. Issues such as the policy around access to education support for children and families and the extent to which they can access and input into their care were explored by the country agents.

Social Care and Child Protection

Children who are in need of social care support, and how this links to pri-mary care services in the community, were investigated by country agents, by extending one of the vignettes developed to describe a child with complex care needs, in this case, a traumatic brain injury. This allowed the country agents to explore the relationship between social care needs and health care needs and how easy it is for children and families to access the correct levels of support. Child protection is an important element of this, and we wished to know if policy allowed easy access to services in a case of vulnerability; the issue of child protection was also investigated in terms of children in foster care and equity (see Chapter 7).

Children with a Long-term (Chronic) Condition

Asthma was the main tracer condition used to identify the extent to which children can self-manage any long-term conditions. The country agents identified areas in which children were able, or not, to manage their own medication (such as in school), access transition from children's services to adult services, and the extent to which policy allows adolescents can seek advice independently and make their own decisions about their care.

Autonomy of Choice

We asked about whether policy allowed children to independently access care, such as in the case of reproductive health or contraception, health advice and education or treatment – or whether the system did not facilitate this without parental or guardian knowledge or payment. The country agents also investigated whether children could override parental decisions about their health, such as in the case of vaccinations.

Use of Apps, Websites and Helplines

Country agents explored the information that is most accessible and attractive to children and young people, namely, that contained in apps, websites and helplines. The extent to which these are regulated for accuracy of advice in each country and the types of data that are collected by the sites were investigated by the country agents.

Home-based Records of Children's Health

We asked about home-based records, the range of their use, means of extending them to children moving into a country and the extent to which parents and older children can contribute to the types of data they collect and whether they can independently record data that will subsequently be used to improve and coordinate services. For more information, see the full report by Deshpande, Rigby, Alexander, and Blair (2018).

Summary

Listening to the views of children and young people is essential in designing and appraising primary care systems to serve them. However, listening is not necessarily an easy task. Children are often necessarily represented by others, which can be beneficial or increase their vulnerability. When the opinions of those representing children are taken into account, care must be taken that they represent their best interests. Research in this area is challenging, but at the same time, vitally important.

The DIPEx findings show that although many children were satisfied with the primary health care services for children, it is not a universally good picture. While some of the needs of the children, young people and their families are complex and beyond the influence of an individual health professional, other concerns are clearly within a health care professional's ability to improve. Careful interpretation and analysis of patients' subjective experiences highlighted what is working well in primary care services for children, what needs to be changed and how to go about making improvements (Alma et al., 2017).

> Tips for health care professionals: try to pay sufficient attention to your patients, and if it is a child, try to explain him or her everything as clear as possible. If the child is older, please evaluate what the child already knows and anticipate. (NL, F, child)

Similarly, the POCHA questionnaire reflects, to a great extent, the perceptions stated by the children in the qualitative interviews about primary care carried out by the DIPEx group. What is interesting, however, is that in Poland and Spain, there seems to be less capacity or cultural acceptance of child autonomy in the management of their health than in Germany, the Netherlands and the United Kingdom (see also Chapter 17).

Indeed, recognising that children grow steadily in understanding, knowledge and the wish to be treated as individuals is a key issue throughout all the work reported in this chapter. It also comes to light in Chapter 10 about children with complex needs and enduring conditions, and in Chapter 14 about E-Health. The wider issues of the growing awareness and autonomy of the child are picked up further in Chapter 19.

In terms of societal reactions to the health care of children, it is clear that issues involving children are emotive and tend to readily provoke national debates. Predominantly, public concerns identified by the MOCHA country agents were directly or indirectly related to health care of children. Some issues became part of public awareness for only a few weeks, such as the national debate about contraception for adolescent girls in France, and others remain in the public consciousness for many years – such as the debates about compulsory vaccination in Italy or the proposed location of the national children's hospital in Ireland. In the MOCHA project, we have tried to elucidate the views of children directly or via actors on their behalf as well as aiming to establish the extent to which children's views are considered important in the policy environment and in the evolution of national primary care services.

References

Alma, M., Mahtani, V., Palant, A., Klůzová Kráčmarová, L., & Prinjha, S. (2017). *Report on patient experiences of primary care in 5 DIPEx countries.* Retrieved from http://www.childhealthservicemodels.eu/publications/technical-reports/

Blair, M., Rigby, M., & Alexander, D. (2017). *Final report on current models of primary care for children.* Retrieved from www.childhealthservicemodels.eu/wp-content/uploads/2017/07/MOCHA-WP1-Deliverable-WP1-D6-Feb-2017-1.pdf

Coyne, I. T. (1997). Sampling in qualitative research. Purposeful and theoretical sampling: Merging or clear boundaries? *Journal of Advanced Nursing, 26,* 623–630.

Deshpande, S., Rigby, M., Alexander, D., & Blair, M. (2018). *Home based records.* Retrieved from www.childhealthservicemodels.eu/wp-content/uploads/R15-Home-Based-Records-Report.pdf

European Parliament and European Council. (2005). Directive 2005/36/EC of the European Parliament and of the council of 7 September 2005 on the recognition of professional qualifications. *Official Journal of the European Union.* L255/22, Article 31. Retrieved from https://eur-lex.europa.eu/LEXUriServ/LexUriServ.do?uri=OJ:L:2005:255:0022:0142:EN:PDF

European Parliament and European Council. (2013). Directive 2013/55/EU of the European Parliament and of the council amending Directive 2005/36/EC on the recognition of professional qualifications and Regulation (EU) No 1024/2012 on administrative cooperation through the International Market Information System ('the IMI Regulation'). *Official Journal of the European Union.* L 354/132. Retrieved from http://eur-lex.europa.eu/legal-content/EN/TXT/PDF/?uri=CELEX:32013L0055&from=EN

Greer, S. L., Kosińska, M., & Wismar, M. (2017). What is civil society and what can it do for health? In S. L. Greer, M. Kosińska, & M. Wismar (Eds.), *Civil society and health, contributions and potential, European observatory on health systems and policies* (p. 12). World Health Organization. Retrieved from www.euro.who.int/en/about-us/partners/observatory/publications/studies/civil-society-and-health-contributions-and-potential-2017

Marshall, M. N. (1996). Sampling for qualitative research. *Family Practice, 13,* 522–525.

Ombudsman for Children's Office. (2012). *Homeless truths: Children's experience of homelessness in Ireland.* Retrieved from www.oco.ie/app/uploads/2017/09/HomelessTruthsWEB.pdf

Riessman, C. K. (2008). *Narrative methods for the human sciences.* Thousand Oaks, CA: Sage.

Rosa, R., & Matysiuk, R. (2013). Ewolucja praw dziecka (aspekty filozoficzne, pedagogiczne i prawne). In E. Jagiełło, & E. Jówko (Eds.), *Dziecko w kulturze współczesnego świata* (pp. 10–33). Siedlce ISBN 978-83-936635-2-1. Retrieved from https://docplayer.pl/4327137-Dziecko-w-kulturze-wspolczesnego-swiata-redakcja-naukowa-ewa-jagiello-ewa-jowko.html

Roth-Cline, M., & Nelson, R. M. (2013). Parental Permission and child assent in research on children. *Yale Journal of Biology and Medicine, 86*(3), 291–301.

Schalkers, I., Dedding, C. H. M., & Bunders, J. F. G. (2014). '[I would like] a place to be alone, other than the toilet' — Children's perspectives on paediatric hospital care in the Netherlands. *Health Expectations, 18*, 2066−2078.

Szczepański, J. (1963). *Elementarne pojęcia socjologii.* Warszawa: PWN.

United Nations Human Rights Office of the High Commissioner (UNHCR). (2018). *Declaration of the rights of the child (1959).* Retrieved from www.ohchr.org/EN/Issues/Education/Training/Compilation/Pages/1DeclarationoftheRightsoftheChild(1959).aspx

van Til, J., Groothuis-Oudshoorn, K., & Boere-Boonekamp, M. (2018). *Public priorities for primary care for children.* Retrieved from www.childhealthservicemodels.eu/wp-content/uploads/member-files/Final-Report-POCHA_14-08-2018.pdf

World Health Organization. (2018). *Child health.* Retrieved from https://www.who.int/topics/child_health/en

Zdunek, K., Schröder-Bäck, P., Rigby, M., & Blair, M. (2018). *The culture of evidence-based practice in child health policy - A report.* Retrieved from www.childhealthservicemodels.eu/wp-content/uploads/Evidence-Based-culture-Report.pdf

Zdunek, K., Schröder-Bäck, P., Alexander, D., Rigby, M., & Blair, M. (2017). *Report on the contextual determinants of child health policy.* Available from http://www.childhealthservicemodels.eu/wp-content/uploads/Context-Culture-Report.pdf

Ziebland, S., & Herxheimer, A. (2008). How patients' experiences contribute to decision making: Illustrations from DIPEx (personal experiences of health and illness). *Journal of Nursing Management, 16*, 433−439.

Chapter 4

Child Centricity and Children's Rights

Kinga Zdunek, Michael Rigby, Shalmali Deshpande and Denise Alexander

Abstract

The child is at the centre of all Models of Child Health Appraised research and indeed all primary care delivery for children. Appraising models of primary care for children is incomplete without ensuring that experiences of primary care, design, treatment, management and outcomes are optimal for the child. However, the principle of child centricity is not implicit in many healthcare systems and in many aspects of life, yet it is extremely important for optimal child health service design and child health. By exploring the changing concept of 'childhood', we understand better the emergence of the current attitude towards children and their role in today's Europe and the evolution of child rights. Understanding child centricity, and the role of agents acting on behalf of the child, allows us to identify features of children's primary care systems that uphold the rights of a child to optimum health. This is placed against the legal commitments made by the countries of the European Union and European Economic Area to ensure that children's rights are respected.

Keywords: Child centricity; child primary care; child rights; socio-cultural context; child value; child agents

Introduction — A Challenge for Policy-makers

The child is at the centre of all Models of Child Health Appraised (MOCHA) research. Appraising models of primary care for children is impossible without ensuring that experiences of primary care, treatment, management and outcomes are optimal for the child. When designing child health systems, it is easy to focus on the population level and on the needs of the majority adult population, but this risks devaluing the status of the child. Children make up a quarter of the population and are frequent users of primary care – not least for preventive services (Blair, Rigby, & Alexander, 2017). The principle of child centricity is not implicit in many healthcare systems and in many aspects of life, yet it is extremely important for optimal child access and child health. This chapter explains the objective and philosophy of child health service provision in MOCHA. Understanding true child centricity is logically an essential prerequisite to the design and provision of optimal child health services. Even certain aspects of the MOCHA mission, in emphasising that children are the future of society, risk a societal utilitarian approach – healthy children are seen as a 'good thing' as they will metamorphose into a healthy adult population, boosting economic and societal strength and gain. The challenge is to make the child the focus, from a local to international level. A child is considered important as a member of society, as evidenced by the European Values Survey (2015) (see Chapter 17), but this is not necessarily represented in societal structures.

The Child in a Socio-cultural Context

How can a child and childhood be considered as the prime value in a child-centric paradigm embedded in the European socio-cultural context? History shows that the attitudes towards the child have changed throughout the ages. These changes are the consequence of socio-cultural shifts in the perception of the child as an intrinsic rather than an extrinsic value. Socio-cultural contexts have altered attitudes towards children and created their value in society, including towards their health. Culture, which is understood as the results of human actions in terms of material and ideal concepts, values and accepted ways of doing things, is objectified and accepted by collectives and transferred to other collectives and next generations (Szczepański, 1963) (see also Chapters 16 and 17). Culture plays a regulatory role towards behavioural aspects in changing multicultural Europe.

The Changing Concept of a Child and the History of Rights Approaches

The concept of the child and childhood has been changing in terms of time, place and space (Garbula & Kowalik-Olubińska, 2012). In Ancient Greece, the child was obliged to yield to his or her father's will. Spartan children were considered to be the property of the state, which was supposed to take care of their physical and military development (Rosa & Matysiuk, 2013), in a system known as *agoge* (Kulesza, 2003). Aristoteles identified the need to care for children's intellectual and physical development and health as it was common that disabled children, or those who were born in an extramarital relationship or orphaned, were often condemned to a life of ostracism and poverty (Rosa & Matysiuk, 2013). In Ancient Rome, the father had the right to decide about the life and death of a child by law (Rosa & Matysiuk, 2013). A change in attitudes towards children came in the Middle Ages. Ariés (1962) describes the Middle Ages as a time when a child was seen solely as a small adult; but this view contrasts with research conducted by other medievalists (Brzezinski, 2012). The perception of a child at that period in Europe was strongly influenced by the image of the child presented in the Christian Bible; expressed, for example, by the privileged access of children to the kingdom of God (Brzeziński, 2012). The child, thus, became an object of value and the family became responsible for his or her social and moral development (Rosa & Matysiuk, 2013). Ibrahim ibn Yaqub, in the tenth century, wrote that in Slavic countries, a soldier was even paid his wages on the day of his child's birth, whether it was male or female. The Renaissance (1350–1700) saw greater appreciation of the personality of a child. Attention was given to poor children, who benefited from public education. Additionally, the idea of Erasmian humanism 'conceived of education as a method for cultivating human potential and dignity to the fullest possible extent' (Parrish, 2013). The enlightenment of the eighteenth century (1685–1815) attached great significance to the institutionalisation of care directed at excluded and marginalised children. John Locke (1632–1704) played a significant role and claimed that 'the child has needs and interests which should be recognised for what they are and that the child should be reasoned with, not simply beaten or coerced into conformity with the ruled of required behaviour' (Archard, 2004). The French Revolution at the end of the eighteenth century marked a point when children were first given rights and parents were obliged to protect the child. Social development, as well as the development of humanism and respect of the individual, was mirrored in the ideas of the French Revolution and the attitudes of the Christian Church claiming that the child has its own rights and lack of respect to them was considered a sin (Jarosz, 2010). However, the industrial era of the nineteenth century in Europe saw new challenges for children. Children suffered high mortality and poor living and working conditions, and they were used as sources of cheap labour (Balcerek, 1986), There was an increased level of juvenile delinquency as the consequence of this lack of care. Initiatives which aimed to care of the homeless and abandoned children, debates on juvenile courts and moral education of children prompted a fundamental change in terms of philanthropic activities in the nineteenth and twentieth centuries in Europe (Balcerek, 1986), which were effectively the first steps in the development of children's rights.

The beginning of twentieth century brought the emergence of protection and educational initiatives directed at children. Organisations such as Save the Children in England, *Rädda Barnen* in Sweden and the International Save the Children Union (UISE) were established to protect and educate children. In 1924, the League of Nations inspired by UISE adapted the Geneva Declaration of the Rights of the Child to protect vulnerable children and victims of the war. We could consider it as a first step in empowering the child as an actor in society; in effect, from this point onwards, it could be argued that this is when the child began to be considered as a value in itself, rather than solely as parents' or state property. This was an important milestone in the recognition of the children rights (see Box 4.1).

Box 4.1.   The Geneva Declaration of the Rights of the Child.

"By the present Declaration of the Rights of the Child, commonly known as "Declaration of Geneva," men and women of all nations, recognizing that mankind owes to the Child the best that it has to give, declare and accept it as their duty that, beyond and above all considerations of race, nationality or creed:

- The child must be given the means requisite for its normal development, both materially and spiritually;
- The child that is hungry must be fed; the child that is sick must be nursed; the child that is backward must be helped; the delinquent child must be reclaimed; and the orphan and the waif must be sheltered and succoured;
- The child must be the first to receive relief in times of distress;
- The child must be put in a position to earn a livelihood, and must be protected against every form of exploitation;
- The child must be brought up in the consciousness that its talents must be devoted to the service of fellow men."

(United Nations, 1924)

Further recognition of a child's rights in the second half of the twentieth century is evidenced by increasing legal recognition of the place of a child in society. Table 4.1 shows the key important events, culminating in the 1989 UN Convention on the Rights of the Child (UNICEF, 1989) which is signed by all MOCHA countries and should inform all aspects of children's health care to this present day.

The Child-centric Paradigm and the Child as an Actor in Health Care

The current recognition of child rights is evidence of the emergence of the concept of the child as an active actor in society. Bronfenbrenner (1979) theorised that development and socialisation of child are affected by linkages on micro-, meso-, exo- and macro-levels. Bronfenbrenner's theory requires the acceptance of the following assumptions:

- Person is an active player, exerting influence on his/her environment.
- Environment is compelling the person to adapt to its conditions and restrictions.
- Environment is understood to consist different size entities that are place one inside another, of their reciprocal relationship and of micro-, meso-, exo- and macro-systems (Bronfenbrenner, 1979; Härkönen, 2007).

Table 4.1. Timeline of increasing awareness and respect for the rights of a child in Europe.

1946	The United Nations International Children's Emergency Fund (UNICEF) and the United Nations Educational, Scientific and Cultural Organization (UNESCO) are created
1948	*The Universal Declaration of Human Rights* is created. Included in article 25 is a statement that makes children's rights equal whether a child is born to married or unmarried parents

- Motherhood and childhood are entitled to special care and assistance. All children, whether born in or out of wedlock, shall enjoy the same social protection.

1948	*Declaration of the Rights of the Child* (United Nations, 2015) supplemented the Geneva Declaration of the Rights of the Child. Two points were added as the consequence of the experiences of the Second World War:

- The child must be protected beyond and above all considerations of race, nationality or creed.
- The child must be cared for with due respect for the family as an entity.
- The child must be given the means requisite for its normal development, materially, morally and spiritually.
- The child that is hungry must be fed, the child that is sick must be nursed, the child that is mentally or physically handicapped must be helped, the maladjusted child must be re-educated, the orphan and the waif must be sheltered and succoured.
- The child must be the first to receive relief in time of distress.
- The child must enjoy the full benefits provided by social welfare and social security schemes, must receive a training which will enable it at the right time to earn a livelihood and must be protected against every form of exploitation.
- The child must be brought up in the consciousness that its talents must be devoted to the services of its fellow men.

Child Rights International Network (2018)

1950	*European Convention on Human Rights*, which in Art 5, states that 'Spouses shall enjoy equality of rights and responsibilities of a private law character between them, and in their relations with their children' (Council of Europe, 1950)
1959	*The Declaration of the Rights of the Child is produced by the United Nations.* This document stresses the importance of child

Table 4.1. (*Continued*)

---

health and in particular the role of the Agents of the Child in the process of care

Principle 4. The child shall enjoy the benefits of social security. He shall be entitled to grow and develop in health; to this end, special care and protection shall be provided both to him and to his mother, including adequate pre-natal and post-natal care. The child shall have the right to adequate nutrition, housing, recreation and medical services.

Principle 5. The child who is physically, mentally or socially handicapped shall be given the special treatment, education and care required by his particular condition.

Principle 6 [...]. He shall, wherever possible, grow up in the care and under the responsibility of his parents, and, in any case, in an atmosphere of affection and of moral and material security; a child of tender years shall not, save in exceptional circumstances, be separated from his mother. Society and the public authorities shall have the duty to extend particular care to children without a family and to those without adequate means of support. [...]

Principle 8. The child shall, in all circumstances, be among the first to receive protection and relief.

(UNICEF, 2003)

1961   *European Social Charter (Council of Europe).* This charter gave recognition to the care of the mother and child: the Right to social protection for mother and child and the Right of children and young persons to protection

(Council of Europe, 1961)

1966   *International Covenant on Civil and Political Rights.* This covenant contained:

Art. 23. Protection of the family

Art. 24. Protection of the rights of the child

(United Nations, 1976)

1976   *International Covenant on Economic, Social and Cultural Rights*

Art. 10.1. Family as the natural and fundamental group unit of society, [...] is responsible for the care and education of dependent children [...].

Table 4.1. (*Continued*)

	Art. 10.3. Special measures of protection and assistance should be taken on behalf of all children and young persons without any discrimination for reasons of parentage or other conditions. [...] Their employment in work harmful to their morals or health or dangerous to life or likely to hamper their normal development should be punishable by law.
	(United Nations Human Rights: Office of the High Commissioner (OHCHR), 1976).
1989	*UN Convention on the Rights of the Child* *Art. 3.*
	1. States Parties undertake to ensure the child such protection and care as is necessary for his or her well-being, taking into account the rights and duties of his or her parents, legal guardians, or other individuals legally responsible for him or her, [...]
	2. States Parties shall ensure that the institutions, services and facilities responsible for the care or protection of children shall conform with the standards established by competent authorities, particularly in the areas of safety, health, in the number and suitability of their staff, as well as competent supervision
	Art. 6.
	1. States Parties recognise that every child has the inherent right to life.
	Art. 24
	1. States Parties recognise the right of the child to the enjoyment of the highest attainable standard of health and to facilities for the treatment of illness and rehabilitation of health. States Parties shall strive to ensure that no child is deprived of his or her right of access to such healthcare services.
	(United Nations, 1989)

We propose to adapt this frame into a child-centric paradigm in health care by:

- considering the child as an active player empowered in the process of healthcare provision but also in defining health policy via the agents of the child;
- the child is embedded in particular environment which requires to adapt and respect the common principles and values; and
- the environment will be understood as the wider context of socio-cultural, structural, external and internal background which will interact between child and its proximal and distant environment on different levels.

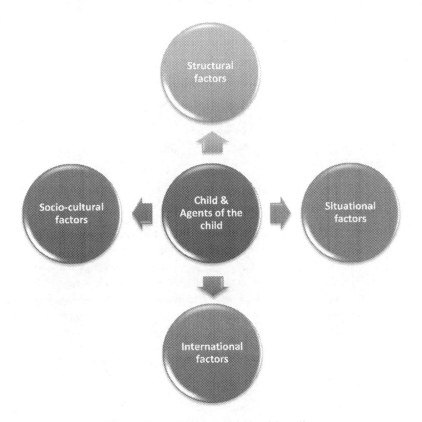

Figure 4.1.   Child-centric health policy.

This is explained in more detail in Figure 4.1.

In order to achieve truly child-centric healthcare systems, it is important not only to consider the individual child, but also to look wider to population measures that benefit the individual. This is where child-centric health policy-making is vital. Policy-making and implementation do not happen in isolation, but are always embedded in a broader societal context which includes both systemic and socio-cultural elements (see Chapter 17). Initiatives in health policy are not only directed *to* the population but also driven *by* the population, including the needs of children (see Chapter 17). Walt and Gilson (1994) applied a triangle framework to describe the paradigm of policy analysis, in which the attention is not only focused on its content, but also on the processes affecting the development and implementation of the change, the context within which policy is created and the actors involved (Walt & Gilson, 1994). Context in our understanding refers to systemic factors (Buse, Mays, & Walt, 2005). It can be considered through the perspective of four factors: situational, structural, (socio)cultural and international (adapted from Buse et al., 2005; Leichter, 1979) (see Figure 4.1). We consider it as extremely useful to child-centric policy-making thus it formed an important part of the MOCHA research on appraisal of primary care systems from a child-centric perspective. Our assumption was to consider the child as an actor in the theatre of child health policy in European countries.

MOCHA research has identified that children are the main object (both direct and indirect) of disputes related to child health care across most European countries in the last decade. In this context, a child as an object of a child-centric health policy is either a well child (embedded in the family context, broadly understood social environment context or preventive care context) or a sick child (with a long-term illness and/or complex healthcare needs). Heterogeneity is expressed also by the differentiation of the child health issues in various age groups (from pre-natal period via infancy to adolescence).

The Concept of an 'Agent' for the Child

In most discussions on child health policy, the child is not an active participant in discussions even though a child is the subject and often the cause of a societal movement or change in policy; in other words, the child is a *causative actor*. As such, the child is surrounded by an extensive network of representatives. These actors are able to act and represent the interest of the child and are thus defined as *executive actors*. These individuals, who may be parents, teachers, nurses, physicians or other adults, can be considered as *agents* of the child in the proximal or distal environment of the child. The proximal environment of the child is defined as the micro-level, or the direct milieu of the child's environment (such as a parent or other family member); distal environments are defined as the indirect surroundings, on the mezzo- and macro-level. The difference between the distal and proximal environment of the child is expressed by the type of relationship. In the proximal perspective, the agents are capable of constructing a direct relationship whereas the agents of the distal environment are generally acting on the basis of indirect contact. This is illustrated by Figure 4.2.

Agents of the Proximal Environment

This group includes parents, close family members and others who have close contact with the child, such as teachers, nurses and physicians. Parents are vocal in their role as a child's representative and, in many situations, are supported by involved caregivers within social care and healthcare services. Parents, more often than other agents, are considered as both causative and executive actors. For instance, policy in Austria concentrates on helping pregnant women and new mothers to cope with the challenges of early childhood (ages 0−6) and puts in place guidance through the health and social care system in that country. Parents are also central in the role of advocating for the rights of their child, in countries where there is compulsory vaccination, parents have raised objections to the potential marginalisation of children who have not been vaccinated; arguments both for and against the policy have featured parent voices very strongly (see Zdunek, Schröder-Bäck, Alexander, Rigby, & Blair, in press) (see Chapters 16 and 17). Agents of the child in the proximal environment may also include other people who closely surround the child, such as family members, acquaintances, friends, neighbours, adults in the

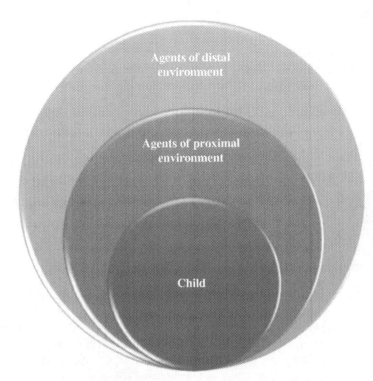

Figure 4.2.   Child as the central actor in the process of shaping child health policy.

school environment as well as general practitioners or other representatives of health care who are the 'listeners' and 'observers' institutionally empowered to act in the name of the child. It was teachers who raised awareness of children in Greece who, as a result of extreme austerity measures in that country, were fainting at school because of hunger, causing a national scandal, and in Spain, schools became part of anti-poverty measures by keeping their canteens open during the summer holidays to ensure children would be able to eat a meal (see Zdunek et al., *in press*).

Agents of the Wider Environment
The distal (wider) environment is where agents of the child become more closely entwined in national policy and population-level perspectives, while being child-centric in outlook. Examples of such agents include healthcare professionals' representative of the healthcare system as a whole, non-governmental organisations (NGOs) and research and media outlets. An institutional voice can take the form of, for example, health inspectorates, professional groups, children's health centres, national agencies and public health institutions. For example, paediatricians' associations were actively involved in the public discussion on changes to vaccination eligibility in Spain, and nursing associations in Norway were active in the introduction of weighing and measuring children at school as an obesity prevention policy (see Zdunek, Schröder-Bäck, Blair, & Rigby, 2017).

NGOs can be the platform for the exchange of views for health professionals, parents and carers and other interested persons who wish to ensure the protection of child health and well-being is protected. For example, in the UK, charities and organisations have strongly criticised the absence of a coordinated response to meet the needs of unaccompanied asylum seeking children in the country (Zdunek, Schröder-Bäck, Blair, & Rigby, 2017). Representatives of government such as the Ministry of Health (MoH) or other national institutions can also act as distal agents of the child. They can play the role of initiator of a policy, or be a mediator or guardian in a debate even though they are, by the definition, the 'voice of the state'.

An important example of a distal agent of the child is that of individual authorities, such as an ombudsman for children's rights. The individuals and their departments directly advocate for children's rights, whether it is in terms of child abuse, disabilities, unaccompanied asylum-seekers or disabled children's rights (for further details, see Zdunek, Schröder-Bäck, Blair, & Rigby, 2017).

A crucial role is also played by research centres and the mass media as sources of information and means of dissemination about certain phenomena. The media, in particular, can play a dual role, in terms of identifying and disclosing information about an issue; they are powerful instruments in public discussion. It was investigative journalism in Romania that exposed a potential scandal in children's residential home, where 12 out of 28 children aged between six and 16 had been administered narcoleptic medication for behavioural disorders, despite the fact that the facility was not a special needs centre, but housed children at risk, or abandoned children (mostly because of family poverty) (Blair et al., 2017). Public outcry led to an investigation that found, in this case, that the medication had been medically prescribed.

Children's Rights to Health

Meanwhile, society can discharge a focus and responsibility for children by acknowledging the need to frame what the child can expect from society as declaration of rights. These are intended both to define the child's interests and to discharge society's duty of care as distal agent. The study of how to collate aspects of children's rights into meaningful service provision-related statements has been led by Michael Rigby and Shalmali Deshpande, linking also to other work such as the World Health Organization's initiatives.

Core Concepts of Children's Right to Health

Recognition of Children's Rights is an important enablement and policy tool which seeks to give authenticity and impact to child centricity. Given that the child, as a legal minor, cannot advocate for themselves, and not every parent or service provider can be guaranteed to act optimally, giving legal underpinning to the rights of children gives a clear framework, and a yardstick against which failures can be judged, and redress applied where appropriate. It is an approach strongly supported at the highest level by the European Commission, through the Fundamental Rights Agency (2018) (which covers all ages) and by the Rights of the Child unit within DG Justice and Fundamental Rights (2018).

However, within this commitment to children's rights, health is a complex paradox. Firstly, there is the definitional problem. An oft cited key principle is the Right of the Child to Health, as enshrined in the United Nations Declaration on the Rights of the Child (United Nations OHCHR, 1959). However, the wording is aspirational and laudable, but lacks any meaningful definition, as being:

> States Parties recognize the right of the child to the enjoyment of the highest attainable standard of health and to facilities for the treatment of illness and rehabilitation of health.

There are no measurable benchmarks or definitions within that aim. Secondly, the provision of health services is a national competence under EU law, and so each country has its own approach to healthcare provision – deepening the measurement challenge as shown throughout the MOCHA project.

As for Health itself, that too is challenging to measure. The Constitution of the World Health Organization (World Health Organization, 1946) provides the authoritative definition, as being:

> Health is a state of complete physical, mental and social well-being and not merely the absence of disease or infirmity.

Clearly, to measure that for children through the life course is a daunting challenge. Though recognising that there are some contributors such as the Health Behaviour of School-aged Children (2018), these are not widespread or detailed enough to provide a systematic monitoring of fulfilment of the Right to Health.

The further challenge to the MOCHA project is that the project focus is on primary care for children. As shown throughout the report, primary care is delivered in different ways in different countries and by different people. There are also many reasons for providing health care – for preventive services, for diagnosis and treatment of a health problem at an early stage and for responding to health emergencies. The Right to Health should apply to all these circumstances, within any country's healthcare system, and regardless of individual circumstance. All countries will claim to provide such services universally to their citizens and usually to their residents, but in practice, there may be variation in provision or in accessibility according to locality or socio-demographic, cultural or ethnic factors, as discussed in Chapter 5. One specific aspect to this complexity concerns primary care provision for migrant and refugee children, and a focussed investigation within MOCHA addressed and researched this in detail and highlighted problematic areas (Hjern & Østergaard, 2017). However, important though rights and equity are for migrant and refugee children, this does not assist with the problem of assessing achievement of the Right to Health for resident children.

Appraisal of the Right to Health

The conclusion of the MOCHA team is that a more meaningful expression of the Right of the Child to Health, not least within primary care, is needed, giving practical operational instantiation to the high-level right. The World Health Organization Regional Office for Europe has previously started an initiative to enable countries to assess whether children are receiving the health care thought appropriate, based on the broad concepts in the United Nations Convention on the Rights of the Child turned into provision-based aspects. A toolkit has been produced with tools aimed at 6−11-year-old children, 12−18-year-old children and separately for management, health professionals and parents and carers (World Health Organization, 2015). These tools assess whether in the respondent's view good practice is being followed in order to facilitate the child's right to health through good primary care, but the questions themselves are only indirectly derived from Rights statements. This initiative builds on a successful initiative looking at Children's Rights in Hospitals and a related toolkit, but so far, the primary care toolkit has only been piloted in two countries in Europe (Guerreiro, Kuttumuratova, Babamuradova, Atajanova, & Weber, 2015). As presented, it is a local use initiative, and there is no infrastructure for comparison between states.

The MOCHA project has looked at assembling a more comprehensive grouping of all children's documented rights relating to health and in accord with enabling and achieving the core Right to Health. There are several relevant treaties or consensus statements which have one or more items relevant to affecting the Child's Right to Health. All the sources selected are legally binding treaties or potentially robust European policy statements which can be analysed as supporting aspects of children's primary healthcare delivery. There is recognised to be a hierarchy of conventions, treaties and agreements. Those which are legally binding international conventions are the strongest in that countries agree at governmental level to ratify them as a nation, after which they are bound to uphold them. Second, within the European Union, Commission Directives are the strongest form of instrument and are arrived at after due process of discussion and agreement and are legally binding on Member States. A third and lower level of impact can be achieved when Ministers of Health meet on a special topic and mutually agree principles. These are not legally binding, but usually are based on sound evidence plus mutual solidarity and can provide useful benchmarks and levers for ensuring that countries keep to agreed principles. These latter types of agreement can be reached globally, or within global regions such as Europe.

Based on this hierarchy, the MOCHA project has identified four instruments which when linked together can give more detailed expression of the Rights of the Child to Health within primary care. These are as follows:

- *International conventions* − there are two which are relevant:
    (1) Universal Declaration of Human Rights (United Nations, 1949); and
    (2) United Nations Convention on the Rights of the Child (United Nations, 1924)

- *EU directives* – none were identified pertaining to children's primary health care;
- *Ministerial convention declarations* – at global level Declaration of Alma-Ata, International Conference on Primary Health Care, 1978 (World Health Organization, 1978); and
- *Ministerial convention declarations* – at European level Tallinn Charter: Heath Systems for Health and Wealth 2008 (World Health Organization Regional Office for Europe, 2008).

Based in decomposition of the child and primary care relevant content of these four agreements, and reassembly in a systematic and integrated manner, the project has synthesised 12 suggested Rights of Children to Primary Health Care, with supporting enabling statements. These are shown in Table 4.2 and are based in statements in the four source documents.

The project has also commenced a process of assembling underpinning evidence from scientific literature to support the approaches, but within the terms of reference and resources of the MOCHA project, it has not been possible to fully complete this work. A hypertext linked presentation has also been developed, enabling automated linkage from any listed Right to the underpinning authorising text and where compiled the related literature.

From this assemblage of the Rights of the Child to Primary Care, it will be possible to assemble means for monitoring policy and provision to achieve these rights. This should enhance the approach already commenced by the WHO European Regional Office.

More work remains to be done on defining and monitoring a Child's Right to Primary Health Care, but this fundamental concept underpins the concept of child centricity and the Right to Health. There is need and opportunity to develop fully and obtain high-level agreement to these rights statements translated into practical service guidelines and to further developing monitoring tools, including child-friendly ones.

Summary

This section of study has traced the change in the perception of the child within society, from being a chattel of the father to being a person who should be nurtured, then from being an economic agent to being a developing person whose value to society will be achieved as a peak of optimal adulthood. Along this route, society has changed its views of the role of children and the duty of care from one of paternal protectionism to one of defining and actively supporting the child's rights. And during that journey, the role of the health sector has moved from one of paternalistic protection, to one of protecting rights to protection and self-determination as an emergent citizen. Child centricity is simultaneously a recognition of the individual child's importance in terms of rights and as a user of services and also

Table 4.2. Rights of children to primary health care.

Child Primary Care Rights Statement	Enabling Service Policy Statements (and Underpinning Source)
1. All children in Europe have the *Right to the Highest Attainable Standard of Health and Health Care, based on Primary Health Care*	1.1 All children have the right to the enjoyment of the highest attainable standard of physical and mental health *UNCRC Art. 24*
	1.2 Primary Health Care is the basis and foundation for preventive and therapeutic health care *AA Art. VI; UNCRC Art. 24*
	1.3 All children have the right to access appropriate facilities for the treatment of illness and rehabilitation of health *AA Art. V*
2. All children in Europe have the *Right to Timely Access to Appropriate Primary Health Care without discrimination of any nature*	2.1 Primary health care services for children should be appropriate, particularly with regard to their age *UNCRC Art. 2 & Art. 24*
	2.2 Such provision should adhere to the principles of Availability, Accessibility, Affordability and Acceptability of services *UDHR Art. 21.2; UNCRC Art. 2 & Art. 24*
	2.3 Such services should be culturally and linguistically appropriate *UNCRC Art. 2*
	2.4 Children are not the creators of their circumstances; services should be equally available to all children within a country, regardless of location, family circumstances, creed, ethnicity or civil status *UDHR Art. 21.2; UNCRC Art. 2 & Art. 22.1*
	2.5 Primary Health Care services, and the need for supporting and related services, should be the subject of specific plans, constructed with input from stakeholder representation including children and resourced appropriately *AA Art. VI & Art. VIII; TC Sec. 13*

Table 4.2. (*Continued*)

3.	All children in Europe have the *Right to Privacy and Confidentiality* in all aspects of seeking or enjoying primary health care service	
	3.1	Consultation should be in private *UDHR Art. 12; UNCRC Art. 16; TC Sec. 13*
	3.2	The fact of seeking or receiving a consultation, or any form of follow-up, should itself be confidential *UDHR Art. 12; UNCRC Art. 16; TC Sec. 13*
4.	All children in Europe have the *Right to a Child-centric Focus* in all aspects of primary health care provision.	
	4.1	Planning and provision of services for children should be focussed first and foremost on the child's (or group of children's) needs *UNCRC Art. 3; TC Sec. 13*
	4.2	In the making of decisions about a treatment, or service provision, the interest of the child or children should be foremost, including their safety *UNCRC Art. 3 & Art. 12*
5.	All children in Europe have the *Right for their Parents or Primary Caregivers to Receive Appropriate Education* and advice to improve the child's health and health behaviours.	
	5.1	Information regarding children's health and health behaviours should be available to parents and caregivers, in accessible form *UNCRC Art. 18 & Art. 24; AA Art. VII*
	5.2	Parents and caregivers should be advised of the availability of appropriate information and how to access it *UNCRC Art. 18 & Art. 24; AA Art. VII*
	5.3	As appropriate, accessible child health-related education including health literacy should be available to parents and caregivers *UNCRC Art. 23 & Art. 24; AA Art. VII*
6.	All children in Europe, or parents acting as agents of younger children, have the *Right to Choice of Primary Health Care Provider*	
	6.1	Choice of provider is important in engendering trust, as well as ensuring appropriateness *AA Art. VII; TC Sec. 6 & Sec. 10*

6.2 Older children may wish to choose a provider other than the one selected by their parents, in order to ensure confidentiality and empathy

UNCRC Art. 24; AA Art. VII; TC Sec. 6 & Sec. 10

6.3 Ability to access specific types of primary care provision is important to maintaining the mental, reproductive and physical health of older children

AA Art. VII; TC Sec. 6 & Sec. 10

7. **All children in Europe have the *Right to Confidentiality and Control of their Primary Health Data***

7.1 Primary health records, and health data, should always be subject to clinical confidentiality.

TC Sec. 13

7.2 Children, or parents acting on their behalf, should be advised when external parties have accessed their record – including hacking

UNCRC Art. 16

7.3 Children who are old enough to understand, and parents acting on behalf of younger children, should have access to their health record and data in line with policy and good practice

UNCRC Art. 12; TC Sec. 13

8. **All children in Europe have the *Right to be Informed about and Participate in their Primary Health Care processes***

8.1 Appropriate to their age and maturity, children have the right to be informed about their health and related health care issues

UNCRC Art. 12; AA Art. VII

8.2 The views and perceptions of the child should be sought and taken into account in health care delivery decision-making

UNCRC Art. 12; AA Art. VII

8.3 To the greatest extent possible, children should be co-producers and co-managers of their own health and health care

UNCRC Art. 12; AA Art. VII

Table 4.2. (*Continued*)

9. Where a longer-term condition necessitates care at home linked to primary care, all children in Europe and their informal care team have the *Right to Coordinated and Appropriate Care*	9.1 The need for ongoing health (and as appropriate related social or other) care should be communicated and documented *UNCRC Art. 12; AA Art. 12* 9.2 Where necessary, a care coordinator should be designated *UNCRC Art. 12; AA Art. VII* 9.3 The overall plan, pathway and objectives of care should be agreed by all parties – child, family carers and professionals *UNCRC Art. 12; AA Art. VII* 9.4 Appropriate respite care, for the benefit of the child and informal carers, should be a part of the plan for children with long-term conditions or where necessitated by carers' needs *UNCRC Art. 12; AA Art. VII; TC Sec. 6 & Sec. 10*
10. When a child's health condition necessitates hospital admission, all children in Europe have the *Right to a Planned, Prepared and Timely Hospital Discharge* linked to Primary Care support	10.1 Discharge planning should commence at the time of admission (whether emergency or planned) *UNCRC Art. 24; AA Art. VII; TC Sec. 10* 10.2 Primary health care services, and community or specialised health and care support as needed, should be involved in planning and informed of the final plan, arrangements and date of discharge *UNCRC Art. 24; AA Art. VII; TC Sec. 10* 10.3 The needs and views of the child, and of family and other informal carers, should be acknowledged, documented and accommodated as far as possible *UNCRC Art. 12; AA Art. VII; TC Sec. 6 & Sec. 10*

11. Older children in Europe with a long-term health condition have the *Right to a Planned Transition to Appropriate Adult Services*, linking specialist and primary care services

11.1 Transition planning should be initiated by the lead specialist, linking with adult service partners and with primary care

UNCRC Art. 23; TC Sec. 10

11.2 The child should be fully involved in preparation of the transition plan and should be considered a co-designer

UNCRC Art. 12 & Art. 23; TC Sec. 10

11.3 Depending on the condition, and on local services, the transition may be before or after the 18th birthday

UNCRC Art. 23; TC Sec. 6 & Sec. 10

11.4 Where children's primary care is provided by dedicated community paediatricians, the double transition of primary and specialist care to adult services should be planned carefully

UNCRC Art. 23; TC Sec. 10

12. All children in Europe have the *Right to Quality and Equity of Primary Health Care Services* (and related services) through Good Governance to enable fulfilment of their Rights

12.1 There should be defined standards for aspects of service structure (including professional skills), access and delivery

UNCRC Art. 3

12.2 All personnel treating children in primary care should be appropriately trained for their role with children

UNCRC Art. 3; AA Art. VII

12.3 There should be open and transparent governance and quality assurance processes, ensuring efficacy and safety of services

UNCRC Art. 3; AA Art. VI; TC Sec. 6

as an agent of societal change. Using the example of children as actors in the creation of child health policy, we have looked at how and to what extent child centricity has been developed in Europe. The extent to which a system has the capacity to be child-centric is an important factor in the appraisal of primary care systems.

References

Archard, D. (2004). *Children. Rights and childhood.* London: Routledge.
Ariès, P. (1962). *Centuries of childhood: A social history of family life.* London: Jonathan Cape.
Balcerek, M. (1986). *Prawa dziecka. Prawa dziecka Wydawnictwo Naukowe.* Warszawa: PWN.
Blair, M., Rigby, M., & Alexander, D. (2017). *Final report on current models of primary care for children.* Retrieved from www.childhealthservicemodels.eu/wp-content/uploads/2017/07/MOCHA-WP1-Deliverable-WP1-D6-Feb-2017-1.pdf
Bronfenbrenner, U. (1979). *The ecology of human development, experiments by nature and design.* Cambridge, MA: Harvard University Press. Retrieved from https://khoerulanwarbk.files.wordpress.com/2015/08/urie_bronfenbrenner_the_ecology_of_human_developbokos-z1.pdf
Brzeziński, W. (2012). Obraz dziecka w perspektywie historyczno-porównawczej. Przeszłość we współczesności, współczesność w przeszłości. *Przegląd Pedagogiczny, 1*(21), 141–153.
Buse, K., Mays, N., & Walt, G. (2005). Making health policy. *Understanding public health.* London: Open University Press.
Child Rights International Network. (2018). *Declaration of the rights of the child 1948.* Retrieved from https://www.crin.org/en/library/un-regional-documentation/declaration-rights-child-1948
Council of Europe. (1950). Convention for the protection of human rights and fundamental freedoms Rome, 4.XI.1950. In *European convention on human rights.* Strasbourg: Council of Europe. Retrieved from https://rm.coe.int/1680063765
Council of Europe. (1961). *European social charter.* Retrieved from https://rm.coe.int/168006b642
European Union Agency for Fundamental Rights. (2018). *About FRA.* Retrieved from http://fra.europa.eu/en
European Values Survey. (2015). *About EVS.* Retrieved from https://europeanvalues-study.eu/
Garbula, J., & Kowalik-Olubińska, J. (2012). Konstruowanie obrazu dzieciństwa w perspektywie psychologicznej i socjokulturowej. *Przegląd Pedagogiczny, 1*(21), 25–34. Retrieved from http://repozytorium.ukw.edu.pl/handle/item/626
Guerreiro, A. I. F., Kuttumuratova, A., Babamuradova, M., Atajanova, Z., & Weber, M. W. (2015). *Assessment and improvement of children's rights in health care: Piloting training and tools in Uzbekistan; Panorama, 1, 3, 2015.* Copenhagen: WHO.
Härkönen, U. (2007). The Bronfenbrenner ecological systems theory of human development. In Slahova, A. et.al. (Ed.), *Scientific articles of V international conference PERSON.COLOR.NATURE.MUSIC. Saule.* Latvia: Daugavpils

University. Retrieved from https://studylib.net/doc/8356343/the-bronfenbrenner-ecological-systems-theory-of-human

Health Behaviour of School-aged Children. (2018). *HBSC*. Retrieved from www. hbsc.org

Hjern, A., & Østergaard, L. S. (2017). *Migrant children in Europe: Entitlements to health care*. Retrieved from http://www.childhealthservicemodels.eu/wp-content/uploads/2015/09/20160831_Deliverable-D3-D7.1_Migrant-children-in-Europe.pdf

Jarosz, E. (2010). Krzywdzenie dzieci-piętno społeczne? (w) "CHOWANNA" 53 (66), T. 1 (34): DZIECIŃSTWO – WITRAŻ BOLESNY.

Kulesza, R. (2003). Starożytna Sparta. Poznańskie Towarzystwo Przyjaciół Nauk, Mała Biblioteka PTPN t. 12, Pozdnań.

Leichter, H. (1979). *A comparative approach to policy analysis: Health care policy in four nations*. Cambridge: Cambridge University Press.

Parrish, J. M. (2013). Education, Erasmian humanism and more's Utopia. In C. Brooke & E. Frazer (Eds.), *Ideas of education: Philosophy and politics from Plato to Dewey*. London: Routledge.

Rosa, R., & Matysiuk, R. (2013). Ewolucja praw dziecka (aspekty filozoficzne, pedagogiczne i prawne). In E. Jagiełło & E. Jówko (Eds.), *Dziecko w kulturze współczesnego świata* (pp. 10–33). Siedlce ISBN 978-83-936635-2-1. Retrieved from https://docplayer.pl/4327137-Dziecko-w-kulturze-wspolczesnego-swiata-redakcja-naukowa-ewa-jagiello-ewa-jowko.html

Szczepański, J. (1963). *Elementarne pojęcia socjologii*. Warszawa: PWN.

UNICEF. (2003). *Declaration of the rights of the child 1959*. Retrieved from https://www.unicef.org/malaysia/1959-Declaration-of-the-Rights-of-the-Child.pdf

United Nations. (1924). *Geneva declaration of the rights of the child*. Retrieved from http://www.un-documents.net/gdrc1924

United Nations. (1949). *Universal declaration of human rights*. New York, NY: United Nations. Retrieved from https://www.jus.uio.no/lm/en/pdf/un.universal.declaration.of.human.rights.1948.portrait.letter.pdf

United Nations. (1976). *International covenant on civil and political rights 1966*. Retrieved from https://treaties.un.org/doc/publication/unts/volume%20999/volume-999-i-14668-english.pdf

United Nations. (1989). *Convention on the rights of the child*. New York, NY: UN. Retrieved from https://downloads.unicef.org.uk/wp-content/uploads/2010/05/UNCRC_united_nations_convention_on_the_rights_of_the_child.pdf?_ga=2.209651665.274437633.1540996300-199092997.1540996300

United Nations. (2015). *Universal declaration of human rights. Illustrated edition*. Retrieved from http://www.un.org/en/udhrbook/pdf/udhr_booklet_en_web.pdf

United Nations Human Rights Office of the High Commissioner (OHCHR). (1959). *Declaration of the rights of the child*. Retrieved from www.ohchr.org/EN/Issues/Education/Training/Compilation/Pages/1DeclarationoftheRightsoftheChild(1959).aspx

United Nations Human Rights: Office of the High Commissioner (OHCHR). (1976). *International covenant on economic, social and cultural rights*. Retrieved from https://www.ohchr.org/en/professionalinterest/pages/cescr.aspx

Walt, G., & Gilson, L. (1994). Reforming the health sector in developing countries. The central role of policy analysis. *Health Policy and Planning, 9*(4), 353–370.

World Health Organization. (1946). *Constitution of the World Health Organization.* New York, NY: WHO. Retrieved from https://www.loc.gov/law/help/us-treaties/bevans/m-ust000004-0119.pdf

World Health Organization. (1978, September 6–12). *Declaration of Alma-Ata. International conference on primary health care.* Alma-Ata, USSR. Geneva: WHO. Retrieved from http://www.who.int/publications/almaata_declaration_en.pdf

World health Organization. (2015). *Children's rights in primary health care series.* Retrieved from http://www.euro.who.int/en/health-topics/Life-stages/child-and-adolescent-health/publications/2015/childrens-rights-in-primary-health-care-series

World Health Organization Regional Office for Europe. (2008). WHO European ministerial conference on health systems – Tallinn Charter: Heath systems for health and wealth. Tallinn: WHO.

Zdunek, K., Schröder-Bäck, P., Rigby, M., & Blair, M. (2017). *Report on the contextual determinants of child health policy.* Available from http://www.childhealthservicemodels.eu/wp-content/uploads/Context-Culture-Report.pdf

Chapter 5

Equity

Mitch Blair and Denise Alexander

Abstract

Equity is an issue that pervades all aspects of primary care provision for
children and as such is a recurring theme in the Models of Child Health
Appraised project. All European Union member states agree to address
inequalities in health outcomes and include policies to address the gradient
of health across society and target particularly vulnerable population
groups. The project sought to understand the contribution of primary care
services to reducing inequity in health outcomes for children. We focused
on some key features of inequity as they affect children, such as the importance of good health services in early childhood, and the effects of inequity
on children, such as the higher health needs of underprivileged groups, but
their generally lower access to health services. This indicates that health services have an important role in buffering the effects of social determinants
of health by providing effective treatment that can improve the health and
quality of life for children with chronic disorders. We identified common
risk factors for inequity, such as gender, family situation, socio-economic
status (SES), migrant or minority status and regional differences in healthcare provision, and attempted to measure inequity of service provision. We
did this by analysing routine data of universal primary care procedures,
such as vaccination, age at diagnosis of autism or emergency hospital
admission for conditions that can be generally treated in primary care,
against variables of inequity, such as indicators of SES, migrant/ethnicity
or urban/rural residency. In addition, we focused on the experiences of
child population groups particularly at risk of inequity of primary care provision: migrant children and children in the state care system.

Keywords: Equity; child health services; primary care; measurement;
children in care; migrants

Introduction

Equity is an issue that pervades all aspects of primary care provision for children and as such is a recurring theme in the Models of Child Health Appraised (MOCHA) project. As outlined in Chapter 1, primary care itself is intended to provide and equitable and accessible service to everyone (see Chapter 1). This chapter outlines the work done in MOCHA specifically on equity.

All European Union (EU) member states have agreed to address inequalities in health outcomes (European Parliament, 2011). This requires policies which include both actions to address the gradient in health across the whole of society and actions which are specifically targeted to those children who face an increased risk due to multiple disadvantage such as Roma children, some migrant or ethnic minority children, children with special needs or disabilities, children in alternative care and street children, children of imprisoned parents as well as children within households at particular risk of poverty, such as single parent or large families. Some of the MOCHA Country Agents explained how specific countries are addressing equity issues. For example, the Greek Country Agent claimed that even at the level of a social worker directly interacting with a young person, there is a culture of trying to 'reduce inequalities' for the children. This equity goal is emphasised not just in strategy planning but is enforced at multiple stakeholder levels. France and Spain reference the social inclusion of vulnerable children as a key focus of their equity goals. Denmark, meanwhile, highlights the 'aim of increasing education and employment rates' for vulnerable children. One interpretation that may be deduced from these inclusions in national strategy is that in these countries, a more holistic attitude towards child health strategy seems to be suggested with greater equity explicitly recognised as a pillar of improved child and adolescent health. The UN Convention on the Rights of the Child (UNCRC) (United Nations, 1989) has been ratified by all members of the United Nations (193 countries), except for the United States. States party to the UNCRC must ensure that its provisions and principles are fully reflected and given legal effect in relevant domestic legislation. One of the general principles of the convention is non-discrimination which is outlined in the second paragraph, all children have the same rights irrespective of social or legal status. Thus, equitable health care is not negotiable for children, it is something that is a duty for countries that have signed this convention.

Defining the Terms

Health differences between economically privileged and underprivileged population groups were initially labelled as 'inequalities' (Black, 1980). Since the mid-1980s, however, the term 'inequity' has been used for the presence of 'systematic and potentially remediable differences among population groups defined socially, economically, or geographically' (Starfield, 2011) and will be used in this sense throughout this chapter. Equity in health implies that ideally everyone could attain their full health potential and that no one should be disadvantaged from achieving this potential because of their social position or other socially determined circumstance (Moore, McDonald, Carlon, & O'Rourke, 2015; Whitehead & Dahlgren, 2006). In other words, no child should be left behind.

Inequity in access to health care can be horizontal or vertical. Horizontal inequity refers to the situation when people with the same needs do not have equal access to the necessary healthcare resources. Vertical inequity exists when people with greater healthcare needs are not provided with resources adequate for their need (Starfield, Gervas, & Mangin, 2012). Horizontal inequity disadvantages particular social or ethnic groups, the poor who cannot afford access (including time poverty as a barrier) or those with a weaker or very dispersed pattern of service; there are also examples of gender-based inequity. Vertical inequity involves a false equity of providing the same time and access resource to all, thus depriving those with greater needs of the additional service intensity necessary to meet their greater need. This is precisely what proportionate universalism aims to achieve (Carey, Crammond, & De Leeuw, 2015; Marmot, 2010). Primary child health services need to be appraised against the degree to which they adopt this approach.

A large body of research shows that inequities in health related to social position in the population are present in a wide range of health outcomes and indicators throughout the life course, already commencing in the intrauterine period. Neighbourhood deprivation, parental lower parental income/wealth, child poverty, income inequality, educational attainment and occupational social class, higher parental job strain, parental unemployment, lack of housing tenure and household material deprivation have been identified as some of the key social factors that explain these inequities in child health and developmental outcomes (Pillas et al., 2014).

There are major differences in both the levels of child poverty in Europe (which tend to follow the general wealth [GDP] of a country) and the degree of income inequality (as measured by the Gini index) (see also Chapter 9). For example, the levels of child poverty in Iceland and Hungary are 13% and 35.7%, respectively, whereas UK and Romania remain among the worst countries in terms of income inequality compared to Czech Republic and Denmark (Eurostat, 2015). Income inequality has particularly detrimental effects on the many dimensions of child well-being and health (Pickett & Wilkinson, 2007).

The Importance of Early Childhood

The period of early childhood, defined as the period between prenatal development to eight years of age, is increasingly recognised as the most crucial period during the life course and the period that is the most highly sensitive to external influences (Britto et al., 2017). During early childhood, the foundations are laid for every individual's physical and mental capacities that influence their subsequent growth, health and development throughout the life course. In certain aspects of child health and development, the potential adverse effects of social and biological influences, such as suboptimal infant brain growth, are likely to be irreversible (World Health Organization Early Childhood Knowledge

Network, 2007). Hence, intervening to improve early childhood health and developmental outcomes is increasingly being suggested as a priority, as potential interventions are expected to have a stronger impact on an individual's life course health and development while also achieving higher returns than later interventions (Moore et al., 2015). In recognition of the importance of early childhood, the World Health Organization (WHO) Commission on Social Determinants of Health in their final report *Closing the Gap in a Generation* (World Health Organization, 2008) suggested that 'equity from the start' should be an essential component of any attempt to improve health outcomes overall and, in particular, to address health inequalities.

In consequence, the quality of health services is particularly important in early childhood, so that the negative effects of poor health on the developing body and mind can be minimised. The Commission recognises that:

> Preventing the transmission of disadvantage across generations is a crucial investment in Europe's future, as well as a direct contribution to the Europe 2020 Strategy for smart, sustainable and inclusive growth, with long terms benefits for children, the economy and society as a whole. (European Commission, 2013)

Effects of Health Inequalities on Child Health

Children in lower social strata, however, have not only more illnesses, but also more severe illnesses (Starfield et al., 2012). Obesity and thinness (Pearce, Rougeaux, & Law, 2015; Ruiz et al., 2016) and adolescent mental health disorders including depression are all commoner in socially disadvantaged and single parent families (Klanšček, Žiberna, Korošec, Zurc, & Albreht, 2014; Varga, Piko, & Fitzpatrick, 2014; Wirback, Möller, Larsson, Galanti, & Engström, 2014). French adolescents who are socially disadvantaged are at risk or multi-morbidities such as substance misuse, suicide, tendency to violence, decreased school performance and obesity (Chau, Baumann, & Chau, 2013). Unemployment of parents leads to much greater risk of small for gestational age infants in Finland (Räisänen, Kramer, Gissler, Saari, & Heinonen, 2014). Dental health is extremely sensitive to social inequalities both at individual and at intercountry level (Tchicaya & Lorentz, 2014). Parental education has been associated with asthma inequality in ten European cohort studies, in other words, the offspring of mothers with a low level of education have an increased relative and absolute risk of asthma compared to offspring of high educated mothers (Lewis et al., 2017) and low socio-economic status (SES) parents more likely to give birth to Small for Gestational Age and Premature babies (Ruiz et al., 2015).

It follows that needs for health care are greater in children in socially disadvantaged families. This indicates that health services have an important role to buffer the effects of the social determinants of health by providing effective treatment that can improve the health and quality of life for children with chronic disorders. Unfortunately, underprivileged groups, despite their higher needs, are often shown to have less access to care than the more privileged, given rise to the concept of 'the inverse care law' first described by Hart (1973) and explored further by Black (1980).

Primary Care and Its Contribution to Addressing Health Inequity

Although inequities in health are primarily caused by social determinants, the health services have an important role in buffering the effects of adverse social determinants. Consequently, the quality of primary care health services is particularly important in early childhood when the negative effects of poor health on the developing body and mind can be minimised.

Primary care systems operate in a wider socio-economic context and the quality of primary care is determined not only by the general wealth in the country and the amount of funding allocated specifically for primary care compared to high-tech hospital medicine but also to key aspects such as the caseloads of doctors and nurses or the availability of equipment or medicines, access and continuity of care (see Chapter 9). This ecosystem and the interrelationships are reflected in the working MOCHA Working Model (Chapter 2).

In a similar vein, Maeseneer, Willems, De Sutter, Van de Geucchte, and Billings (2007) describe a number of features at the macro (public policy)-, meso (community)- and micro (individual patient and health system and provider)-levels which can influence the effectiveness of the primary care system in addressing inequity. At the micro-level, utilisation of a service is determined by the individual's risk of a health issue (socially patterned) which in turn is recognised as a perceived need by that individual. That perception will be influenced by their health beliefs, predisposing factors (e.g. pain threshold or symptom severity or response to medication) and contextual factors (e.g. family concern or inability to work). Utilisation of a service requires that individual to express the need which itself may be influenced by financial resources, insurance, logistics attitude and so on. Similarly, utilisation will be influenced on the healthcare provider side by knowledge skills and attitude towards the individual including socio-cultural, socio-economic or socio-demographic factors and similar features of the healthcare system in terms of administrative or physical access (Maeseneer et al., 2007). Healthcare utilisation was the focus of the scientists working on equity in the MOCHA group. We also looked for known risk factors of inequity and healthcare utilisation, to establish if these were reflected in the research.

Healthcare Utilisation and Equity for Child Health

We found that diverse indicators of healthcare utilisation were employed in the literature, including use of telephone services, visits to general practitioner (GP), use of mental health services, use of emergency health services, use of school health services, drug prescription patterns, missing school and hospital admission in children with asthma and physician visits in children with recurrent abdominal pain. The studies we found covered all ages of children. However, only four studies adjusted the analysis of healthcare utilisation to an indicator of healthcare need; these included the perceived health status in the use of primary care physicians in Spain (Berra et al., 2006), physical and mental health in Catalonia (Palacio-Vieira et al., 2013), morbidity load in Aragon, Spain (Calderon-Larrañaga et al., 2011), and a measure of mental health (SDQ) in use of somatic and mental health services in Germany (Wölfle et al., 2014).

Common Risk Factors for Inequity.

We searched for known risk factors of inequity, to see if research had focused on these in relation to healthcare utilisation. The risk factors identified were gender, family situation, SES, migrant or minority status and regional differences.

Gender
Of the research identified, there was no conclusive gender influence on inequity, although 12 of the identified studies had reported patterns of healthcare use by gender. In northern Norway, Turi, Bals, Skre, and Kvernmo (2009) reported a much higher use of school health services and also a higher use of GPs among 15–16-year-old girls compared to boys, a pattern that was shown also in use of general practice in 5–14-year-olds in Catalonia, Spain, by Berra et al. (2006) and by Ivert, Torstensson-Levander, and Merlo (2013) for use of mental health care in teenagers in the south of Sweden. In contrast, 11–18-year-old boys and girls were found to have quite similar use of general practice in Greece (Giannakopoulos, Tzavara, Dimitrakaki, Ravens-Sieberer, & Tountas, 2010) and of GP and primary care paediatrician in 0–17-year-old children in Germany (Rattay et al., 2014).

Family Situation
Ivert et al. (2013) reported a twofold increase in use of mental health care in children in single parent households in two studies in southern Sweden, but otherwise, family situation was not reported in relation to healthcare use in the reviewed studies.

Socio-economic Status
Many different indicators of SES were used in the studies identified. These included: parental education, income, parental occupation and the socio-economic composition of the neighbourhood often expressed as deprivation quintiles/quartiles. SES patterns differed considerably between countries. We found that in some countries (research from Greece, Norway and Germany), there was higher use of primary care (general practice) in families with high SES compared to families with low SES. Although in the German research, it was found that families of higher SES used the primary care paediatrician services

and those from the lower SES group used GP services (Rattay et al., 2014), while Wölfle et al. (2014) described a higher use of somatic health care, but a lower use of mental health care in families of low SES compared to families with a higher SES, after adjusting the analysis for a mental health measure (SDQ). Two Spanish studies (Berra et al., 2006; Palacio-Vieira et al., 2013) reported generally equitable healthcare utilisation by children aged 5–14 years and 8–18 years, after adjusting for indicators of healthcare needs. In southern Sweden, Mangrio, Hansen, Lindstrom, Kohler, and Rosvall (2011) described a higher use of general practice in preschool children from families with low SES, compared to those with high SES and Ivert et al. (2013) found a similar pattern in adolescent use of mental health care. In Scotland (UK), Wilson, Hogg, Henderson, and Wilson (2013) reported that families used GP services as a source of information for their children similarly despite their SES background.

In the United Kingdom, telephone advice is provided by the health service (see Chapter 14). Patterns of use for the advice service were reported by two studies. Cooper et al. (2005) found that families from less deprived areas used this service more often in the age group 5–14 years, while the use of the service was more equitable during the preschool years. These findings were followed up by Cook, Randhawa, Large, Guppy, and Chater (2012), who found that deprivation patterns differed by the gender of the child. More deprived families of girls used this service more often, but for boys, the more deprived families used the services less.

In the only study identified of children diagnosed with asthma, Austin, Selvaraj, Godden, and Russell (2005) found that children from more deprived neighbourhoods in Scotland (UK) were more often admitted to hospital and missed school because of their asthma condition compared with children from less deprived areas.

Migrants/Minorities
A range of categorisations were used to identify minority and migrant children in the identified research chapters. One such categorisation was that of foreign-born children compared to foreign-born parents. Fadnes, Moen, and Diaz (2016) reported that children who were foreign-born used less primary and emergency hospital care, while the opposite was true for children born in Norway to foreign-born parents. In Spain, children with foreign-born parents in the region of Aragon were found to visit primary care less often (Gimeno-Feliu, Armesto-Gomez, Macipe-Costa, & Magallon-Botaya, 2009) and be prescribed drugs less often (Gimeno-Feliu et al., 2009), compared to children with Spanish-born parents. In a register study by Calderon-Larrañaga et al. (2011) from the same region, adjustment for a morbidity indicator normalised this association, suggesting that the earlier finding could be explained by better health in the migrant children.

Ivert et al. (2013) described the barriers to using mental healthcare services by adolescents with foreign-born parents in Stockholm (Sweden), and a further study (2013) in southern Sweden found this to be particularly pertinent for children with foreign-born parents who originated from low- and middle-income countries, but not for those with parents originating from other high-income countries. We found only one study on undocumented children, which was based in Germany. Wenner, Razum, Schenk, Ellert, and Bozorgmehr (2016) found that migrant children without residency used emergency health services more than twice as frequently compared to children in migrant families who had been granted residency.

Regional Differences

Two German studies describe the difference in healthcare utilisation between the former East and West Germany. Children in the former East Germany used more healthcare services, in particular family physicians in primary care, while children in the former West Germany were more likely to visit a primary care paediatrician (Hintzpeter et al., 2015; Rattay et al., 2014). According to Rattay et al. (2014), this pattern has been consistent between 2003–2006 and 2009–2012.

Quality Indicators of Primary and Evidence of Inequity

We investigated five indicators representing the quality of primary care for children, as defined in administrative data from healthcare services (see Chapter 6) in relation to equity of provision. In line with the agenda of the World Health Organization's Social Determinants of Health (World Health Organization, 2008), we prioritised indicators of preventive health care and early childhood.

Preventive Care

- Percentage of population vaccinated before two years of age with at least one shot of measles-containing vaccine (MCV): reports of recent measles outbreaks in Europe (Muscat, 2011) showed that marginalised populations with poor access to health care, such as the Roma and traveller populations, have been particularly susceptible to measles. This underlines the importance of equitable access to preventive health care.
- Age at operation for cryptorchidism (in those operated 0–17 years of age): (1) percentage operated before 12 months of age and (2) percentage operated before three years of age.
- Age at first diagnosis of autism spectrum disorder in native-born children according to diagnosis in specialised/hospital care.

Curative care.

- Yearly incidence of (1) hospital admissions and (2) emergency room care with a diagnosis of viral or unspecific gastroenteritis in native-born 1–5-year-olds. Viral gastroenteritis is a tracer condition for care of acute conditions in primary care. Viral gastroenteritis is a common acute disorder in preschool children, particularly because pre-schools and other day care centres are a common setting for transmission of these viruses (Ethelberg et al., 2006). Day care attendance tends to vary little by SES in northern Europe (Hjern, Haglund, Rasmussen, & Rosen, 2000), as a result, major differences in incidence of viral gastroenteritis by SES seem unlikely (Olesen et al., 2005).

- Yearly incidence of (1) hospital admissions and (2) emergency room care with an asthma diagnosis in 6–15-year-olds. Hospital admission for asthma in schoolchildren is a tracer condition for primary care quality of chronic disorders.

(Hjern, Arat, & Klöfvermark, 2017).

We searched for data that included at least one link to an indicator of SES, migrant/ethnicity or urban/rural residency. Data were required to be nationally representative, but data on regional populations were accepted when national data were unavailable. Only eight countries were able to provide such data and none for all of the desired indicators: Austria, Denmark, Finland, Iceland, Ireland, Spain, Sweden and the United Kingdom (England) (see also Chapter 6; Hjern et al., 2017)

- Austria: hospital admissions asthma, cryptorchidism and age at diagnosis of autism;
- Denmark: MMR vaccinations, cryptorchidism, asthma and gastroenteritis;
- Finland: vaccination data, cryptorchidism, asthma and gastroenteritis;
- Iceland: vaccinations via electronic health records (see Chapter 14);
- Ireland: MMR1, hospital admissions, cryptorchidism, asthma and gastroenteritis;
- Spain: vaccinations;
- Sweden: DPT and MMR1 vaccinations, cryptorchidism, asthma, gastroenteritis and age at first diagnosis of autism; and
- United Kingdom (England): MMR1 vaccinations, hospital admissions cryptorchidism, asthma and gastroenteritis.

Findings

Vaccinations

Finland, Iceland and Denmark (random sample only) were able to provide individual data from comprehensive national registers. Complete national data were available with area-based linkage from Ireland. Individually linked regional total population data were available from Sweden and regional small area-based population data from Spain (Catalonia). UK (England-only) data were provided from 1,200 nationally representative English general practices. The Swedish and Danish data were older (2010–2011) than the more recent data provided by the other countries. Regional data and data on ethnicity were only available from three countries (Sweden, Finland and Iceland).

We found minimal differences by gender for MCV (generally MMR1), but girls were slightly more likely to be vaccinated in England and Denmark, and boys more often in Finland. In Finland and Ireland, there were no clear differences between SES groups, but in Spain, uptake of MMR was lower in children from higher SES groups. In Denmark, families in lower SES groups had lower vaccination uptake, as was the case in England.

Age at Operation for Cryptorchidism
Six countries provided data on age at operation for cryptorchidism. Despite the presence of clear guidelines, these were adhered to poorly in all the responding countries. Denmark and Finland had the highest proportion operated aged under 12 months (in line with the guidelines) at 21% and 25%, and the UK (England) had the highest proportion operated before three years of age (78%). Sweden showed a consistent pattern of later operation for disadvantaged children (by family income as well as parental country of birth). Only minimal differences were found between urban and rural areas, again with Sweden as the exception with children in rural areas more often being operated before three years of age than those living in the larger cities.

Age at Diagnosis of Autism
Only three countries provided data on age at the first diagnosis of autism (defined as ICD-10 code F84.0) in the available patient databases, and only two, Finland and Sweden, included social stratification. The long follow-up time needed for this indicator implies that this information reflects clinical practices that may have changed considerably in recent years. There were no clear differences between social groups in Sweden and Finland.

Ambulatory Care-sensitive Conditions:
Hospital care for viral gastroenteritis in preschool children. Data on hospital admissions for viral gastroenteritis were provided by six countries, five of whom also provided data stratified by a SES indicator. Denmark had the highest incidence of hospital admissions, followed by Austria and the UK (England). There was a graded social pattern in Finland, Ireland, Sweden and England, with socially disadvantaged children having the highest incidences of hospital admissions. In Sweden, this gradient also included children of foreign-born parents compared with Swedish-born parents. Denmark was the exception, having high admission rates and relatively small differences between income categories.

In Finland and the United Kingdom, vaccination has taken place against rotavirus (in 2009 and 2013, respectively), which is the main cause of hospital admission for gastroenteritis in high-income countries (Van Damme et al., 2006). Sweden was the only country that could provide outpatient data on emergency care for gastroenteritis. For more details, see Hjern et al. (2017).

Hospital Care for Asthma in Schoolchildren. Six countries provided data on hospital admissions for asthma, five of which provided data stratified by a SES indicator. Four of these six countries participated in the international ISAAC study 2000−2003 into asthma (Lai et al., 2009). Incidence rates of admissions differed greatly between countries, with a 10-fold difference between the highest rates in the United Kingdom (England) and the lowest in Sweden. Despite these differences in incidence rates, gender patterns and the social patterns were similar between countries, with children in more disadvantaged families/areas having higher rates of admissions. When incidence rates were stratified by age groups, England has particularly high rates for 13–15-year-olds, and the difference between the countries with the lowest incidence (Sweden and Austria) and the United Kingdom (England) is almost 20-fold for this age group.

Relationship of Equity Indicators and Model Types

In general, no specific relationship between indicators of equity and the different model types was observed in the MOCHA study, suggesting that other factors contribute to these particular incidence.

Lead Practitioner

Four countries in this study have systems led by primary care paediatricians (Austria, Germany, Greece and Spain). Data from Spain seem to indicate an equitable primary care model for children but there are indicators of a considerable degree of inequity in the literature reviews in the other three countries in terms of healthcare utilisation as well as vaccinations. In Germany, there exist considerable regional differences within the country. The former East Germany relies more on GPs as the principal primary care physicians for children, and the former West Germany relies more on paediatricians (Rattay et al., 2014). Uptake of vaccination rates were higher in the former East compared to the former West Germany, while the SES patterns for access to curative care were similar, suggesting that there are other factors than the lead practitioner in primary care that affect the quality of primary care for children and equity of provision of care in this country.

Regulatory, Financial and Service Provision Classifications

Data from this study showed that primary healthcare organisations based on the professional non-hierarchical model (Austria, Belgium, France and Germany) seem to be associated with considerable regional differences in access to health care (Hjern et al., 2017). In Austria and Germany, there were also indications of considerable socio-economic differences in uptake of preventive health services and for Germany also in access to care.

Reform of many National Health Service-based systems is taking place in Europe, including in the United Kingdom, Spain and Sweden (Saltman, Allin, Mossialos, Wismar, & Kutzin, 2012). An increase in the proportion of private providers, application of market-based mechanisms, the promotion of a patient-choice agenda and changes to resource allocation systems are common features of the reform. Studies in adult populations in these countries show that such changes led to increased inequity in utilisation of primary care (Burstrom,

Burstrom et al., 2017; Burstrom, Marttila, Kulane, Lindberg, & Burstrom, 2017). The consequences of these changes for children should be monitored.

Vulnerable Populations

The MOCHA project has focused on two particularly vulnerable populations to see how existing primary care services address their specific needs. The groups identified for in-depth research are migrant children and children in the state care system.

Migrant Children's Entitlements to Health Care

Children from asylum-seeking families and newly settled refugee children have high rates of stress-related mental health problems during the first years after resettlement, with unaccompanied minors having the highest rates of symptoms. Infectious diseases and poor dental health are more common in these children than in settled European populations and many have an accumulated need of preventive and basic health. Thus, access to health care is a major concern for migrant children (Hjern & Østergaard, 2016).

We investigated the legal entitlements that migrant children have to health care in the EU and European Economic Area (EEA) countries using data from the MOCHA Country Agents and knowledge from the scientific and expert literature. In this report, it was only possible to identify the legal situation as defined by the host country; and it is likely that there are differences between this and the actual delivery 'on the ground' in each country. We found that there exists considerable inequity of legal provision to this vulnerable group (Hjern & Østergaard, 2016).

Table 5.1 summarises the entitlements to care for the different categories of migrant children in the EU and EEA countries. It seems that a migrant child who is legally categorised as an asylum-seeker is more likely to be entitled to health care on equal terms with a resident child than other migrant children without permanent residency. Twenty out of the 30 states have a policy to care for an asylum-seeking child in the same way as they do for the host population. Only 11 states have similar arrangements for irregular migrant or undocumented children from non-EU/EEA countries (see Table 5.1). Eight countries have similar entitlements for asylum-seeking children to that of the host population in a parallel primary care organisation outside of the general primary health care. Healthcare policies in the EU/EEA frequently do not address the rights of migrant families from other EU countries, who have overstayed the three-month period of free mobility or who lack identification. These migrants fall outside the defined categories of a migrant in many national as well as European policies.

A number of key points were identified in the MOCHA research:

- Twelve countries state that unaccompanied children have broader entitlements to health care than accompanied children. This is certainly beneficial

Table 5.1. Levels of equality regarding entitlements to health care for three groups of migrant children compared to national children. (No data = no data were available)

Key:
Entitlements equal to nationals regarding coverage and cost and included in same health care system
Entitlements equal to nationals regarding coverage and cost but enrolled in parallel health care system
Entitlements restricted compared to nationals/No legal entitlements
Unclear legal provision

	Equality Dimension		
	Child Asylum Seekers	Children of Irregular Third-country Migrants	Children of Irregular Migrants from Other EU Countries
Austria			
Belgium			
Bulgaria			
Croatia			No data
Cyprus			No data
Czech Republic			No data
Denmark			
Estonia			No data
Finland			
France			
Germany			
Greece			
Hungary			
Iceland			
Ireland			
Italy			
Latvia			No data
Lithuania			
Luxembourg			
Malta			No data
Netherlands			
Norway			
Poland			
Portugal			
Romania			

Table 5.1. (*Continued*)

Slovakia			
Slovenia			
Spain			
Sweden			
UK		No data	

for this group, but it is also a policy that discriminates migrant children by family status. Germany and Slovakia are the only countries that have policies that restrict health care for asylum-seeking children as well as for irregular migrant children originating outside of the EU/EEA area. In Germany, health care to irregular migrants is tied to a reporting duty.

- Different systems of funding health care for migrant children exist − some countries have a tax-based system while others are funded by health insurance. The insurance-based system is more administratively complicated, but identified successful solutions to this challenge in some insurance-funded countries, such as France and the Netherlands, show that there is no obvious relationship between the funding system and healthcare policy for migrant children in Europe.
- A number of countries define entitlements using concepts such as 'basic', 'necessary' or 'emergency' care. This lack of clarity can make access to health care and, in particular primary and psychological care, arbitrary and dependent upon the judgement of individual healthcare providers, and thereby fosters inequity.
- In all but four countries in the EU/EEA, there are systematic health examinations of newly settled migrants of some kind. In most eastern European countries and Germany, this health examination is mandatory; while in the rest of western and northern Europe, it is voluntary. All countries that have a policy of health examination aim to identify communicable diseases, so as to protect the host population.

Children in the State Care System

For decades, studies from Europe, North America and Australia have consistently reported that children entering and residing in societal out-of-home care (OHC) have radically more health problems and more healthcare needs than other children in national populations (Vinnerljung & Hjern, 2018). The MOCHA project explored how the primary care systems in the EU and EEA addressed the needs of these children, and whether the health system targets this population as having extra need, or if no extra provision is provided (see Chapter 15; Vinnerljung & Hjern, 2018).

A detailed study within the MOCHA project asked the Country Agents to provide data about how the EU and EEA countries address health care for children in OHC. This was combined with research knowledge and the results of an international seminar held in Sweden. The resulting report found a number of key points:

- Administrative responsibility for children in the state care system varies, between local, regional, national or combinations of different government levels.
- In all countries, children in OHC have similar access to care as other children in the population, but in some countries, such as in Ireland, there is prioritised access to somatic, dental and mental health care.
- All countries include and cover children by the national health or national health insurance systems.
- The MOCHA Country Agents reported that provision of health care to these children can vary substantially between regions within the same country.
- There is variation between national guidelines and legislation on health assessment and health monitoring of children in OHC. Half of the countries have some form of legally mandated rules for health assessment of children in the care system, but a standard practice for doing this is less common.
- Despite known high rates of mental health morbidity in these children and young people, only two countries (Spain and the United Kingdom) have legislation or a standard practice for assessment and monitoring of the mental health of children in OHC.
- No country has guidelines specifically concerning the sexual health of youth in OHC, for example, sex education and access to contraceptives.
- Only one country (United Kingdom) monitors immunisations for this population group.

(Vinnerljung & Hjern, 2018).

What Europe Can Do to Address Child Health Inequity in Primacy Care Health Systems

Our research findings support many of the recommendations made by the European Commission to strengthen primary care systems to address the needs of disadvantaged children (European Commission, 2013). These include the following:

- Improved universal coverage of preventive and health promotion activities, especially in the early years;
- Addressing the many obstacles children and families living in such circumstances face, such as cost, cultural and linguistic barriers and lack of information, as was investigated in Chapter 10, in the case of assisting families whose children have complex care needs and are at risk of considerable equity.
- Adequate planning and funding of primary health care, especially where workforce density and skill mix are less developed, and ensuring good inter-sectoral action for health by connecting primary care with community groups working with disadvantaged communities, for example the coordination

between the non-governmental organisations working with children who have complex health (see Chapter 10) or social care needs (see Chapter 15) are strategies which can help (Gilson, Doherty, Loewenson, & Francis, 2007). Training of the primary care health workforce to recognise inequity, the effects of the social determinants of health and empowering them to address these issues (see Chapter 13) will go some way to addressing the problem.

• Improved data availability on key risk factors for inequity, such as gender, SES, family composition, migrant status and regional differences, will facilitate the monitoring of pro-equity initiatives in primary care (see also Chapters 5 and 6; Shadmi, Wong, Kinder, Heath, & Kidd, 2014).

The European Parliament has now built on earlier recommendations of the Commission (European Commission, 2013) and has mandated the Directorate General Employment and Social Justice to assess the feasibility of a Child Guarantee (European Parliament, 2018) to ensure provision of and access for all at-risk children to:

> free healthcare, free education, free early childhood education and care, decent housing and adequate nutrition.

Echoing the findings of the MOCHA project, the target at-risk groups in the Child Guarantee proposal are as follows: children living in precarious family situations (including single parenthood, severe poverty, and Roma), children residing in institutions, children of recent migrants and refugees and children with disabilities and other children with special needs. This Child Guarantee, if endorsed, would provide a framework for availability of European funds to address these target groups' needs and strengthening of the specified core services. While a distance removed from the core MOCHA study, it is a practical initiative to address specific inequities affecting children in Europe. MOCHA evidence and expertise is being drawn into this feasibility study.

Future Directions

Primary care has an important role, but not the only role, in improving health and access to services for children who are at risk of inequity. There is great influence of social determinants of health and the economic situation of the country on health service provision. The MOCHA project has identified areas of inequity, or potential inequity throughout its work (see Chapters, 3, 6, 7, 8, 9, 10, 11, 13, and 14), and in addition, the project has attempted to identify the areas of particular risk of equity in children and young people, such as in areas of autonomy of access for young people, the experience of migrant children and children in the care systems of EU and EEA countries. In addition, we have tried to gather statistical evidence of inequity in terms of vaccinations, age at operation of cryptorchidism, two ambulatory care-sensitive conditions and age at diagnosis of autism to illustrate equity or inequity in the various primary care systems. This investigation has identified a gap in the data availability to assess inequity of provision and also to evaluate any changes in service in terms of equity measures (see also Chapters 6 and 7). We found no clear relationship to the principle models of primary child health care and equity for vulnerable groups. However, highly specialised services for vulnerable children supported by national legislative frameworks or established multi-professional practice networks show promise. Action to address inequalities in primary care to children and young people must be primarily at the national level, as this is where the competency base for health and welfare services is sited. However, the exploration at European Commission level of means of targeting European funds is a welcome signal and endorsement as to the importance of this challenge to children.

References

Austin, J. B., Selvaraj, S., Godden, D., & Russell, G. (2005). Deprivation, smoking, and quality of life in asthma. *Archives of Disease in Childhood, 90*(3), 253–257. doi:10.1136/adc.2004.049346

Berra, S., Borrell, C., Rajmil, L., Estrada, M. D., Rodríguez, M., Riley, A. W., … Starfield, B. (2006). Perceived health status and use of healthcare services among children and adolescents. *European Journal of Public Health, 16*(4), 405–414. doi:10.1093/eurpub/ckl055

Black, D. (1980). *Inequalities in health: Report of a research working group*. London: Deparment of Health and Social Security.

Britto, P. R., Lye, S. J., Proulx, K., Yousafzai, A. K., Matthews, S. G., Viavada, T., … Bhutta, Z. A. et al. (2017). Nurturing care: Promoting early childhood development. *Lancet, 389*(10064), 91–102. doi:10.1016/S0140-6736(16)31390-3

Burstrom, B., Burstrom, K., Nilsson, G., Tomson, G., Whitehead, M., & Winblad, U. (2017). Equity aspects of the primary health care choice reform in Sweden – A scoping review. *International Journal for Equity in Health, 16*(1), 29. doi:10.1186/s12939-017-0524-z

Burstrom, B., Marttila, A., Kulane, A., Lindberg, L., & Burstrom, K. (2017). Practising proportionate universalism – A study protocol of an extended postnatal home visiting programme in a disadvantaged area in Stockholm, Sweden. *BMC Health Services Research, 17*(1), 91. doi:10.1186/s12913-017-2038-1

Calderón-Larrañaga, A., Gimeno-Feliu, L. A., Macipe-Costa, R., Poblador-Plou, B., Bordonaba-Bosque, D., & Prados-Torres, A. (2011). Primary care utilisation patterns among an urban immigrant population in the Spanish National Health System. *BMC Public Health, 11*, 432. doi:10.1186/1471-2458-11-432

Carey, G., Crammond, B., & De Leeuw, E. (2015). Towards health equity: A framework for the application of proportionate universalism. *International Journal for Equity in Health, 14*, 81. doi:10.1186/s12939-015-0207-6

Chau, K., Baumann, M., & Chau, N. (2013). Socioeconomic inequities patterns of multi-morbidity in early adolescence. *International Journal for Equity in Health, 12*(1), 65. doi:10.1186/1475-9276-12-65

Cook, E. J., Randhawa, G., Large, S., Guppy, A., & Chater, A. (2012). A UK case study of who uses NHS direct: Investigating the impact of age, gender, and deprivation on the utilization of NHS direct. *Telemedicine and E-Health, 18*(9), 693–698. doi:10.1089/tmj.2011.0256

Cooper, D., Arnold, E., Smith, G., Hollyoak, V., Chinemana, F., Baker, M., & O'Brien, S. (2005). The effect of deprivation, age and sex on NHS Direct call rates. *British Journal of General Practice, 55*(513), 287–291.

Ethelberg, S., Olesen, B., Neimann, J., Schiellerup, P., Helms, M., Jensen, C., Böttiger, B., Olsen, K. E., Scheutz, F., Gerner-Smidt, P., & Mølbak, K. et al. (2006). Risk factors for diarrhea among children in an industrialized country. *Epidemiology, 17*(1), 24–30.

European Commission. (2013). *Investing in children: Breaking the cycle of disadvantage.* Report no. 2013/112/EU. Retrieved from https://eur-lex.europa.eu/legal-content/EN/TXT/PDF/?uri=CELEX:32013H0112&from=EN

European Parliament. (2011). *Resolution of 8 March 2011 on reducing health inequalities in the EU* (2010/2089(INI)) 2011. Retrieved from http://www.europarl.europa.eu/sides/getDoc.do?pubRef=-//EP//TEXT+TA+P7-TA-2011-0081+0+DOC+XML+V0//EN

European Parliament. (2018). *Parliamentary questions 24th August, 2018. Answer given by Ms Thyssen on behalf of the European Commission.* Retrieved from http://www.europarl.europa.eu/doceo/document/E-8-2018-003679-ASW_EN.html?redirect

Eurostat. (2015). http://appsso.eurostat.ec.europa.eu/nui/show.do?dataset=ilc_di12

Fadnes, L. T., Moen, K. A., & Diaz, E. (2016). Primary healthcare usage and morbidity among immigrant children compared with non-immigrant children: A population-based study in Norway. *BMJ Open, 6*(10), e012101. doi:10.1136/bmjopen-2016-012101

Giannakopoulos, G., Tzavara, C., Dimitrakaki, C., Ravens-Sieberer, U., & Tountas, Y. (2010). Adolescent health care use: Investigating related determinants in Greece. *Journal of Adolescence, 33*(3), 477–485. doi:10.1016/j.adolescence.2009.06.003

Gilson, L., Doherty, J., Loewenson, R., & Francis, V. (2007). *Challenging inequity through health systems – Final report knowledge network on health systems.* WHO Commission on Social Determinants of Health. Retrieved from http://www.who.int/social_determinants/resources/csdh_media/hskn_final_2007_en.pdf

Gimeno-Feliu, L. A., Armesto-Gomez, J., Macipe-Costa, R., & Magallon-Botaya, R. (2009). Comparative study of paediatric prescription drug utilization between the Spanish and immigrant population. *BMC Health Services Research, 9,* 225. doi:10.1186/1472-6963-9-225

Hart, J. T. (1971). The inverse care law. *Lancet, 1*(7696), 405–412. doi:10.1016/S0140-6736(71)92410-X

Health Organisation Commission on Social Determinants of Health. (2008). *Closing the gap in a generation Health equity through action on the social determinants of health.* Geneva: WHO, 2008.

Hintzpeter, B., Klasen, F., Schon, G., Voss, C., Holling, H., Ravens-Sieberer, U., & BELLA Study Group. (2015). Mental health care use among children and adolescents in Germany: Results of the longitudinal BELLA study. *European Child and Adolescent Psychiatry, 24*(6), 705–713. doi:10.1007/s00787-015-0676-6

Hjern, A., & Østergaard, L. S. (2016). *Migrant children in Europe: Entitlements to health care.* Retrieved from http://www.childhealthservicemodels.eu/wp-content/uploads/2015/09/20160831_Deliverable-D3-D7.1_Migrant-children-in-Europe.pdf

Hjern, A., Arat, A., & Klöfvermark, J. (2017). *Report on differences in outcomes and performance by SES, family type and migrants of different primary care models for children.* Retrieved from http://www.childhealthservicemodels.eu/wp-content/uploads/2017/12/20171214_Deliverable-D12-7.2-Report-on-differences-in-outcomes-and-performance-by-SES-family-type-and-migrants-of-different-primary-care-models-for-children-v1.1.pdf

Hjern, A., Haglund, B., Rasmussen, F., & Rosen, M. (2000). Socio-economic differences in daycare arrangements and use of medical care and antibiotics in Swedish preschool children. *Acta Paediatrica, 89*(10), 1250–1256.

Ivert, A., Torstensson-Levander, M., & Merlo. (2013). Adolescents' utilisation of psychiatric care, neighbourhoods and neighbourhood socioeconomic deprivation: A multilevel analysis. *PLoS One, 8*(11). doi:10.1371/journal.pone.0081127

Klanšček, H. J., Žiberna, J., Korošec, A., Zurc, J., & Albreht, T. (2014). Mental health inequalities in Slovenian 15-year-old adolescents explained by personal social position and family socioeconomic status. *International Journal for Equity in Health, 13*(1), 26. doi:10.1186/1475-9276-13-26

Lai, C. K., Beasley, R., Crane, J., Foliaki, S., Shah, J., Weiland, S., the ISAAC Phase Three Study Group (2009). Global variation in the prevalence and severity of asthma symptoms: Phase three of the International Study of Asthma and Allergies in Childhood (ISAAC). *Thorax, 64*(6), 476–483. doi:10.1136/thx.2008.106609

Lewis, K. M., Ruiz, M., Goldblatt, P., Morrison, J., Porta, D., Forastiere, F., ... Pikhart, H. (2017). Mother's education and offspring asthma risk in 10 European cohort studies. *European Journal of Epidemiology, 32*(9), 797–805. doi:10.1007/s10654-017-0309-0

Maeseneer, M., Willems, S., De Sutter, M., Van de Geucchte, I., & Billings, M. (2007). *Primary health care as a strategy for achieving equitable care: A literature review commissioned by the Health Systems Knowledge Network.* Retrieved from http://www.who.int/social_determinants/resources/csdh_media/primary_health_care_2007_en.pdf

Mangrio, E., Hansen, K., Lindstrom, M., Kohler, M., & Rosvall, M. (2011). Maternal educational level, parental preventive behavior, risk behavior, social support and medical care consumption in 8-month-old children in Malmo, Sweden. *BMC Public Health, 11*, 891. doi:10.1186/1471-2458-11-891

Marmot, M. (2010). *Fair society, healthy lives: The Marmot review.* London: Strategic Review of Health Inequalities in England post-2010. Retrieved from http://www.instituteofhealthequity.org/resources-reports/fair-society-healthy-lives-the-marmot-review/fair-society-healthy-lives-full-report-pdf.pdf

Moore, T. G., McDonald, M., Carlon, L., & O'Rourke, K. (2015). Early childhood development and the social determinants of health inequities. *Health Promotion International, 30*(Suppl 2), ii102–ii115. doi:10.1093/heapro/dav031

Muscat, M. (2011). Who gets measles in Europe? *Journal of Infectious Diseases, 204*(Suppl 1). S353–S365.

Olesen, B., Neimann, J., Bottiger, B., Ethelberg, S., Schiellerup, P., Jensen, C., Helms, M., Scheutz, F., Olsen, K. E. P., Krogfelt, K., Petersen, E., Mølbak, K. & Gerner-Smidt, P. (2005). Etiology of diarrhea in young children in Denmark: a case-control study. *Journal of Clinical Microbiology, 43*(8), 3636–3641. doi:10.1128/JCM.43.8.3636-3641.2005

Palacio-Vieira, J. A., Villalonga-Olives, E., Valderas, J. M., Herdman, M., Alonso, J., & Rajmil, L. (2013). Predictors of the use of healthcare services in children and adolescents in Spain. *International Journal of Public Health, 58*(2), 207—215. doi:10.1007/s00038-012-0360-2

Pearce, A., Rougeaux, E., & Law, C. (2015). Disadvantaged children at greater relative risk of thinness (as well as obesity): A secondary data analysis of the England National Child Measurement Programme and the UK Millennium Cohort Study. *International Journal for Equity in Health, 14*(1), 61. doi:10.1186/s12939-015-0187-6

Pickett, K. E., & Wilkinson, R. G. (2007). Child wellbeing and income inequality in rich societies: Ecological cross sectional study. *BMJ, 335*(7629), 1080. doi:10.1136/bmj.39377.580162.55

Pillas, D., Marmot, M., Naicker, K., Goldblatt, P., Morrison, J., Pikhart, H. (2014). Social inequalities in early childhood health and development: A European-wide systematic review. *Pediatric Research, 76*(5), 418—424. doi:10.1038/pr.2014.122

Räisänen, S., Kramer, M. R., Gissler, M., Saari, J., & Heinonen, S. (2014). Unemployment at municipality level is associated with an increased risk of small for gestational age births — A multilevel analysis of all singleton births during 2005-2010 in Finland. *International Journal for Equity in Health, 13*(1), 95. doi:10.1186/s12939-014-0095-1

Rattay, P., Starker, A., Domanska, O., Butschalowsky, H., Gutsche, J., Kamtsiuris, P., KiGGS Study Group et al. (2014). Trends in the utilization of outpatient medical care in childhood and adolescence. Results of the KiGGS study — A comparison of baseline and first follow up (KiGGS Wave 1). *Bundesgesundheitsblatt-Gesundheitsforschung-Gesundheitsschutz, 57*(7), 878—891. doi:10.1007/s00103-014-1989-1

Ruiz, M., Goldblatt, P., Morrison, J., Kukla, L., Švancara, J., Järvelin, M.-R., … Pikhart, H. (2015). Mother's education and the risk of preterm and small for gestational age birth: A DRIVERS meta-analysis of 12 European cohorts. *Journal of Epidemiology and Community Health, 69*(9), 826—833. doi:10.1136/jech-2014-205387

Ruiz, M., Goldblatt, P., Morrison, J., Porta, D., Forastiere, F., Hryhorczuk, D., … Pikhart, H. (2016). Impact of low maternal education on early childhood overweight and obesity in Europe. *Paediatric and Perinatal Epidemiology, 30*(3), 274—284. doi:10.1111/ppe.12285

Saltman, R., Allin, S., Mossialos, E., Wismar, M., Kutzin, J.Ie. (2012). Assessing health reform trends in Europe. In J. Figueras & M. McKee (Eds.), *Health systems, health, wealth and societal well-being assessing the case for investing in health systems* (pp. 209—246). London: European Observatory on Health Systems and Policies. McGraw Hill Open University Press. Retrieved from http://www.euro.who.int/__data/assets/pdf_file/0007/164383/e96159.pdf

Shadmi, E., Wong, W. C., Kinder, K., Heath, I., & Kidd, M. (2014). Primary care priorities in addressing health equity: Summary of the WONCA 2013 health equity workshop. *International Journal for Equity in Health, 13*, 104. doi:10.1186/s12939-014-0104-4

Starfield, B. (2011). The hidden inequity in health care. *International Journal for Equity in Health, 10*, 15. doi:10.1186/1475-9276-10-15]

Starfield, B., Gervas, J., & Mangin, D. (2012). Clinical care and health disparities. *Annual Review of Public Health, 33*, 89—106. doi:10.1146/annurev-publhealth-031811-124528

Tchicaya, A., & Lorentz, N. (2014). Socioeconomic inequalities in the non-use of dental care in Europe. *International Journal for Equity in Health, 13*(1), 7. doi:10.1186/1475-9276-13-7

Turi, A. L., Bals, M., Skre, I. B., & Kvernmo, S. (2009). Health service use in indigenous Sami and non-indigenous youth in North Norway: a population based survey. *BMC Public Health, 8*(9), 378. doi:10.1186/1471-2458-9-378

United Nations. (1989). *Convention on the rights of the child*. New York, NY: United Nations. Retrieved from https://downloads.unicef.org.uk/wp-content/uploads/2010/05/UNCRC_united_nations_convention_on_the_rights_of_the child.pdf?_ga=2.209651665.274437633.1540996300-199092997.1540996300

Van Damme, P., Van der Wielen, M., Ansaldi, F., Desgrandchamps, D., Domingo, J. D., Sanchez, F. G., ... Rose, M. (2006). et al. Rotavirus vaccines: Considerations for successful implementation in Europe. *Lancet Infectious Diseases, 6*(12), 805–812. doi:10.1016/S1473-3099(06)70657-0

Varga, S., Piko, B. F., & Fitzpatrick, K. M. (2014). Socioeconomic inequalities in mental well-being among Hungarian adolescents: A cross-sectional study. *International Journal for Equity in Health, 13*(1), 100. doi:10.1186/s12939-014-0100-8

Vinnerljung, B., & Hjern, A. (2018). *Health care in Europe for children in societal out-of-home care*. Retrieved from http://www.childhealthservicemodels.eu/wp-content/uploads/Mocha-report-Children-in-OHC-May-2018.pdf

Wenner, J., Razum, O., Schenk, L., Ellert, U., & Bozorgmehr, K. (2016). Health status and use of health services of children with insecure residence status in Germany. *European Journal of Epidemiology, 30*, S226–S227.

Whitehead, M., & Dahlgren, G. (2006). *Concepts and principles for tackling social inequities in health. Levelling up Part 1*. Copenhagen: WHO Europe. Retrieved from. http://www.euro.who.int/__data/assets/pdf_file/0010/74737/E89383.pdf

Wilson, C., Hogg, R., Henderson, M., & Wilson, P. (2013). Patterns of primary care service use by families with young children. *Family Practice, 30*(6), 679–694.

Wirback, T., Möller, J., Larsson, J.-O., Galanti, M. R., & Engström, K. (2014). Social factors in childhood and risk of depressive symptoms among adolescents – A longitudinal study in Stockholm, Sweden. *International Journal for Equity in Health, 13*(1), 96. doi:10.1186/s12939-014-0096-0

Wölfle, S. 1., Jost, D., Oades, R., Schlack, R., Hölling, H., & Hebebrand, J. (2014, Sep). Somatic and mental health service use of children and adolescents in Germany (KiGGS-study). *European Child and Adolescent Psychiatry, 23*(9), 753–764. Retrieved from https://doi.org/10.1007/s00787-014-0525-z.

World Health Organization. (2008). *Commission on social determinants of health: Closing the gap in a generation* (p. 247). Retrieved from https://www.who.int/social_determinants/thecommission/finalreport/en/World.

World Health Organization Early Child Development Knowledge Network, (ECDKN). (2007). *Early child development: A powerful equalizer*. Final report of the Early Childhood Development Knowledge Network of the Commission on Social Determinants of Health. Geneva: WHO.

Chapter 6

The Limited Inclusion of Children in Health and Health-related Policy

Mitch Blair, Michael Rigby, Arjun Menon,
Michael Mahgerefteh, Grit Kühne and Shalmali Deshpande

Abstract

Whilst nations have overall responsibility for policies to protect and serve their populations, in many countries, health policy and policies for children are delegated to regions or other local administrations, which make it a challenging subject to explore at a national level. We sought to establish which countries had specific strategies for child and adolescent health care, and whether primary care, social care and the school–healthcare interface was described and planned for, within any policies that exist. In addition, we established the extent to which a child health strategy and meaningful reference to children's records and care delivery exist in an e-health context. Of concern in the Models of Child Health Appraised (MOCHA) context is that 40% of European Union and European Economic Area countries had reported no health strategy for children, and more than a half had no reference to supporting delivery of children's health in their e-health strategy.

We investigated the differences in ownership and leadership of children's policy, which was a range of ministry input (health, education, labour, welfare or ministries of youth and family); as well as cross-ministerial involvement. In terms of national policy planning and provider planning, we investigated the level of discussion, consultation and interaction between national healthcare bodies (including insurance bodies), providers and the public in policy implementation. The MOCHA project scrutinised the way countries aim to harness the latest technologies by means of e-health strategies, to support health services for children, and found that some had no explicit plans whereas a few were implementing significant innovation. Given that children are a key sector of the population, who by very nature have a need to rely on government and formally governed services for their well-being in the years when they cannot themselves seek or advocate for services, our findings are particularly worrying.

Keywords: Health policy; children; adolescent; child primary care; e-health; strategy

Introduction

In trying to ascertain the details of child and adolescent health strategy across Europe, Models of Child Health Appraised (MOCHA) project researchers designed a questionnaire which was distributed to the 30 country agents, of which 27 responded. A challenge when undertaking this type of policy research is that in many countries (and not solely formally federated ones), many aspects of policy for operational services are delegated to regions or other local administrations; for instance, in France, Finland, Spain and the UK, there were reported issues with universal acceptance or adoption of plans when regional governments were involved. In this chapter, in all cases, replies are aggregated and analysed to the Member State level.

The Existence of National Child and Adolescent Health Strategies

The first aspect looked to ascertain whether countries have specific strategies for child and adolescent health care, whether these are included within other broader strategies, or simply do not exist at all. Countries were also asked details about the inclusion of primary health care, social care and the school–health-care interface within their planning. Further to this, questions assessed the process of such planning, including key stakeholder involvement, the format of relevant discussions and when these take place.

Of the 27 countries responding, 17 country agents (63%) responded that there was a specific strategy, while 10 (37%) replied that their countries did not have one. Of the 17 countries with a specific child and adolescent health strategy, 16 (94%) include primary healthcare planning for children within this, representing 59% of all countries surveyed. Only Norway does not have primary healthcare planning for children included within its specific child health strategy, although its standalone primary healthcare strategy accounts for children and adolescents. Thus, only half of European children live in a country which has a specific strategy for their health and health care.

Of the 10 countries that do not have a specific child and adolescent strategy, eight reported that they have primary healthcare planning included elsewhere. Malta and Hungary are the only two countries, out of all those who responded, that have neither primary healthcare planning nor specific child health strategies.

Of the 27 respondents, 21 (78%) reported that social planning is included in the planning of their strategies. However, different countries have different attitudes towards social care legislation with respect to child and adolescent health care. Five countries (Bulgaria, Denmark, France, Greece and Portugal) seem to focus on improving the lives of children with chronic health conditions and disabilities. Meanwhile, preventative healthcare services and health promotion are emphasised in seven countries (France, Germany, Greece, Iceland, Netherlands, Spain and the UK). Mental healthcare services are a primary aim of social care planning in six countries (Estonia, Greece, Italy, Latvia, Netherlands and the United Kingdom).

Of note, 10 countries (33%) address equity issues specifically in their strategies. Reducing social inequality in health is the focus in four countries (Greece, Norway, Portugal and Romania). Meanwhile, there is a notable focus on protecting vulnerable groups of children in 6 countries (Czech Republic, Denmark, France, Romania, Spain and Greece).

Ownership and Leadership of Children's Policies

The Ministry of Health is involved in the strategic planning of child policy in 24 (89%) countries, with the UK agent not responding to this question, while Slovenia and Malta claimed hardly any from the Ministry of Health. Further to this, the Ministry of Health assumed the clear lead ministerial role in strategy development for 17 (63%) of the countries who responded. Other ministries that were also commonly quoted as being involved in the strategic planning were the Ministry of Education (14 countries), the Ministry of Labour (including Welfare and Social Affairs ministries) (12 countries) and the Ministry of or concerning Family (11 countries) – this includes countries who had ministries covering Youth, Children, Family and/or Sports.

Estonia and Germany had the largest amount of cross-ministerial involvement, with eight and six ministries involved respectively. In contrast, seven (26%) countries reported single ministry involvement in the development of such strategies; these countries are Greece (Ministry of Health), Iceland (Ministry of Health), Lithuania (Ministry of Health), Malta (Ministry of Family, Social Solidarity and Children), Norway (Ministry of Health), Poland (Ministry of Health) and Romania (Ministry of Health). Of these countries, solely the respondent from Norway claimed that there is an open consultation process with key stakeholders before the ratification and implementation of a policy.

Relationship between National Policy Planning and Provider Planning

On the whole, countries generally described some level of discussion between national healthcare bodies and providers before the implementation of a strategy. In 20 (74%) countries, healthcare professionals, scientific institutions or healthcare associations are described as being involved in the consultation process for strategy development. In France, Finland and Spain, it is seen that the implementation of national directives remains under the control of regional health authorities. In the UK meanwhile, the governments of each of the four 'Home Countries' (England, Northern Ireland, Scotland and Wales) are responsible for both the planning and the implementation of strategies within their respective 'countries'. This contrasts with Denmark, Netherlands and Norway, where national policies are developed and subsequently issued as directives to be followed by municipalities, with relevant guidance on directing and financing care at the local level.

Insurance bodies are involved in strategy discussions in a variety of countries, such as Bulgaria, Czech Republic and Lithuania. However, in Bulgaria and Czech Republic, it was found that there is government representation on the boards of the insurance companies. In Cyprus, the national health insurance fund will feature in strategy discussions once established in 2020. This is different to Hungary and Iceland where the national health insurance funds do not impact the content of the policies whatsoever, but are simply involved in the reimbursement process.

In several countries, draft legislation is created and then heavily discussed by key stakeholders before being passed on to parliament for approval. These countries include Bulgaria, Ireland, Latvia, Malta and Poland. In Croatia, the agent reported that it is difficult for interministerial strategic discussions to progress past initial stages, as there is 'no clearly defined institutional responsibility for each ministry involved'.

Public involvement in the development of child and adolescent health strategy seems to be low across Europe. Only in one part of one country, namely, Scotland within the UK, was it reported that young people are involved in policy discussions on child and adolescent health, through the Scottish Youth Parliament. The Austrian country agent made mention of the involvement of Patient Associations in the development of strategy.

Issues in Health Policy Planning for Children's Services

There appears to be no evident correlation between the date of accession to the European Union (EU) and the likelihood of having a strategy. For example, Germany and France, founding members of the EU, respectively, do and do not have a specific child and adolescent health strategy; similarly, Romania and Portugal, who both joined the EU at similar times, respectively, did and did not have a specific strategy either.

Cross-ministerial involvement heavily features in the development of child and adolescent healthcare strategies across Europe. Some country agents found that strategy planning for children engages a broad mix of ministries. Health ministries, while regularly involved, were not the only ministry needed for strategy planning. Education ministries were regularly cited for their involvement in the development of health education curricula, as well as for ensuring an appropriate interface between healthcare services and schools.

Estonia and Germany both described the largest cross-ministerial involvement in strategic planning. Interestingly, both these countries also benefit from broad stakeholder involvement in developing strategies, in keeping with their willingness for multi-organisational and multi-stakeholder input.

Universal adoption is also not guaranteed in countries where the powers of policy planning are devolved to regional governments. This goes to show that regardless of structure, federal countries can have difficulties in the planning and implementation of policy.

Even though key stakeholders were often involved in the consultation process for strategy development, youth involvement was a consistently lacking aspect of the strategy planning. However, an apparent exception to the lack of youth involvement in strategy or policy formation was the situation in Scotland, as described by the country agent from the UK. In this case, 'Members of the Children's Parliament and the Scottish Youth Parliament attended the 2017 [Scottish government] cabinet meeting. Issues raised included school and teachers, safety, bullying, children's rights, mental health and Europe'. This is the only cited clear example of very high-level engagement between youth and legislators in this area of questioning. Until now, The Scottish Youth Parliament has continued to be involved in contributing to the aspects of health strategy, with a further meeting with the Scottish government cabinet took place in 2018 (Scottish Youth Parliament, 2018).

Interestingly, in the 2017 meeting, Scottish Youth Parliament members requested a specific 'Young People's Mental Health Strategy' for 16–25-year-olds due to the 'transitional phase' in young people's lives at this stage.

Identification of Children's Interests in e-Health Strategies

Very much separate in many ways from the issue of health strategies is that of e-health strategies. Here, the focus is on how a government and health system will harness the very new technologies to support the health of its citizens and, in particular, how those new technologies will support healthcare delivery. And within this field, electronic health records (EHRs) and special functionalities within EHRs are major opportunity to ensure each child is looked after optimally (see Chapter 14). At the same time, because of their means of accessing health services, their need for advocacy in their early years and the special data sets and actions regarding children's health, special functionality and data items need to be provided for children in an e-health setting.

Given its central importance to future healthcare delivery, the MOCHA project had a specific focus on e-health, including assessing the degree of focus on children's interests within national e-health plans. One line of approach within this was to examine every country's e-health strategy and the degree of recognition this had of children's needs. This was included in a formal project (Kühne & Rigby, 2016) and in a publication (Rigby et al, 2017).

In early 2016, the MOCHA country agents were asked about national e-health strategies, thus ensuring local analysis in national languages. Replies were received regarding 30 countries – of these 14 countries, that is Bulgaria, Cyprus, Denmark, France, Germany, Hungary, Ireland, Latvia, Lithuania, Norway,

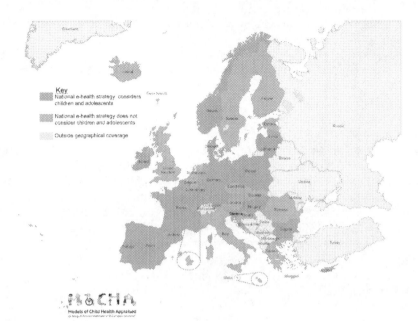

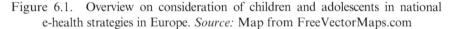

Figure 6.1.   Overview on consideration of children and adolescents in national e-health strategies in Europe. *Source:* Map from FreeVectorMaps.com

Poland, Portugal, Slovenia and Spain, mentioned that their countries' e-health strategy contained considerations on children and adolescents. Sixteen countries replied that their national e-health strategy did not consider children and adolescents. The details as of that time are shown in a map in Figure 6.1.

Of the countries which did refer to children, a number of innovative initiatives were identified by countries which should have a very positive effect on health care and on individual children's health – for details see the cited deliverable and published chapter. This shows the contrast between the 16 out of 30 countries that had no specific mentions of children's healthcare and delivery needs in their e-health strategy and those countries that were focussing on specific innovation for the benefit of children.

Summary

In looking at Appraisal of Models of Child Health, two specific policy areas seemed worthy of specific study – existence of a children's health strategy and existence of meaningful reference to children's records and care delivery in an e-health context. Of concern in the MOCHA context is that 40% of EU and EEA countries had no health strategy for children, and more than a half had no reference to supporting delivery of children's health in their e-health strategy. The Czech Republic, Finland, Greece, Luxembourg, Malta and parts of the UK have reported neither health strategies for children nor children's health in their e-health strategy. Given that children are key sector of the population, who by very nature have a need to rely on government and formally governed services for their well-being in the years when they cannot themselves seek or advocate for services, this is particularly concerning.

References

Kühne, G., & Rigby, M. (2016). *Description and analysis of current child health electronic record keeping across Europe.* Retrieved from http://www.child-healthservicemodels.eu/wp-content/uploads/2015/09/Description-and-analysis-of-current-child-health-electronic-records.pdf

Rigby, M. J., Kühne, G., Majeed, A., & Blair, M. E. (2017). Why are children's interests invisible in European National E-Health Strategies? In R. Randell, R. Cornet, C. McCowan, N. Peek, & P. J. Scott (Eds.), *Informatics for health: Connected citizen-led wellness and population health series studies in health technology and informatics* (pp. 58–62, Vol. 235). iOS press e books.

Scottish Youth Parliament. (2018). *Children and young people take part in second historic meeting with the Scottish Cabinet.* Retrieved from https://www.syp.org.uk/children_and_young_people_take_part_in_second_historic_meeting_with_the_scottish_cabinet

Chapter 7

The Invisibility of Children in Data Systems

Michael Rigby, Shalmali Deshpande, Daniela Luzi,
Fabrizio Pecoraro, Oscar Tamburis, Ilaria Rocco,
Barbara Corso, Nadia Minicuci, Harshana Liyanage,
Uy Hoang, Filipa Ferreira, Simon de Lusignan,
Ekelechi MacPepple and Heather Gage

Abstract

In order to assess the state of health of Europe's children, or to appraise the systems and models of healthcare delivery, data about children are essential, with as much precision and accuracy as possible by small group characteristic. Unfortunately, the experience of the Models of Child Health Appraised (MOCHA) project and its scientists shows that this ideal is seldom met, and thus the accuracy of appraisal or planning work is compromised. In the project, we explored the data collected on children by a number of databases used in Europe and globally, to find that although the four quinquennial age bands are common, it is impossible to represent children aged 0–17 years as a legally defined group in statistical analysis. Adolescents, in particular, are the most invisible age group despite this being a time of life when they are rapidly changing and facing increasing challenges. In terms of measurement and monitoring, there is little progress from work of nearly two decades ago that recommended an information system, and no focus on the creation of a policy and ethical framework to allow collaborative analysis of the rich anonymised databases that hold real-world people-based data. In respect of data systems and surveillance, nearly all systems in European society pay lip service to the importance of children, but do not accommodate them in a practical and statistical sense.

Keywords: Data; indicators; child health; primary care; database; children; medical record system; computerised

Counting and Understanding Infants, Children and Adolescents

In order to assess the state of health of Europe's children, or to appraise the systems and models of healthcare delivery, data about children are essential, with as much precision by small group characteristic, and accuracy of data, as possible. Unfortunately, the experience of the Models of Child Health Appraised (MOCHA) project and its scientists shows that this ideal is seldom met, and thus, the accuracy of appraisal or planning work is compromised. Indeed, the opening paragraph of Chapter 1 was not able to put an exact figure on the number of children in Europe as children aged 0–17 years inclusive are not a recognised statistical demographic grouping; similarly, it could not accurately identify the proportion of health activity performed by primary care as primary care activity is not a healthcare activity statistic despite primary care being set as the core component of health care. These challenges neatly summate the problems facing all who seek to study child health or related healthcare activity, as this involved measuring the unquantified.

Within the 30 European Union (EU) and European Economic Area (EEA) countries, the total reported population in 2017 was 514 million. Of this, there are roughly 97 million children younger than 18 years, accounting for around 19% of the total EU and EEA population (United Nations Population Division, 2017). The fact that we cannot even state definitively the total number of children in Europe starts to highlight the problem. Children form a large, important population group who have specific health needs. Non-communicable diseases present as the highest morbidities within this age group, while injuries and accidents account for the highest mortalities. These diseases and health events are largely preventable. But if we cannot count them, let alone by health or other characteristic, Europe is going to fail them.

Basic Registration Data

Population data within the European Region are collected through vital statistics registrations, national surveys and other government records. These data are available through published secondary databases, allowing the public to access information through simple online interfaces. Databases include the WHO Health for All (HFA) database, the Health Behaviours in School-aged Children (HBSC) portal, the Eurostat statistics database and the Global Burden of Disease (GBD) results tool, among others, and these are considered in more detail in following sections.

However, most current literature for child health data only focuses on mortality rates for children younger than five years of age. Meanwhile, little if any comparable data are present for children and adolescents (5–17 years of age). Further, there is sparse systematic data collection on the burden of disease (fatal and non-fatal) and injuries in this age group, even though these are some of the leading causes of child and adolescent morbidity (Global Burden of Disease, 2016). Lastly, public access means to routine vital statistics collected to ascertain mortality rates for children and adolescents are also partial or missing completely. The absence of this data has an impact on aspects of health service provision (health expenditure, workforce, etc.), which leads to suboptimal health care for children.

In an effort to reduce morbidity and mortality, achieving universal health coverage (UHC) has been a significant goal of WHO, and progress within the WHO European Region has involved the expansion of coverage of essential interventions for children. Though there has been progress, further improvement is still needed in order to avoid deaths from preventable causes. It is evident that further refinement of existing and introduction of improved health-promoting and health-protecting policies and interventions are required to reduce risky behaviours and to promote healthy habits (World Health Organization Regional Office for Europe, 2014; World Health Organization Regional Office for Europe, 2016).

In order to introduce the most effective policies to improve quality of care, WHO recommends implementing evidence-based guidelines for patient management. Their guidance emphasises that healthcare provision should adhere to an evidence base, and that treatments should be based on guidelines that follow international scientific evidence (World Health Organization Regional Office for Europe b, 2016). In this case, information and data are an essential resource for healthcare systems and health services. To supplement this, epidemiological data and vital statistics are central to policymaking and guidelines. Accurate information and a wide range of core indicators separated into age, gender, geographical and socio-economic status (SES) components can improve health status monitoring over time (World Health Organization Regional Office for Europe, 2017).

A specific focus on collecting child and adolescent health data is required so that policies and interventions may correctly target the health needs of this population group. Clinicians, policymakers and researchers need top class evidence to support decision-making in child health. Many databases are available and present this type of data on simple online interfaces. This includes the WHO HFA database, the HBSC portal, the Eurostat statistics database and the GBD results tool, among others. Separately, these databases provide rich data on specific aspects of child health at different ages throughout childhood and adolescence. However, none of these databases contain data on the full spectrum of child health indicators as determined by the 'Child Health Indicators of Life and Development' (CHILD) Project, which in 2002 recommended a set of indicators that cover health determinants, health status and the well-being of children with specific definitions for each indicator (Rigby & Köhler, 2002; Rigby, Köhler, Blair & Mechtler, 2003). It is difficult to combine data from these different sources to present a holistic picture of child health, since all databases use different methodologies. Investigations into these databases show that children are largely unaccounted for, and where there are data, they are not present for all ages.

The Databases Available and Included Child Health Indicators

WHO Health for All Explorer
Access to explorer via https://gateway.euro.who.int/en/hfa-explorer/
The WHO European HFA explorer was launched in 2016 as an easy tool to access health data and information, where the information tool allows the user to select indicators and view data from the last 36 years. This information tool is

available on the 'European Health Information Gateway' and consists of three datasets: European HFA dataset, European Mortality Indicator dataset (MDB) and European database on human and technical resources (HRes) for health dataset. The HFA dataset includes indicators on basic demographics, health status, health determinants and risk factors. The MDB presents age-specific and gender-specific analyses of trends by broad disease groups, as well as disaggregated to 67 specific causes of death. The HRes dataset provides statistics on HRes for health and offers data on healthcare resources (World Health Organization Regional Office for Europe, 2017; World Health Organization Regional Office for Europe, 2018a). Combined, these three datasets offer information on 1,503 indicators for the 53 countries of the WHO European Region. Population-weighted averages are also available for specific groups of countries, if more than 80% of the countries in the group have data available in the given year. Some data can also be sorted by gender.

Although the WHO HFA explorer is an extremely rich information source, there are some noticeable problems particularly for the child population. Firstly, the database does not allow the user to sort indicator data by small age groups (e.g. 1−4 years, 5−9 years, 10−14, and so on). In considering child health, this is a fundamental flaw since the available data cannot accurately represent the numbers or health status of children, since the accepted international definition is of those between birth and their 18th birthday. Put simply and starkly − the HFA explorer cannot explore the numbers or health of children in Europe as it cannot compute them as a statistical group. For example, child mortality data are presented as either crude rates for 0- and 1−4-year-olds or age-standardised rates for 0−14-, 1−19- or 5−14-year-olds. Moreover, these data are only present for certain causes of death. Secondly, there are not enough child health indicators included in the database to provide comprehensive information on the health of children in the European Region to make informed policy decisions. The user can access some population data, mortality data, immunisation coverage and one socio-economic indicator (Table 7.1).

Lastly, although these health indicators are present in the data explorer, much of the data are missing or are not recent. Further indicators are available through the 'European Health Information Gateway' website under the Child and Adolescent Health dataset World Health Organization Regional Office for Europe, 2018b). The database includes the indicators mentioned in Table 7.1 and also includes the following:

- child immigrant population of 0−14-year-olds;
- child population at risk of poverty or social exclusion of 0−15-year-olds;
- minimum age of criminal responsibility;
- potential criminal liability for children;
- HPV vaccine coverage; and
- tuberculosis cases in children.

Table 7.1. Overview of child health indicators available on the WHO Health for All explorer.

Child Health Indicator	Source
Life expectancy at age 1	HFA
Life expectancy at age 15	HFA
Population aged 0-14 years	HFA
Probability of dying before age 5	HFA
Proportion of children of official primary school age not enrolled	HFA
Neonatal and perinatal mortality	HFA
Proportion of infants vaccinated against invasive disease due to Haemophilus influenzae type b	HFA
Proportion of children vaccinated against measles	HFA
Proportion of children vaccinated against diphtheria	HFA
Proportion of children vaccinated against hepatitis B	HFA
Proportion of children vaccinated against mumps	HFA
Proportion of children vaccinated against pertussis	HFA
Proportion of children vaccinated against poliomyelitis	HFA
Proportion of children vaccinated against rubella	HFA
Proportion of children vaccinated against tetanus	HFA
Proportion of children vaccinated against tuberculosis	HFA
Certain cause specific crude mortality data for 0-year-olds	MDB
Certain cause specific crude mortality data for 1-4-year-olds	MDB
Certain cause specific standardised mortality data for 0-14-year-olds	MDB
Certain cause specific standardised mortality data for 1-19-year-olds	MDB
Certain cause specific standardised mortality data for 5-14-year-olds	MDB

Similarly, for these indicators, the user cannot disaggregate data in small age groups. Lastly, there are incomplete data for these indicators, too. For example, the HPV vaccine coverage data only contain 18 values from 18 different countries, over six years. Most of the countries report only one value, but for different years.

The issues with this database are important since they directly affect a major database used by policymakers, health professionals and researchers. The sparse and incomplete child health dataset does not provide substantial information, in order to make a well-informed, evidence-based health policy.

Health Behaviour in School-aged Children (HBSC) Data Portal
Access to portal via http://hbsc-nesstar.nsd.no/webview/

A second database for child health is the WHO/Europe collaboration with the HBSC survey, which collects information on health, well-being, social environment and health behaviour. This survey is conducted in 41 European countries and regions using a standardised questionnaire, allowing for the collection of common data from all participating countries for cross-national comparisons (World Health Organization Regional Office for Europe, 2018c). The survey collects information on 11-, 13-, and 15-year-old children since these ages have been reported as a time of increasing autonomy, which influences the development of their health and health-related behaviours (Health Behaviour in School-aged Children, 2018).

Findings from the survey are published every four years, and the data are presented in an online data portal. Presently, data on the portal are available from 2001/2002, 2005/2006, 2009/2010 and 2013/2014, allowing analysis of trend data (HBSC Data portal, 2018). This data are also available through the Child and Adolescent Health dataset on the 'European Health Information Gateway'. The HBSC portal allows disaggregation of data into gender, school grade, birth month or year, age or age category, country of birth and parental country of birth. The portal allows the user to compile data into a table, adding as many child health indicators as desired. The child health indicators are separated into health behaviours, health outcomes, risk behaviours, social context and social inequity (Figure 7.1).

This dataset is unique, in that it focuses on behaviours established during childhood that may continue into adulthood and have an impact on health outcomes. Additionally, the study focuses on young people in their social context at home, at school and with their family and friends. The combination of these factors, individually and together, is studied as influencers of young people's health from childhood into young adulthood (HBSC Data portal, 2018). The findings from the study help to monitor young people's health, understand the determinants of health and to improve health interventions.

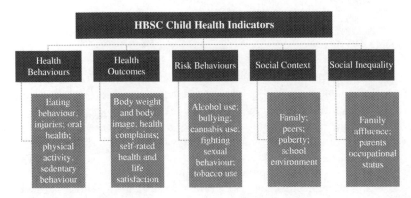

Figure 7.1.   Overview of child health indicators available through the HBSC portal.

Although this dataset is widely praised and used by the WHO European Region, there are some limitations that should be pointed out. Firstly, although the remit of HBSC is to investigate HBSC only, the lack of investigations of these health behaviours in younger children and for all ages (e.g. 10-, 12- and 14-year-olds) presents a gap in the evidence base. Although it is possible to assume that health behaviours might be similar to 11-, 13- and 15-year-olds, this assumption is not robust for evidence-based policymaking. Secondly, the survey methods are designed such that the study takes place every four years, and so data are not collected for the years in between. It is difficult to generate comprehensive trend data in order to monitor policy development and child health research.

A third point concerning this dataset is over the sampling techniques used to identify the specific schools to partake in the survey. Overall, cluster sampling is used to choose school class or schools, in the absence of a sampling frame of classes. Cluster sampling tends to provide less precision than other sampling methods, such as simple random sampling or stratified sampling (Roberts et al., 2009)

Fourthly, the questionnaire is also subject to some criticism, namely, self-reported answers and changes in questions over time. Though subtle, there are some questions and choices for questions that have changed from survey to survey, for example, the variation in questions asked around tobacco use. Further, since the collected responses are self-reported, the reliability of data can be questioned, since certain questions may provoke emotions leading to the young person answering differently to the truth.

Lastly, the emphasis on lifestyle, social and behavioural child health indicators means data on child health systems and policy data, and child health status and well-being data, are missing. Thus, this database too does not provide data on a full range of child health indicators for evidence-based policy action.

Eurostat

Access to database via https://ec.europa.eu/eurostat/data/database

A third database is provided by Eurostat, the statistical office of the EU which provides high-quality, comparable statistics at European level. Data are collected, verified and analysed by Member States and consolidated by Eurostat using a harmonised methodology to ensure data are comparable. The Member States and Eurostat work together to define a common methodology when collecting national data. Data are collected for nine different themes: general and regional statistics; economy and finance; population and social conditions; industry, trade and services; agriculture and fisheries; international trade; transport; environment and energy; and science, technology and digital society (Eurostat, 2018a). Health data are present within the theme 'population and social conditions'.

Eurostat presents European health statistics on both objective and subjective parts of population health. The data are presented in a data navigation tree, which allows the user to choose variables and create tables on the portal. Data for public health (health status, health determinants, health care, morbidity,

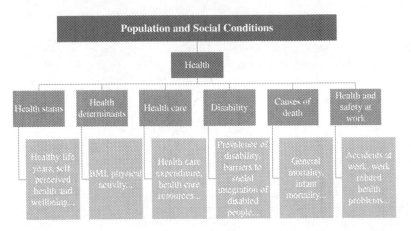

Figure 7.2.   Overview of health indicators available through the Eurostat database.

disability and causes of death) and for health and safety at work (accidents at work and occupational diseases) are available in Eurostat (Figure 7.2).

Data are regularly updated with a few health indicators having undergone a recent update to include data from 2017. Health status and health determinant indicators consist mainly of self-reported data, which are associated with response bias. Depending on the indicator chosen, the data can be disaggregated into age, gender, country, labour status, degree of urbanisation, educational attainment and others. This information is useful since it allows comparisons between specific groups within countries, as well as among countries. However, it should be noted that this level of disaggregation is only available for certain indicators and is not available for child health at all.

When it comes to child health indicators, this database seems to disregard this population group completely. Unfortunately, though data for these health indicators can be sorted by age group, the youngest available age group is 15—19-year-olds, suggesting that data on childhood and early adolescence are not collected. Youth are allocated a specific section under 'population and social conditions' and within this category, youth health is present. There are nine indicators present under youth health that incorporate some information on health status, health determinants and causes of death (Table 7.2).

This 'folder' dedicated to youth health suggests that this topic and this population group have been considered and studied. However, the indicators available in youth health, yet again, do not account for any person under the age of 15, representing a lack of child morbidity data. In spite of this, there is one health indicator that does present data for children younger than 15 years: causes of death. Data on causes of death provide information on mortality patterns and data are presented in five-year age groups, which allows meaningful comparisons between countries and regions (Eurostat, 2018b), but not for the totality of childhood. There are 86 listed causes of death available through

Table 7.2. Overview of child health indicators on the Eurostat database.

Child Health Indicator	Variables Available to Sort By
Daily smokers of cigarettes	Gender, age, educational attainment level, income quintile
Body mass index	Gender, age, educational attainment level, income quintile
Crude death rate by suicide of young people	Gender, age
Psychological distress of young people	Gender, age
Persons reporting an accident resulting in injury	Gender, age, educational attainment
Self-reported unmet needs for medical examination	Gender, age, main reason declared, income quintile
Self-perceived health	Gender, age, income quintile
People having along-standing illness or health problem	Gender, age, income quintile
Self-perceivedlong-standinglimitationsin usualactivitiesduetohealthproblem	Gender, age, income quintile

Eurostat, sorted by ICD10, and mortality data are available as absolute numbers, crude death rates and age-standardised rates. Therefore, comprehensive mortality data are available for children and adolescents. This includes data on injuries and NCDs, two of the most common causes of mortality and morbidity in children and adolescents, respectively.

Global Burden of Disease (GBD) Results Tool
Access to results tool via http://ghdx.healthdata.org/gbd-results-tool
A further database is the GBD results tool developed by the Global Health Data Exchange (GHDx) as a part of the Institute for Health Metrics and Evaluation (IHME), which launched in July 2007. The IHME is a population health research centre based at the University of Washington that provides morbidity and mortality data on the health status of the global population and is funded by the Bill & Melinda Gates Foundation (Institute for Health Metrics and Evaluation, 2018a).

The GHDx comprises information from surveys, censuses, vital statistics and other health-related databases, which is available for analysis and comparison through the results tool. GHDx aims to provide the best information on population health in order to improve health outcomes. This portal allows the user to build tables of information while selecting from nine different variables. The database contains data for 335 causes of morbidity and mortality, 84 risk factors, 19 aetiological factors and 39 impairment factors. In addition to this, the database can also present data on disability-adjusted life years (DALYs), years

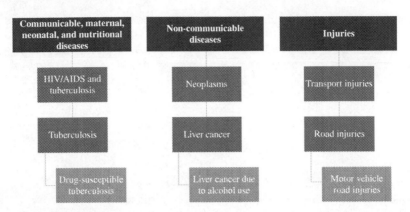

Figure 7.3.   Example of the four levels of hierarchy for causes of mortality.

lived with disability (YLDs), years of life lost (YLLs), prevalence, incidence, life expectancy and maternal mortality ratios, among others (Institute for Health Metrics and Evaluation, 2018b). In other words, the database can paint a very clear picture of the burden of disease across the world.

The data are categorised using a self-specified 'cause hierarchy' separating causes of mortality into four levels (Figure 7.3). Top level categories include the following:

- communicable, maternal, neonatal and nutritional diseases;
- non-communicable diseases; and
- injuries.

It is apparent that there is a large range of data that can be sorted to reveal a very fine level of detail. This type of data is not only useful for establishing burden of disease and rates of mortality, but also for monitoring health policies and interventions and evaluating their impact.

From child health perspective, data are available for children of all age groups, from 195 countries and territories, and are available from 1990 to 2016. Child data can be disaggregated in 11 age groups:

(1) early neonatal;
(2) late neonatal;
(3) post-neonatal;
(4) under 1 year;
(5) 1–4 years;
(6) under 5;
(7) 5–9 years;
(8) 5–14 years;
(9) 10–14 years;
(10) 15–19 years; and
(11) under 20 years.

This database provides the most complete picture of child morbidity and mortality of all the databases available for public use. Data on the most common causes of child and adolescent mortality and morbidity (injuries, NCDs, mental health and substance abuse) are also available from this database. This information is very useful for tracking the health status of European children; however, still absent is data for SES, behavioural or country policy stances. This makes it difficult to attribute reasons for trends in mortality rates and to draw a comprehensive overview of children's health.

An addition enigma with the GBD tables is that there is a strong drive for completeness of data to enable comprehensive comparative analyses; therefore, the process computes missing value to create a putative complete dataset. However, some of this computation can be opaque, though the team are open about the principle (Leach-Kemon & Gall, 2018). Users may, however, be concerned that they may not know which data are real facts and which are assumptions

World Bank Open Data and DataBank
Access to portal via https://data.worldbank.org/

The World Bank understands the need for good data in order to 'set baselines, identify effective public and private actions, set goals and targets, monitor progress, and evaluate impacts' (World Bank, 2018a). Resultantly, it provides a database that focuses on delivering good-quality statistical data for Member countries. There are 189 Members countries in the World Bank, who govern the World Bank Group. Data are obtained from the statistical system of a country, and therefore, the quality is dependent on the performance of a country's national systems. In order to maintain a high quality, the Development Data Group, within World Bank, coordinates with other organisations to improve the capacity of Member countries to produce and use statistical information. In addition, professional standards are followed for the collection, compilation and dissemination of data to ensure data quality and integrity.

World Bank Open Data allows the public free and open access to global developmental data (World Bank, 2018b). These data can be browsed by countries and economies or by indicators. When searching by country, the database presents data for individual countries, as well as groupings such as region, income levels, small states and so on. When looking through indicators, data are categorised into 21 indicators, of which 'health' is one (Figure 7.4).

Investigation into the health section reveals 52 indicators including data on population rates, vital statistics, mortality rates, life expectancy, incidence and prevalence of infectious diseases and so on (see Table 7.3). The information is presented in a clear online format and can also be downloaded via an online visualisation tool or as a spreadsheet.

Although a wide range of indicators are available, this database provides data for the set indicator only and does not allow the user to sort data, for example by age groups. Furthermore, of the 52 indicators available, just over a quarter mention some form of child health or involve data for children within

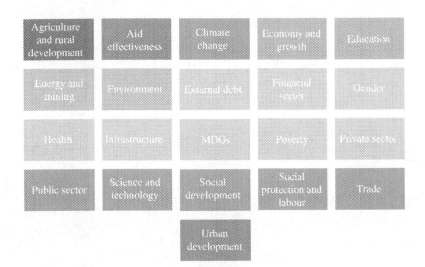

Figure 7.4.   Overview of indicators available through World Bank Open Data database.

the 0−18 years age range, but even then not specifically for that legal childhood definition.

These data are also available through the World Bank DataBank, an analysis and visualisation tool that holds time series data and comprises 71 databases (2018c). Upon searching for 'health', seven databases are presented: Gender Statistics, Health Nutrition and Population Statistics, Population estimates and projections, Service Delivery Indicators, UHC and Human Capital Index. A few further indicators are available through these databases, where, for example through the 'Health, Nutrition and Population Statistics' database, information is available on children and HIV, diarrhoea treatment, population stratified by quintile age groups and gender, school enrolment and vitamin A supplementation coverage rate. However, it still does not allow disaggregation of data into small age groups.

Central Intelligence Agency − The World Factbook
Access to Factbook via https://www.cia.gov/library/publications/the-world-factbook/

The Central Intelligence Agency (CIA) of the US government presents a World Factbook that is a resource containing summary information on demographic, geographic, governmental, economic and military data on each of the 267 world entities (Central Intelligence Agency, 2018) − in this context, entities comprise independent countries, Taiwan, the EU, dependencies and areas of special sovereignty, Antarctica and places in dispute and the world and the oceans. Although this information is primarily designed for the use of US government officials, it is open to the public as a research resource. Information is available for each country on a profile and includes a map of the country, the flag, as well

Table 7.3. List of health indicators available through World Bank Open Data database.

Adolescent fertility rate (birthsper1,000women ages 15–19)

Age dependency ratio (% of working-age population)

Birth rate, crude (per 1,000 people)

Births attended by skilled health staff (% of total)

Causeofdeath, by communicable diseasesandmaternal,prenatalandnutrition conditions(%oftotal)

Cause of death, by injury (% of total)

Cause of death by non-communicable diseases (% of total)

Completeness of birth registration (%)

Completeness of death registration with cause-of-death information (%)

Contraceptive prevalence, any methods (% of women ages 15–49)

Death rate, crude (per 1,000 people)

Diabetes prevalence (% of population ages 20–79)

Fertility rate, total (births per woman)

Hospital beds (per 1,000 people)

Immunisation, DPT (% of children ages 12–23 months)

Immunisation, measles (% of children ages 12–23 months)

Incidence of tuberculosis (per 100,000 people)

International migrant stock, total

Life expectancy at birth, female (years)

Life expectancy at birth, male (years)

Life expectancy at birth, total (years)

Maternal mortality ratio (modelled estimate, per 100,000 live births)

Mortality caused by road traffic injury (per 100,000 people)

Mortality rate, infant (per 1,000 live births)

Mortality rate, neonatal (per 1,000 live births)

Mortality rate, under 5 (per 1,000 live births)

Net migration

Number of surgical procedures (per 100,000 population)

Population ages 0–14 (% of total)

Population ages 15–64 (% of total)

Population ages 65 and above (% of total)

Population growth (annual %)

Population, female (% of total)

Table 7.3. (*Continued*)

Population, total
Pregnant women receiving prenatal care (%)
Prevalence of HIV, female (% ages15–24)
Prevalence of HIV, male (% ages15–24)
Prevalence of HIV, total (% of population ages 15–49)
Prevalence of anaemia among children (% of children under 5)
Prevalence of overweight, weight for height (% of children under 5)
Prevalence of severe wasting, weight for height (% of children under 5)
Prevalence of stunting, height for age (% of children under 5)
Prevalence of undernourishment (% of population)
Prevalence of underweight, weight for age (% of children under 5)
Prevalence of wasting, weight for height (% of children under 5)
Refugee population by country or territory of asylum
Refugee population by country or territory of origin
Risk of catastrophic expenditure for surgical care (% of people at risk)
Risk of impoverishing expenditure for surgical care (% of people at risk)
Specialist surgical workforce (per 100,000 population)
Teen age mothers (% of women ages 15–19 who have had children or are currently pregnant)
Unmet need for contraception (% of married women ages 15–49)

as an introduction to the country's history. Additional information is available on the geography, the people and society, the government, the economy, energy, communications, transportation, military and security, terrorism and transnational issues.

The most relevant section for the MOCHA project is 'people and society'. Within this, information on 31 indicators is available, of which thirteen indicators are directly related to health. This includes data on birth and death rates, maternal and infant mortality ratios, life expectancy data, health expenditure, physician and hospital bed density, HIV/AIDS and obesity prevalence rates. Aside from infant mortality ratio and school life expectancy, there are no other child-related indicators available.

Organisation for Economic Cooperation and Development – OECD.Stat Web Browser
Access to web browser via https://stats.oecd.org/index.aspx?DataSetCode= HEALTH_STAT

The Organisation for Economic Cooperation and Development (OECD) focuses on policies that improve economic and social well-being of people, among its member states globally — these are mainly larger economies. These policies are based on facts and real-life experiences such as economic drivers, social and environmental change, taxation and social security, leisure time and so on (OECD, 2018a).

The OECD collects data on member countries and for some outside the OECD membership, especially though an understanding with the European Commission, and analyses this data for discussions and policy decisions. Data are available for 26 topic areas, of which one is health. This section has data on health outcomes and health system resources, as well as healthcare policies, in an effort to improve health systems within the OECD area. Within the health section, there are 13 areas that OECD focuses on, including ageing and long-term care, mental health and public health (OECD, 2018b). Notably, there is no section available on child health.

This data are available through reports, but also through OECD.Stat, a database explorer where users can search the statistical databases and easily build tables with different variables and extract data to be downloaded into MS Excel. Information on methodology and data sources is also available through this interface (OECD, 2013).

Within health, there are 12 themes: health expenditure and financing, health status, non-medical determinants of health, healthcare resources, health work-force migration, healthcare utilisation, healthcare quality indicators, pharmaceutical market, long-term care resources and utilisation, social protection, demographic references and economic references (OECD, 2018c).

Although these themes are comprehensive and inclusive of several aspects of health, there is no specific focus on child health. The child-related indicators available are infant health, maternal and infant mortality and immunisation, which do not focus on children above five years of age and do not cover the breadth of topics that are important in child health.

Discussion of Key Points on Data Sources

The information available from seven key databases shows that data for child health and policies surrounding their well-being are not widely available. The databases show little congruency between the level of information available for child health indicators and only one database allows disaggregation of data into small age groups for morbidity and mortality. The disparity in statistics and the availability of child health indicators is evident in all databases.

However, of the seven databases, Eurostat and GBD show the most accord-ance for child health indicators, such as mortality rates for small age groups. The GBD database can provide data on 335 causes of morbidity and mortality and gives the most comprehensive coverage for data on child health morbidity and mortality indicators. Nonetheless, data related to and around obesity for children and adolescents are missing, even though this is one of the leading causes of morbidity in this population group. Only some obesity data are available through HBSC though it is self-reported and therefore open to issues surrounding response bias.

These current positions of these databases show that although there is some data available for children in data and policy systems, they are largely missing. Efforts to improve health status and health outcomes within this population group will require a wider range of child health indicators and a systematic and robust database that allows manipulation of data. Not least, as Chapter 5 shows, measurement of the important and recognised significant field of Equity is greatly hampered by lack of relevant child-specific data − it is very difficult to act effectively on a societal priority if there are not the data to show what action and where is needed.

Invisibility of Children in Quality Measures

Since the early 1990s, attention has been drawn to the invisibility of children as individual entities (Chapple & Richardson, 2009; Rees, Bradshaw, Goswami, & Keung, 2006), often subsumed within statistics about parents, families and households. This issue has been often highlighted by other authoritative organisations, such as the OECD (2009), UNICEF (2009) and WHO (2010), which raise the question of scarcity of available data, poor data quality and the need for data harmonisation. Although efforts in this direction are increasing (Wolfe, 2014), children's statistical invisibility still limits the breadth of the analysis and therefore the evaluation of childcare, especially in the view of cross-country comparison.

The main goal of focussed work the team from CNR Italy undertook within the MOCHA project was to identify potential measures through the exploration of a continuum of feasible measures. The team sought clinical, health status and satisfaction perspectives that could be used effectively by the stakeholders within diverse structural models (across countries) and paediatric settings to quantify the impact of the paediatric care (Minicuci et al., 2017). To achieve this challenging goal, measures available in international open-accessible databases on child health-related issues as well as those used by the MOCHA countries in their evaluation of childcare were analysed. This analysis contributes to the identification of potential feasible and already available measures and at the same time helps in identifying gaps that hinder a multidimensional approach of the evaluation of primary care systems for children.

The MOCHA Analysis

All international databases that were open access and dealt with a broad spectrum of child health-related issues were searched. Scrutinised sources came from organisations, agencies, research networks and observatories. Ongoing and complete research projects on child health care were also investigated.

In parallel, an ad hoc designed questionnaire was developed and administered to Country Agents (CAs) to gather information on:

- agencies/organisations in charge of the evaluation of quality of care at national and/or local level and/or devoting a specific part of quality assessment to childcare; and
- measures used to evaluate childcare.

Among the 30 MOCHA countries, 27 CAs responded to the questionnaire. Two CAs (Poland and Romania) reported that their assessment of healthcare system is based on accreditation procedures, while two other CAs (Greece and Malta) did not provide any measures devoted to child health care. Therefore, our analysis considered 23 countries that reported a system in place to assess the quality of child health care and also provided the measures adopted.

The development of a conceptual map of domains, further detailed in a two-level hierarchy of subcategories, helped the classification and the comparative analysis of the data collected.

Additionally, to analyse whether the child's psychophysical development is considered within the available measures, the results were also analysed considering the coverage of child age range, to capture the level of child invisibility in both sources of information. To balance the need of granularity with the choice of standardised age ranges and with the intent of capturing the most common ones (but also the less frequent), the following age ranges have been adopted: 0−11 months and 1−4, 5−9, 10−17 and >17 years.

Moreover, an analysis of measures related to diseases was carried out to investigate whether and to what extent they adequately capture child-centric health issues and well-being.

In the following, two main aspects of child invisibility are analysed focusing on age and disease-related measures available in international databases as well as those used by the MOCHA countries, as reported by the CAs.

Analysis of Age-related Measures

International Databases

Among the 207 measures identified in the international databases, 157 (76%) are age-related, and among them, 86 measures fall within the identified age groups, while the rest cover more than one age class (Table 7.4).

Two age groups are most frequently covered:

(1) the child aged less than one year (40 measures); and
(2) the child aged 10−17 years (42 measures).

The first age group (children aged younger than one year) focuses, in particular, on the different types of vaccine administration (14 measures), on neonatal and infant mortality (eight measures) and, to minor extent, on breastfeeding (three measures) and preterm and low birth weight (three measures). Measures considering adolescents (10−17 years) are frequently related to school performance taking advantages of yearly international surveys (nine measures related to

Table 7.4. Distribution of measures by age ranges in international databases.

<1	[1–4]	[5–9]	[10–17]	>17
40 (25%)	3 (2%)	1 (1%)	42 (27%)	0
18 (11%)				
12 (8%)				
19 (12%)				
			14 (9%)	
			7 (4%)	
	1 (1%)			

PISA (Program for International Student Assessment), three to PIRLS (Progress in International Reading Literacy Study) and two to TIMSS (Trends in International Mathematics and Science Study)), and also consider health-related behaviour such as addiction related to tobacco smoking and alcohol consumption and nutrition, concerning fruit and vegetable consumption and weight problems. The 1–4 and 5–9 age groups are covered by a limited number of measures exclusively pertaining to family expenditures on education, leaving out other aspects that could measure this important child developmental life course.

Measures considering more than one age range are generally designed to capture disease distribution, hospitalisation, health and school health service' expenditures. They are generally related to diseases classified by ICD.

Responses by the MOCHA Country Agents
Among the 352 measures reported by the CAs, 122 (35%) are age-related. The most frequently considered single age range is the neonatal period (29 measures), while the majority of measures (88, 72%) tend to combine more than one interval, shown in Table 7.5.

This is evident by the high number of measures ($N = 51$; 42%) that cover the 0–17 year period of life and seven measures (6%) that cover the whole spectrum of age ranges.

Focusing on 29 measures related to the neonatal period, particular emphasis is posed on birth and delivery (nine measures) and mortality (eight measures) and to a minor extent on breastfeeding (two measures) and health issues such as low weight newborns (one measure) and malfunctions (one measure). It is worth noting that within these measures, despite only being sparsely adopted by the

Table 7.5. Distribution of measures by age ranges according to Country Agent responses.

<1	[1–4]	[5–9]	[10–17]	>17
29 (24%)	2 (2%)	0	2 (2%)	1 (1%)
4 (3%)				
6 (5%)				
51 (42%)				
7 (6%)				
		4 (3%)		
	7 (6%)			
		8 (6%)		
		1 (1%)		

MOCHA countries, there are some attempts to evaluate the preventive functions of paediatric primary care measuring the number of neonatal children being screened during well-child visits (one measure adopted by Ireland and the other by Austria, Finland, Greece, Ireland and Portugal).

Focusing on the consistent number of measures covering the entire range of age groups, the majority of them (37 measures out of 58) consider childhood and adolescence as a whole period, without making any age group distinction. These measures are generally related to hospitalisation rates due to pathologies or track the prevalence/proportion of certain diseases. Moreover, the large majority of these measures are heterogeneously and sparsely distributed among the 23 countries, with the highest peak of eight countries using the same type of measure.

Analysis of Disease-related Measures

International Databases

Fifty-eight out of 207 measures (23%) are disease-related, covering 30 different pathologies, as shown in Figure 7.5. Eleven measures provide a wide spectrum of diseases using the ICD classification focusing mainly on hospitalisation (discharge and length of stay, four measures) and mortality (two measures). The three measures related to health expenditures distributed by ICD provide data about a limited number of countries: a maximum of five EU/EEA countries provide data to international databases.

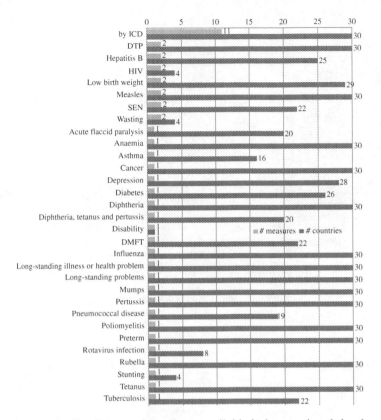

Figure 7.5.   Distribution (*n*) of measures available in international databases by disease − total number of countries providing data for at Least One measure related to the specific disease.

Similar to the age-related measures, the remaining measures are mainly focused on immunisations (17 measures) and morbidity (10 measures). However, data on morbidity only unevenly cover all the EU/EEA countries, especially when they are related to specific diseases such as HIV or severe wasting (four countries covered). Also in diseases common in childhood, such as asthma, national data available in international databases partially cover the MOCHA countries (16 countries report the prevalence of asthma in children ages 6−7 or 13−14).

Responses by Country Agents
About 173 out of 352 (49%) measures reported by CAs are related to diseases covering 50 different pathologies. Data gathered by CAs allowed us to analyse them under different perspectives. First, to explore whether a set of measures are commonly used across countries to evaluate child health care related to diseases. This analysis provided indications on the frequency of use across

countries (i.e. the number of countries using the same or similar measures). It also highlighted whether there is a convergence in the evaluation on certain aspects of child health care (types of diseases analysed). Second, we investigated the number of measures that are used to evaluate a specific aspect of child health care. This indicates the efforts of an in-depth evaluation through the selection of different measures that capture detailed aspects that contribute to a more comprehensive analysis. In the case of diseases, this may also indicate countries' concerns on specific child disorders, whose prevalence needs particular monitoring efforts.

Figure 7.6 shows that countries' assessment on children diseases tends to use a higher number of measures concentrated on a limited number of diseases, while a consistent number of diseases are analysed by one measure generally within a single country.

Asthma is the most frequently analysed illness in terms of both the number of measures reported by the CAs ($N = 22$; 13%) and the number of countries that focus part of the quality assessment on the basis of such measures ($N = 14$, 61.0%). Similar results are provided for diabetes (16 measures and nine countries, respectively, 9% and 39%) and for mental health (16 measures and 13 countries, respectively, 9% and 57%). However, if we consider commonalties across countries for the analysis of these diseases, there is a peak of six countries using hospitalisation rates due to asthma and five countries adopting the incidence rate of Diabetes Type 1 and Type 2.

Considering the overall distribution by country, there is a remarkable variation. A limited number of countries use the same or similar measures. The highest convergence is once again on immunisation rates for MMR (nine countries), DPT3 (eight countries) and meningitis (eight countries). The remaining measures are unevenly distributed between the countries, in some cases indicating particular attention on the analysis of specific diseases. For instance, Denmark uses 11 measures to report laboratory test values on diabetic children, and 12 to analyse the different aspects of asthma treatment ranging from primary care visits to hospitalisations and drug consumption. It is also the only country that monitors ADHD with eight different measures that comprise various types of visits performed and use of drugs.

Quality Measures Key Points

The analysis of measures related to age and disease available in international databases and resulting from CAs' responses provide a first snapshot of children's invisibility. If we consider the age-related measures, the major focus is on maternal and prenatal health and on the first years of childhood. This is especially the situation at country level, where the attention on age groups is not so diffused (35% of measures applying this distinction). Conversely, international databases tend to consider also adolescents mainly under the perspective of healthy behaviour and school performance. Infant age and early childhood (1-4 years and 5-9 years) are the most invisible ones, even if often included in

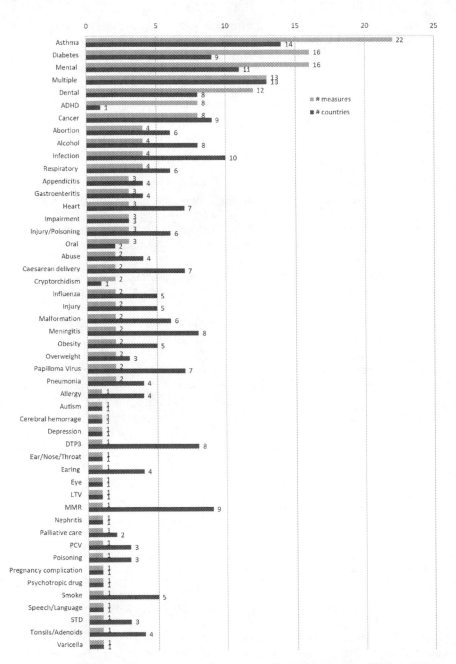

Figure 7.6.   Distribution (n) of measures provided by CAs by disease. Total number of CAs reporting at least one measure related to the specific disease.

measures that cover the whole period, making it difficult to track important stages of children's psychophysical development.

Age-related measures are generally focused on immunization, mortality and hospitalisation and this trend is confirmed also in the analysis of disease-related measures, leaving out other important aspects of childcare. At country level, as reported by CAs, there is a particular attention on asthma, diabetes and mental health, however analysed under different perspectives, making country comparison very difficult. The scattered presence on other disease-specific measures lets us presume that other morbidities may be included in the evaluation of care. There is little attention on the increasing number of children with non-communicable diseases (Wolfe, 2013), or disability that pose crucial challenges for services provision (not only health-related) in a perspective of mitigating and enhancing quality of life of both children and their families.

Finally, and this is evident considering the whole range measures analysed (Minicuci et al., 2017), only a limited number of countries evaluate aspects connected with the provision of services, including health promotion and prevention activities or types and access to primary care child-centric services.

Seeking Children's Data in Records-based Research Databases

A third approach innovated by a team within the MOCHA project was to assess the potential of collaborative research using the considerable and much vaunted use of anonymised health databases drawn from record systems. This has been written up in the scientific literature (Liyanage, Hoang, Ferreira, & de Lusignan, 2018). By utilising the local knowledge in each country of the CAs, and the specially designed MOCHA International Research Opportunity Instrument (MIROI) tool, a total of over 150 data repositories has been identified. Details of these, with metadata on custodianship, access and broad contents, were collated and stored securely on a health data cataloguing website. All the databases gave informed consent to these details being recorded, with the aspiration that comparative research could be undertaken on healthcare and health outcomes for the child patients recorded. Given the recognised importance of research on utilising real-world data from health care and actual patients, and the potential interest of all these databases, it was hoped that significant study could be undertaken of children's health care and outcomes for selected tracer conditions.

In the event, this vision did not materialise. As reported, there were significant problems of resourcing access (many database holders did not have time or financial resources to undertake even small one-off analyses, as these were not within the organised resource framework of the data-holding organisation). Secondly, there is no means of mutually recognising ethical approval or research validity across European countries (unlike within country, where there often is mutual recognition). Thirdly, data were not necessarily recorded in compatible ways or for the same aspects.

So the MOCHA project hit another child data barrier. Even where potentially rich data were held and there was willingness to use these for service
appraisal studies, the logistics meant that these data were in practice inaccessible, even though the foundational work of creating the downloaded database
had already been undertaken. The child data repository was visible, but the data
were inaccessible.

Data: Financial Environment and Spending

From an economics perspective, the starting point for analysing the focus on
children in healthcare provision at a national level would be by exploring the
data on healthcare expenditure. This would incorporate scrutiny of variables
such as total healthcare expenditure per child, proportions that are publicly versus privately financed, the extent of out-of-pocket (OOP) expenditures by par-
ents/carers and the distribution of expenditure (as a reflection of access to health
care). Data on these variables, however, are not generally available. While some
information is provided at the national level, and collated by international organisations such as the World Bank and the World Health Organization, it is not
disaggregated to show the proportions of expenditure on children and young
people, or how expenditure is distributed between primary and secondary care.

Total health expenditure per capita, public and private health spending per
capita and OOP expenditure on health are shown in Table 7.6 for the MOCHA
countries, providing some indication of how much each country spends in the
area of health overall and how it is financed. Lags exist, however, in the compilation of these data such that those available may be some years out-of-date.
Population size and the numbers of children and young people are also included,
but little can be inferred from this about how much health care is absorbed by
children without further detail on the age distribution of the whole population
and relative expenditures across all age groups. It is likely that expenditure on
older people is disproportionately high such that expenditure on children cannot
be assumed to be a simple percentage of health expenditure equivalent to the
proportion of children in the population. Hence, children are 'invisible' in
national figures.

The major determinant of overall health expenditure in any country is its
wealth, traditionally measured by its Gross Domestic Product (GDP) per capita.
For the purposes of international comparisons, GDP is standardised to a common Purchasing Power Parity based on the US dollar. Significant variability in
GDP per capita and health expenditures are apparent across the MOCHA countries with implications for the levels of healthcare provision, including for children. GDP per capita is an average figure and does not take account of the
distribution of resources within countries which may be quite inequitable.
National data are available on the proportions of children at risk of poverty but
the relationship between income levels and access to health care cannot be established from the available data (Table 7.6).

Table 7.6. National data on health expenditure and financing and for the MOCHA countries.

Countries	GDP Per Capita: PPP Current International $ (2015)[a]	Total Health Expenditure % of GDP (2014)[b]	Population Total (2016)[c]	% of Population 19 Years and Under (2016)	Private Health Expenditure % of THE (2014)[b]	Public Health Expenditure % of THE (2014)[b]	Out-of-Pocket Payments % of THE (2014)[b]	% of Children 18 Years and Under at Risk of Poverty/Social Isolation (2016)[b]
Austria	43,893	11.21	8,712,137	19.22	22.14	77.86	16.15	20.00
Belgium	41,138	10.59	11,358,379	22.57	22.13	77.87	17.81	21.60
Bulgaria	16,956	8.44	7,131,494	18.27	45.43	54.57	44.19	45.60
Croatia	20,430	7.80	4,213,265	20.28	18.13	81.87	11.21	26.60
Cyprus	30,310	7.37	1,170,125	23.44	54.77	45.23	48.71	29.60
Czech Republic	29,805	7.41	10,610,947	19.43	15.46	84.54	14.33	17.40
Denmark	43,415	10.80	5,711,870	22.83	15.24	84.76	13.36	13.80
Estonia	26,930	6.38	1,312,442	20.57	21.18	78.82	20.72	21.20
Finland	38,643	9.68	5,503,132	21.81	24.69	75.31	18.23	14.70
France	37,306	11.54	64,720,690	24.11	21.79	78.21	6.34	22.60
Germany	44,053	11.30	81,914,672	18.05	23.01	76.99	13.20	19.30
Greece	24,617	8.08	11,183,716	19.33	38.34	61.66	34.86	37.50
Hungary	24,474	7.40	9,753,281	19.48	34.02	65.98	26.59	33.60
Iceland	42,449	8.86	332,474	26.64	18.96	81.04	17.48	14.40

Table 7.6. (*Continued*)

Countries	GDP Per Capita: PPP Current International $ (2015)[a]	Total Health Expenditure % of GDP (2014)[b]	Population Total (2016)[c]	% of Population 19 Years and Under (2016)	Private Health Expenditure % of THE (2014)[b]	Public Health Expenditure % of THE (2014)[b]	Out-of-Pocket Payments % of THE (2014)[b]	% of Children 18 Years and Under at Risk of Poverty/ Social Isolation (2016)[b]
Ireland	51,899	7.78	4,726,078	27.57	33.94	66.06	17.66	27.30
Italy	33,587	9.25	59,429,938	18.31	24.39	75.61	21.19	33.20
Latvia	22,628	5.88	1,970,530	19.46	36.82	63.18	35.13	24.70
Lithuania	26,397	6.55	2,908,249	20.19	32.13	67.87	31.27	32.40
Luxembourg	93,553	6.94	575,747	22.40	16.07	83.93	10.60	22.70
Malta		9.75	429,362	19.83	30.84	69.16	28.86	24.00
Netherlands	46,374	10.90	16,987,330	22.53	13.00	87.00	5.22	17.60
Norway	64,451	9.72	5,254,694	24.06	14.51	85.49	13.61	14.90
Poland	24,836	6.35	38,224,410	19.90	29.02	70.98	23.46	24.20
Portugal	26,690	9.50	10,371,627	19.13	35.18	64.82	26.84	27.00
Romania	19,926	5.57	19,778,083	20.75	19.60	80.40	18.87	49.20
Slovakia	27,394	8.05	5,444,218	20.44	27.49	72.51	22.54	24.40
Slovenia	28,942	9.23	2,077,862	19.33	28.27	71.73	12.07	14.90
Spain	32,814	9.03	46,347,576	19.34	29.12	70.88	23.99	32.90

Sweden	45,296	11.93	9,837,533	22.46	15.97	84.03	14.06	19.90
United Kingdom	38,658	9.12	65,788,574	23.30	16.86	83.14	9.73	27.20

Sources: [a]World Bank, International Comparison Program database.
[b]World Health Organization Global Health Expenditure database.
[c]United Nations, Department of Economic and Social Affairs, Population Division (2017). World Population Prospects.
Notes: GDP – gross domestic product; PPP – purchasing power parity; THE – total health expenditure.
Definition of Health Expenditure and Financing Variables.
Total health expenditure is the sum of public and private health expenditure. It covers the provision of health services (preventive and curative), family planning activities, nutrition activities and emergency aid designated for health but does not include provision of water and sanitation.
OOP expenditure is any direct outlay by households, including gratuities and in-kind payments, to health practitioners and suppliers of pharmaceuticals, therapeutic appliances and other goods and services whose primary intent is to contribute to the restoration or enhancement of the health status of individuals or population groups. It is a part of private health expenditure.
Private health expenditure is the share of current health expenditures funded from domestic private sources. Domestic private sources include funds from households, corporations and non-profit organisations. Such expenditures can be either prepaid to voluntary health insurance or paid directly to healthcare providers.
Public health expenditure is the share of current health expenditures funded from domestic public sources for health. Domestic public sources include domestic revenue as internal transfers and grants, transfers, subsidies to voluntary health insurance beneficiaries, non-profit institutions serving households (NPISH) or enterprise financing schemes as well as compulsory prepayment and social health insurance contributions. They do not include external resources spent by governments on health.
Like GDP per capita, health expenditure figures are average spends per individual in the population and allocation to primary vs secondary care, or by age or income group are difficult to isolate.

Conclusion

There are many aspects to the collation of necessary data about children's health, the provision of services to children and understanding of the environmental and services context. But a strong theme to emerge in this chapter is the invisibility of children. Despite the universal use of the United Nations Convention on the Rights of the Child, children as correctly therein defined are invisible in almost all data systems. The four quinquennial age bands are common, as is also sometimes analysis for the first year of life. But children as a legally defined group, and as a group with clear service needs, do not feature in Europe's or the world's data systems. A further complication is added by those system policies, or legislative rules, that make 16 years a watershed age, as this too is universally ignored statistically.

The outcome of this is that children overall cannot be represented in statistical or policy analyses in a way matching that of other population groups. Secondly, it means that the analyses and policies that are produced are subject to an imprecision, and to potential argument about their data and framing, because the statistical margins are not fixed. A particular consequence is that adolescents, themselves at a rapidly changing and sometimes personally challenging stage of their life course, are the most invisible age group. To say that this is unsatisfactory would be a gross understatement.

Finally, though, this chapter unfortunately is a definition of how nearly all systems in European society and policy pay lip service to the importance of children, but do not really accommodate them. Nearly all data sources in Europe are now digitised at the point of data capture, so the subsequent aggregation and analysis is software driven, and rightly. But this also means that the effort of adjusting software to produce a split of the 15–19 years age group and producing a further analysis for children, would be minimal. It is regularly and easily done when analysing by country, with aggregates for instance for the early EU 15, the current EU 28, the future EU 27 or the whole of geographical Europe. But similar effort for the children who live in Europe does not happen.

Similarly, other good intents or policy visions are not followed through in children's interests. This ranges from the low policy response to the recommended monitoring datasets for children from the CHILD project, (Rigby & Köhler, 2002) commissioned by an initiative which envisaged development of an information system which would have a children's dashboard view, but 16 years later is in effect ignored, through to lack of creation of a simple policy and ethical framework which would enable collaborative analysis of the rich anonymised databases which hold real-world people-based data. Overall, this is a disappointing statement and demonstration of children's low value in policy terms in Europe.

References

Central Intelligence Agency. (2018). *The world factbook*. Retrieved from https://www.cia.gov/library/publications/resources/the-world-factbook/

Chapple, S., & Richardson, D. (2009). *Doing better for children*. Paris: OECD Publishing.

Eurostat. (2018a). *European statistics, overview.* Retrieved from https://ec.europa.eu/eurostat/about/overview

Eurostat. (2018b). *European statistics, database.* Retrieved from https://ec.europa.eu/eurostat/data/database

Global Burden of Disease. (2016). Pediatrics collaboration, global and national burden of diseases and injuries among children and adolescents between 1990 and 2013: Findings from the global burden of disease 2013 study. *The Journal of the American Medical Association- Pediatrics, 170*(3), 267–287.

HBSC Data Portal. (2018). Retrieved from http://hbsc-nesstar.nsd.no/webview/

Health Behaviour in School-aged Children. (2018). *About HBSC.* Retrieved from http://www.hbsc.org/about/index.html

Institute for Health Metrics and Evaluations (IHME). (2018a). *About IHME.* Retrieved from http://www.healthdata.org/about

Institute for Health Metrics and Evaluations (IHME). (2018b). *Global health data exchange (GHDx), GBD results tool.* Retrieved from http://ghdx.healthdata.org/gbd-results-tool

Leach-Kemon, K., & Gall, J. (2018). *Why estimate?* Retrieved from http://www.healthdata.org/acting-data/why-estimate?utm_source=IHME+Updates&utm_campaign=c062742ac8-Weekly_Email_Sep_6_2018&utm_medium=email&utm_term=0_1790fa6746-c062742ac8-422568873

Liyanage, H., Hoang, U., Ferreira, F., & de Lusignan, S. (2018). *Report of measures of quality and outcomes derived from large datasets.* Retrieved from http://www.childhealthservicemodels.eu/wp-content/uploads/Deliverable-D14-5.2-Report-of-Measures-of-Quality-and-Outcomes-derived-from-large-data-sets.pdf

Minicuci, N., Corso, B., Rocco, I., Luzi, D., Pecoraro, F., & Tamburis, O. (2017). *Innovative measures of outcome and quality of care in child primary care models.* Retrieved from http://www.childhealthservicemodels.eu/wp-content/uploads/2015/09/D7-Identification-and-Application-of-Innovative-Measures-of-Quality-and-Outcome-of-Models.pdf

OECD. (2009). *Doing better for children.* Paris: OECD. Retrieved from www.oecd.org/els/social/childwellbeing

Organisation for Economic Cooperation and Development (OECD). (2013). *OECD. Stat Web browser user guide.* Retrieved from https://stats.oecd.org/Content/themes/OECD/static/help/WBOS%20User%20Guide%20(EN).PDF

Organisation for Economic Cooperation and Development (OECD). (2018a). *About us.* Retrieved from www.oecd.org/about/

Organisation for Economic Cooperation and Development (OECD). (2018b). *Health.* Retrieved from www.oecd.org/health/

Organisation for Economic Cooperation and Development. (2018c). *OECD.Stat Web browser.* Retrieved from https://stats.oecd.org/index.aspx?DataSetCode=HEALTH_STAT

Rees, G., Bradshaw, J., Goswami, H., & Keung, A. (2006). Understanding children's well-being: A national survey of young people's well-being. *The Children's Society.* Retrieved from https://www.childrenssociety.org.uk/sites/default/files/tcs/research_docs/Understanding%20children%27s%20wellbeing.pdf

Rigby, M., & Köhler, L. (2002). *Child health indicators of life and development (CHILD): Report to the European Commission. European Commission Health*

Monitoring Programme. Retrieved from https://ec.europa.eu/health/ph_projects/ 2000/monitoring/fp_monitoring_2000_frep_08_en.pdf

Rigby, M. J., Köhler L. I., Blair, M. E., & Mechtler, R. (2003). Child health indicators for Europe — A priority for a caring society. *European Journal of Public Health, 13*(3 Supplement), 38–46.

Roberts, C., Freeman, J., Samdal, O., Schnohr, C. W., de Looze, M. E., Nic Gabhainn, S., … International HBSC Study Group et al. (2009). The health behaviour in school-aged children (HBSC) study: Methodological developments and current tensions. *International Journal of Public Health, 54,* S140–S150. doi:10.1007/s00038-009-5405-9

The World Bank. (2018a). *About us.* Retrieved from https://data.worldbank.org/about

The World Bank. (2018b). *Open data, indicators.* Retrieved from https://data.worldbank.org/indicator

The World Bank. (2018c). *DataBank, health nutrition and population statistics database.* Retrieved from http://databank.worldbank.org/data/source/health-nutrition-and-population-statistics

UNICEF. (2009). *The state of the world's children: Maternal and newborn health.* Retrieved from https://www.unicef.org/sowc09/

United Nations Population Division. (2017). *European population counter.* Retrieved from http://www.worldometers.info/world-population/europe-population/

Wolfe, I. (Ed.). (2014). *European child health services and systems: Lessons without borders.* Retrieved from http://www.euro.who.int/__data/assets/pdf_file/0003/ 254928/European-Child-Health-Services-and-Systems-Lessons-without-borders.pdf

World Health Organization Regional Office for Europe. (2014). *Investing in children: The European child and adolescent health strategy 2015–2020.* Copenhagen. Retrieved from http://www.euro.who.int/__data/assets/pdf_file/0010/253729/64wd12e_ InvestCAHstrategy_140440.pdf?ua=1)

World Health Organization Regional Office for Europe. (2016). *Improving the quality of care for reproductive, maternal, neonatal, child and adolescent health in the WHO European Region: A regional framework to support the implementation of Health 2020.* Copenhagen. Retrieved from http://www.euro.who.int/__data/assets/ pdf_file/0009/330957/RMNCAH-QI-Framework.pdf?ua=1

World Health Organization, Regional Office for Europe. (2017). *Child and adolescent health, data and statistic.* Retrieved from http://www.euro.who.int/en/health-topics/Life-stages/child-and-adolescent-health/data-and-statistics

World Health Organization, Regional Office for Europe. (2018a). *European health information gateway, health for all explorer.* Retrieved from https://gateway.euro. who.int/en/hfa-explorer/

World Health Organization, Regional Office for Europe. (2018b). *Child and adolescent health dataset.* Retrieved from https://gateway.euro.who.int/en/datasets/cah/. Accessed on October 15, 2018.

World Health Organization, Regional Office for Europe. (2018c). *Child and adolescent health, health behaviour in school-aged children (HBSC).* Retrieved from http://www.euro.who.int/en/health-

World Health Organization. (2010). *Monitoring the building blocks of health systems: A handbook of indicators and their measurement strategies.* Retrieved from http:// www.who.int/healthinfo/systems/WHO_MBHSS_2010_full_web.pdf

Chapter 8

The Conundrum of Measuring Children's Primary Health Care

Ilaria Rocco, Barbara Corso, Daniela Luzi, Fabrizio Pecoraro, Oscar Tamburis, Uy Hoang, Harshana Liyanage, Filipa Ferreira, Simon de Lusignan and Nadia Minicuci

Abstract

Evaluating primary care for children has not before been undertaken on a national level, and only infrequently on an international level, an adult-focused perspective is the norm. The Models of Child Health Appraised (MOCHA) project explored the evaluation of quality of primary care for children in a nationally comparable way, which recognises the influence of all components of child well-being and well-becoming. Using adult-focused metrics fails to account for children's physical and psycho-social development at different ages, differences in health and non-health determinants, patterns of disease and risk factors and the stages of the life course. To do this, we attempted to identify comparable measures of child health in the European Union and European Economic Area countries, we aimed to perform a structural equation modelling technique to identify causal effects of certain policies or procedures in children's primary care and we aimed to identify and interrogate large datasets for key tracer conditions. We found that the creation of comparative data for children and child health services remains a low priority in Europe, and the largely unmet need for indicators covering all the healthcare dimensions hampers development of evidence-based policy. In terms of the MOCHA project objective of appraising models of child primary health care, the results of this specific work show that the means of appraisal of system and service quality are not yet agreed or mature, as well as having inadequate data to fuel them.

Keywords: Quality of care; child primary care; measurement; data; indicators; structural equation modelling

Efforts Towards a Comprehensive Populated Framework for the Appraisal of the Child Healthcare System

Assessment of the quality of overall health systems is most frequently undertaken at international level. The need to develop child-focused and child-centric healthcare system quality measurements has been claimed since the 1990s (Peoples-Sheps et al., 1998) and was taken forward systematically in the European Union by the Child Health Indicators of Life and Development (CHILD) project (Rigby, Köhler, Blair, & Mechtler, 2003). However, the evaluation of primary care for children across countries is not so widely explored, especially at European level, nor is a common agreed optimum model of care encompassing all components that influence child well-being and well-becoming. Although efforts in this direction are increasing (Wolfe et al., 2013), cross-country comparisons tend to be based on disease incidence (Cattaneo, Cogoy, Macaluso, & Tamburlini, 2012), on a limited number of countries (Kavanagh, Adams, & Wang, 2009), on specific aspects, such as poverty (Ortiz, Daniels, & Engilbertsdóttir, 2012) or policy (Chapple & Richardson, 2009).

Moreover, the multidimensional approach adopted to evaluate child care strongly support the acknowledgement that a simple extrapolation of adult metrics should be avoided taking instead into account children's physical and psycho-social development at all age, differences in health and non-health determinants and patterns of diseases and risk factors, recognising the stages of the life course (World Health Organization Regional Office for Europe, 2005a; World Health Organization Regional Office for Europe, 2014). A framework as to what information was needed for child health service strategic planning was created to link with policy development (World Health Organization Regional Office for Europe, 2005b).

The need for a defined framework for the healthcare evaluation that is suitable for children still remains despite the earlier work. Creation of comparative data for children and child health services still remains a low priority, and the largely unmet need for indicators covering all the healthcare dimensions and available for the totality of the Models of Child Health Appraised (MOCHA) countries is shown up as hampering development of evidence-based policy. This is explained in detail in Liyanage, Hoang, Ferreira, and de Lusignan (2018).

Recognising the lack of centrally published relevant and sensitive indicators, and with the aim of identifying measures specifically relevant to child healthcare, the leaders of the MOCHA Working Groups had the assignment to scrutinise the answers received during the rounds of Country Agents (CAs) questions and provide relevant measures for the mapping of models of provision in MOCHA countries in a way which it was planned would permit the assessment of quality at the system level. The gathered measures were analysed by an expert group that identified a limited number of categories within which all the measures could be classified. The selected categories were as follows: Context, Access, Coordination and Governance.

Due to the close link among categories, the process of classification of the measures was particularly time-consuming to result in the univocal classification of each measure. However, this was tackled, and the subject experts within MOCHA proceeded with the examination of each measure:

- verifying whether the interpretation of the measure meaning was univocal, that is not ambiguous with respect to the direction of changes in the pertinent category; and
- transforming the measure into score ranging from 1 (weak primary care) to 3 (strong primary care), based on literature and experts' expertise. For example, if a country indicated having a Child Public Health EHR System using e-health records, which is one of the measures belonging to the Coordination category, for both immunisation and screening, then the country scored a '3' on that measure, meaning a feature of strong coordination.

Since the above-mentioned requirements constitute a precondition to compute a category-specific score, the experts' judgement pointed out which measures were not univocally interpretable. Let's consider, for example, the measure 'Number of physicians/paediatric per 100,000 population', classified in the Access category. Would a higher number of physicians/paediatrician produce a higher accessibility to care (univocal interpretation)? In the literature, there was no evidence of an optimal rate of the number of physicians/paediatrician per 100,000 population and consequently the MOCHA experts could not reach an agreement about its univocal interpretability towards the best efficiency in the access to care.

Therefore, this measure could not have been included in the computation of the category-specific (Access) score.

This verification, along with the issue of missing data encountered for some measures, has strongly restricted the potential analysis of the models of provision in MOCHA countries.

However, the Coordination category did fulfil the required criteria and the following example shows the methodology employed to produce the category-specific score.

Identification of the Measures Related to the Category

Among the measures provided by MOCHA WP-leaders, those classified in the Coordination category, which met the univocal interpretation precondition, are listed in the table below (Table 8.1). Two measures, (C3 and C5) are quantitative, while the remaining three are categorical.

Transformation of the Measures into Scores

The measures belonging to the Coordination category were transformed into scores ranging from 1 (weak coordination) to 3 (strong coordination) (Table 8.2).

Observing the scores assumed in the Coordination measures by the 30 MOCHA countries (Table 8.3), it emerged that Lithuania has the lowest scores

Table 8.1. Measures identified by WP-leader related to coordination and assumed values.

Measures Identified by WP-leader Related to Coordination	Possible Values
C1. Procedures to refer the child from primary to secondary care	• PC prescribes the visit • PC prescribes and refers the visit • PC prescribes, refers and books the visit
C2. Formal link between social care and primary care health services	• No framework • A policy framework or a legal framework • Both a policy and a legal framework noted, or single entity in charge of both health and social care
C3. EHR usage in primary care	• Percentage of practices using EHRs in primary care for children [0-100]
C4. Child public health EHR system in use e-health records (primary care EHR/immunisation registration)	• No child public health EHR system in use; • CPH EHR system for immunisation or screening; • CPH EHR for immunisation and screening, passive; • CPH EHR for immunisation and screening, active for defaults or appts.
C5. e-health infrastructure for sharing with other sectors	• Number of partner organisation types with whom structure share data [0−6]

(minimum score for all the measures), while Italy has the highest scores (maximum score for all the measures).

Analysis of the Correlation between Measures Belonging to the Same Category

The analysis of the correlation among the measures classified in the Coordination category showed all positive associations (Table 8.4), confirming that the scores attributed to the measures have the same direction. In particular, although the low number of countries, the Kendall's (1938) correlations among the C3, C4 and C5 measures resulted statistically significant. Consequently, only the three EHR measures, significantly correlated, were considered for the analysis. Given the nature of these measures, the category 'Coordination' will be subsequently referred as 'e-coordination'.

Table 8.2. Measures identified by WP-leader related to coordination and attributed scores.

Measures Identified by WP-leader Related to Coordination	Scores
C1. Procedures to refer the child from primary to secondary care	• PC prescribes the visit • PC prescribes and refers the visit • PC prescribes, refers and books the visit
C2. Formal link between social care and primary care health services	• No framework • A policy framework or a legal framework • Both a policy and a legal framework noted, or single entity in charge of both health and social care
C3. EHR usage in primary care	• No or limited use (<25%) EHRs in primary care for children • 25%–75% of practices use EHRs • over 75% of practices use EHRs
C4. Child public health EHR system in use e-health records (primary care EHR/immunisation registration)	• No child public health EHR system in use; • CPH EHR system for immunisation or screening; • CPH EHR for both immunisation and screening
C5. e-health infrastructure for sharing with other sectors	• no structure for data exchange; • structure for sharing with one partner organisation type; • with two or more partner organisation type

Countries Coordination Level

Based on these three measures, the e-coordination scores were calculated using a confirmatory factor analysis. Then, the countries were grouped according to their e-coordination score: the limits of weak – medium – strong level were determined by the tertiles of valid country scores (Table 8.5).

The last step consisted in the linkage between the strength of the e-coordination and two selected measures: the national expenditure on 'Governance and health system administration' and the Current Health Care Expenditure. Tables 8.6 and 8.7 report descriptive statistics of these

Table 8.3. Scores assumed in the coordination measures by the MOCHA countries.

Country	C1	C2	C3	C4	C5
Austria	2	2	3	1	1
Belgium	3	.	3	.	.
Bulgaria	2	2	3	2	1
Croatia	3	3	3	3	1
Cyprus	3	1	1	1	1
Czech Republic	.	2	3	3	2
Denmark	.	2	3	3	1
Estonia	3	2	2	3	3
Finland	2	3	3	3	3
France	2	.	3	2	2
Germany	2	1	3	.	1
Greece	1	2	1	1	1
Hungary	.	1	3	3	1
Iceland	3	1	3	3	3
Ireland	2	3	3	3	2
Italy	3	3	3	3	3
Latvia	2	2	1	1	1
Lithuania	1	1	1	1	1
Luxembourg	.	.	3	.	.
Malta	2	1	2	3	1
Netherlands	1	2	3	3	2
Norway	2	3	3	3	2
Poland	2	2	1	1	1
Portugal	3	2	3	2	2
Romania	2	1	3	3	3
Slovakia	.	.	2	2	1
Slovenia	.	.	.	.	.
Spain	3	3	3	3	2
Sweden	2	1	3	3	2
United Kingdom	.	3	3	3	2

Table 8.4. Kendall's correlation matrix (*$p < 0.05$).

	C1	C2	C3	C4	C5
C1	1.000	0.174	0.217	0.272	0.304
	$n = 23$	$n = 21$	$n = 23$	$n = 21$	$n = 22$
C2	0.174	1.000	0.275	0.23361	0.259
	$n = 21$	$n = 25$	$n = 25$	$n = 24$	$n = 25$
C3	0.217	0.275	1.000	0.614*	0.416*
	$n = 23$	$n = 25$	$n = 29$	$n = 26$	$n = 27$
C4	0.272	0.234	0.614*	1.000	0.556*
	$n = 21$	$n = 24$	$n = 26$	$n = 26$	$n = 26$
C5	0.304	0.259	0.416*	0.556*	1.000
	$n = 22$	$n = 25$	$n = 27$	$n = 26$	$n = 27$

Table 8.5. Countries distribution by e-coordination strength.

Weak	Medium	Strong
Austria	Croatia	Finland
Bulgaria	Czech Republic	Iceland
Cyprus	Denmark	Italy
France	Estonia	Romania
Greece	Hungary	
Latvia	Ireland	
Lithuania	Malta	
Poland	Netherlands	
Portugal	Norway	
Slovakia	Spain	
	Sweden	
	United Kingdom	

Table 8.6. National expenditure on 'Governance and health system administration' by e-coordination strength (Euro Per Inhabitant, 2015).

Weak (n = 10) (as per Table 8.5)	Medium (n = 9)	Strong (n = 4)
Mean (SD) = 55 (74)	Mean (SD) = 69 (49)	Mean (SD) = 34 (18)
Median (Q2) = 25	Median (Q2) = 59	Median (Q2) = 38
Q1 = 14	Q1 = 29	Q1 = 20
Q3 = 32	Q3 = 85	Q3 = 48
	Data missing for: Estonia, Ireland, Malta	

Table 8.7. Current health care expenditure by e-coordination strength (Euro Per Inhabitant, 2015).

Weak (n = 10) (as per Table 8.5)	Medium (n = 11)	Strong (n = 4)
Mean (SD) = 1,598 (1,289)	Mean (SD) = 3,175 (2,092)	Mean (SD) = 2,599 (1,560)
Median (Q2) = 1,167	Median (Q2) = 3,912	Median (Q2) = 3,028
Q1 = 718	Q1 = 1,003	Q1 = 1,422
Q3 = 1,557	Q3 = 4,938	Q3 = 3,775
	Data missing for: Malta	

measures according to the strength of the e-coordination as classified in Table 8.5.

Countries with low expenditure, both on governance and health system administration and on health care, belong to the weak e-coordination group; on the other hand, countries with the highest expenditures have a medium level of strength for e-coordination, which could be interpreted by potential ongoing ICT investments to reach a better e-coordination.

Conclusions on Analysing Children's Primary Health Systems

The MOCHA effort to create a harmonised dataset has contributed to the categorisation of 'e-coordination' in three levels of strength and showed how this can be linked to selected measures. The findings presented in this chapter will be then further elaborated with statistical modelling techniques (see Chapter 14) in order to provide an example on how this harmonised dataset can be used to investigate the relationships across measures such as:

- the country immunisation coverage;
- the presence of mandatory child vaccination policies in the country;
- the national economic context; and
- the availability, at national level, of electronic health records as well as e-health infrastructures.

A Structural Equation Modelling Approach Applied to MOCHA

Healthcare systems are a very pertinent example of complex systems, both in lay terms by its complicated design and in scientific terms by its non-linear, dynamic, and unpredictable nature. One of the most commonly accepted notions of complexity is the interrelatedness of components of a system (Simon, 1962, 1973, 1996), that is the mutual influence that system components have on each other. Researchers interested in the healthcare systems interrelatedness among multiple factors cannot reach their research objectives resorting to classical statistical methodologies, for example, regression analysis. A statistical solution suitable for dealing with the mutual relationships among variables is the Structural Equation Modelling (SEM).

SEM is a very general statistical modelling technique, widely used in the behavioural sciences, which combine the strengths of factor analysis and multiple regression in a single model that can be tested statistically. Consequently, this statistical modelling technique provides two advantages:

(1) It includes, in the model, both manifest (or observed) variables and latent factors.
(2) It analyzes the interrelatedness of the factors considered, estimating both the direct effect that a certain factor has on the outcome of interest and the effect mediated by other factors (indirect effect).

The exploration of available measures focused on child health care showed a high variability in the use of diverse measures across countries, outlining a patchy and disperse way in the evaluation of quality of child care (Minicuci et al., 2017). Measures are generally focused on immunisation, mortality and hospitalisation, leaving out other important aspects of child health care (see Chapter 7).

Earlier in this chapter, we have illustrated the Italian CNR Team's efforts within towards the identification of a comprehensive populated dataset for the investigation of the child healthcare system. In particular, due to the presence of a small number of measures within each of the identified category (Context, Access, Coordination and Governance), the computation of the category-specific score was possible only for a subset of the Coordination measures (e-coordination, see Chapter 7) and, therefore, the investigation of the relationship across the four categories was not feasible. Moreover, the presence of missing values reduced the number of records available for the analysis.

Bearing in mind these limitations, an application of the SEM methodology was performed, as described below, in order to exemplify its potentiality in the investigation of complex research questions.

Example of SEM Model Applied to the MOCHA Dataset

The following gives an example of how we would analyse the interrelatedness of four factors across the MOCHA countries:

(1) the country immunisation coverage;
(2) the presence of mandatory child vaccination policies in the country;
(3) the national economic context; and
(4) the availability, at national level, of electronic health records as well as e-health infrastructures.

If we assume we are interested in the following research questions:

• Do the countries with mandatory national vaccination have a higher immunisation coverage?
• Are the countries with a high adoption of primary care records and e-health infrastructures facilitated in monitoring the individual immunisation status and, consequently, leading to a higher immunisation rate?
• Does the national economic context influence:
 (a) whether the child vaccination is mandatory
 (b) the adoption of primary care records and e-health infrastructures?
• Does the national economic context indirectly influence the country immunisation coverage?

The path diagram (Figure 8.1) shows how the above relationships can be described graphically.

Immunisation Coverage

Immunisation is an essential component for reducing under-five mortality. Immunisation coverage estimates are used to monitor coverage of immunisation services and to guide disease eradication and reduction. It is a good indicator of health system performance (Bos & Batson, 2000).

In our example, we focused on the Diphtheria, Tetanus and Pertussis (DTP) vaccine, which conveys immunity to three different infectious diseases. In particular, we considered the percentage of infants who have received first dose of the combined diphtheria, tetanus toxoid and pertussis vaccine in 2017 (DPT1 coverage).

Mandatory Vaccination

All countries in the European Union have a long tradition of implementing vaccination programmes. In the presence of such a large variety of vaccines on

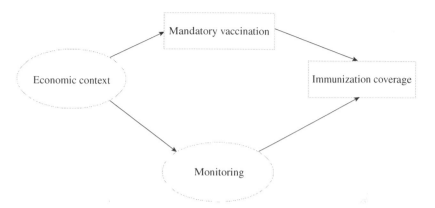

Figure 8.1.   Path diagram of the relationships across the research questions.

offer, the way immunisation is organised differs considerably between countries. There are also large differences in whether vaccinations included in the national programmes are recommended or mandatory.

In our example, we compared the countries where DTP vaccines were mandatory and the countries where these vaccines were recommended.

The following definitions were used:

- recommended: a vaccination included in the national immunisation programme for all or some specific groups independent of being funded or not; and
- mandatory: a vaccination that every child must receive by law without the possibility for the parent to choose to accept the uptake or not, independent of whether a legal or economical implication exists for the refusal (Haverkate et al., 2012).

Economic Context Factor
The national economic context factor was measured using three variables:

- the Gini coefficient, a measure of inequality of income or wealth (Gini, 1936). A Gini coefficient of zero expresses perfect equality, where everyone has the same income. A Gini coefficient of 1 expresses maximal inequality among values, where only one person has all the income and all others have none;
- the child relative income poverty rate, defined as the percentage of children (0–17 year-olds) with an equivalised household disposable income (i.e. an income after taxes and transfers adjusted for household size) below the poverty threshold. The poverty threshold is set here at 50% of the median disposable income in each country; and
- the child material deprivation, defined as the average number of household amenities and goods that a child does not have access to. The household amenities and goods considered are: (1) a washing machine, (2) a colour TV,

(3) a telephone and (4) a personal car, and on the household having the ability to (5) keep the household adequately warm, (6) pay utility bills, (7) meet mortgage or rent payments, (8) eat meat, chicken or fish at least every second day and (9) pay its necessary expenses generally.

The higher the score in this factor the more unfavourable economic context the country has. For this reason, we will refer to this factor as 'Unfavourable economic context'.

Monitoring Factor

The measures identifying the 'e-coordination' factor were used to define the availability of e-health infrastructures. They are as follows:

- EHR usage in primary care (C3);
- Child Public Health EHR System in Use e-health records (primary care EHR/immunisation registration) (C4); and
- e-health infrastructure for sharing with other sectors (C5).

Since the score of this factor increases with the increase in the availability of e-health infrastructures, we will refer to this factor as 'Monitoring strength'.

The identified model is shown in Figure 8.2.

The results of this SEM modelling are reported in Table 8.8.

The national economic context results to influence the country monitoring strength, highlighting the negative effect (−0.0609) of an unfavourable economic context on the strength in the monitoring.

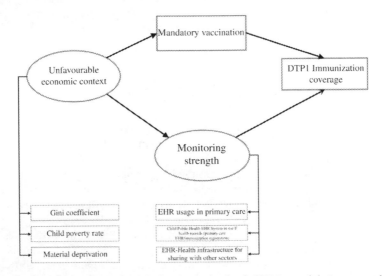

Figure 8.2. Path diagram of the hypothesised SEM model (structural and measurement models).

Table 8.8. Decomposition of the effects estimated by the hypothesised SEM model.

Effects	Direct	Indirect	Total
On 'Mandatory vaccination' (Yes vs No)			
Unfavourable economic context	0.1079	–	0.1079
On 'Monitoring strength'			
Unfavourable economic context	−0.0609*	–	−0.0609*
On 'DTP1 immunisation coverage'			
Mandatory vaccination (Yes vs No)	−0.4638	–	−0.4638
Monitoring strength	−0.0402	–	−0.0402
Unfavourable economic context	–	−0.0476	−0.0476

Note: *p < 0.10.

The DTP1 immunisation coverage results not to be influenced by neither the obligatory vaccine (the direct effect (−0.4638) is not statistically significant), the strength of the monitoring system (the direct effect (−0.0402) is not statistically significant), nor the economic context (the indirect effect (−0.0476) is not statistically significant). This means that even if a country has a mandatory vaccination, or a strong monitoring system or favourable economic context, its immunisation coverage is not higher than that reported in a country where these three conditions are not fulfilled. If other relevant measures had been available, it would have been possible to identify other potential factors influencing the immunisation rate.

Despite of the limits of this exemplifying SEM model, it clearly shows the potentiality of this statistical technique to simultaneously estimate complex relationships among factors, allowing the decomposition of the total effects of a factor on another one in direct and indirect effect.

Since the indirect effects represent how the influence of a factor on an outcome of interest is mediated by other factors, the SEM approach allows a deeper comprehension of complex mechanisms and, consequently, being able to go beyond the lack of data, it would be a valid instrument to use in further research on child health care.

Service Quality Measurement

Quality Measures

Separate from the assessment of the quality of the healthcare system for children is the assessment of the quality of care delivered within the system, in an operational context. Health Care Quality is a multidimensional concept, since it encompasses a number of aspects to be evaluated. Scientific research as well as the extended vision by the World Health Organization has progressively enlarged the concept of health including other important aspects of the individual's life related to life style, well-being as well as contextual factors such environmental, economics and socio-cultural. Under a child-centred perspective, scientific evidence underlines that the criteria used to evaluation quality of care for adults cannot be directly translated to children. As reported by Rigby et al. (2003), health determinants, disease patterns, preventive and therapeutic health services and data sources are all different for children compared to adults.

The focussed work the team from CNR Italy undertook within the MOCHA project sought to identify potential quality measures through the exploration of a continuum of feasible measures, from the clinical, health status and satisfaction perspectives, that could be used effectively by the stakeholders within diverse structural models (across countries) and paediatric settings to quantify the impact of the paediatric care.

The main objectives of the analysis were to:

- provide an overview of the measures available in internationally open-accessible databases;
- develop an ad-hoc questionnaire to collect information on the availability and utilisation of measures to evaluate the quality of the child care in each of the 30 countries;
- provide an overview of the measures adopted in each of the 30 countries for the evaluation of child care; and
- explore whether the Patient-reported Experience Measures (PREMs) and the Patient-reported Outcome Measures (PROMs) are used in the evaluation of paediatric care in each of the 30 countries.

The MOCHA Analysis

Provided that monitoring child health status and monitoring the quality of child health care are likely to produce different findings, the initial approach taken aimed to distinguish between the measures used to evaluate the child health status, as collected by the international databases, and the measures used to evaluate the quality of the child health care, as reported by the MOCHA CAs (see Chapter 1) through an ad-hoc designed questionnaire applied in each country.

All international databases that were open-access and dealt with a broad spectrum of child health-related issues were searched. Scrutinised sources came from organisations, agencies, research networks and observatories. Ongoing and ended research projects on child care were also investigated. In parallel, an ad-hoc designed questionnaire was developed and administered to the CAs to gather information on:

- agencies/organisations in charge of the evaluation of quality of care at national and/or local level;
- coverage of quality evaluation specifically devoted to child care;

- topics covered in the evaluation of child primary healthcare services; and
- measures used to evaluate child care.

In addition to these objective measures, gathering the perspective of patients has been proved to provide a deeper insight as to their experience facing illnesses as well as their interaction with health services. This information is hard to capture through other evaluation systems of quality of care and highlights the difference between measuring children's 'objective' health status using scales and, on the other hand, their 'subjective' perception of their quality of life. Thus, the questionnaire included a section on PREMs and PROMs aimed at identifying to what extent these recently introduced tools were adopted across countries as well as applied to child care. In this, a core challenge is that many measures cannot easily be applied to children's services, while proxy respondents to data gathering such as parents may not always take the child's or a child-centric view.

Measures' Classification
To facilitate the analysis, measures collected from the two groups of sources were classified and organised within a schema that represents the principal areas, further detailed in a two-level hierarchy of subcategories (hereafter called topic and subtopic).

The top-down and the bottom-up approach used to classify the measures helped the identification of five main areas that comprise both healthcare and non-healthcare determinants: (1) Structure; (2) Process; (3) Outcome; (4) Social, political, economic and environmental context; and (5) Health-related behaviour. The complete schematic diagram is shown in Figure 8.3.

The finer operationalisation of the 22 identified topics led to a selection 19 subtopics for the 'Structure' area, 23 subtopics for the 'Process' area, 19 subtopics for the 'Outcome' area, 27 subtopics for the 'Social, political, economic and environmental context' area, and no sub-topic for the 'Health-related behaviour' area.

A comprehensive piece of work to map the different indicators, both those from databases and those in use by countries as reported by the MOCHA CAs, was completed as a MOCHA deliverable and is available on the web site (Minicuci et al., 2017). This includes detailed reporting and mapping of availability of quality-related measures by country. A brief summary is given here.

International Databases
Almost half of the measures fall into the Social, political, economic and environmental context (49%). The second most representative area concerns the Outcome (19.2%) area, whereas the remaining measures are approximately equally distributed among the other three areas. For all countries, the Social, political, economic and environmental context area is the most represented. With regard to the three areas possessing the strongest links with the healthcare system, that are Structure, Process and Outcome, only Cyprus has more than

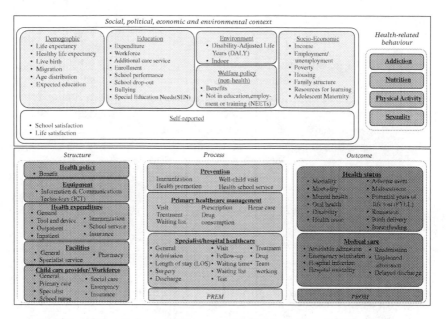

Figure 8.3.   Schematic diagram for the measures classification.

half of its measures (52%) classified in these areas, while Ireland is the country in which these areas are less represented (29.4%).

The distribution of the collected measures among the topics covered by the international databases shows that education is the most represented topic (18.3% of the measures), followed by health status (17.8%) and welfare policy (non-health) (13.9%). Within the process area, one PREM was found concerning self-reported unmet needs for medical examination, while within the outcome area, three PROMs regarding self-perceived health and limitations were present.

Country Agents Questionnaire

Twenty-six countries out of the 30 involved in the project provided answers to the questionnaire on local use of quality measures. Considering the measures reported by CAs, in two countries (Poland and Romania), quality assessment is mainly carried out using healthcare accreditation procedures, relating to the functioning of hospitals and primary health care as well as specialist outpatient care and treatment of addictions, while Greece and Malta have no system in place for quality assessment. Therefore, these countries were excluded from the analysis.

The majority of the measures are related to the Process (50.9%) and to the Outcome (33%) of care. These two areas are covered by the remaining 24 countries (96%) but only six countries (Austria, Germany, Finland, Northern Ireland, Ireland and Latvia) cover all the five areas of the map. About 10.2% of the measures fall in the Structure area, which is covered by 72% of the countries. The remaining two areas account for a 3.1% (Social, political, economic and environmental context area) and a 2.8% (Health-related behaviour area), with a coverage of 68% and 40% of countries, respectively.

The most analysed topic is the health status considering both the number of measures (25%) and the coverage among countries (92%). Another important part of the quality assessment is related to three topics of the process area: specialist/hospital health care (24%), prevention (14%) and primary healthcare management (12%). These results are also confirmed analysing the distribution by country where both the prevention and the health status are analysed in 23 countries (92%) while the primary healthcare management is studied in 20 countries (80%).

PREMs and PROMs

Five countries (Estonia, Germany, Italy, Poland and England) have implemented surveys for both PROMs and PREMs. Austria reported only outcome measures, while Czech Republic, Lithuania, Norway, Republic of Ireland and Spain use only PREMs for their quality evaluation. In Denmark, the same national survey described presents both PROMs- and PREMs-related aspects. Other national surveys, specifically focused on the evaluation of patients' experiences, have been implemented in Croatia, Norway, Republic of Ireland and England.

Comparison between International Databases and Country Agents Coverage

This comparison pertains to the potential use of feasible and already available measures collected through open-access databases by acknowledging that the considered measure is being used by some European countries, as reported by the CAs, to evaluate the quality of the child health care. Considering the five areas of the map, International databases collect the majority of the measures on the Social, political, economic and environmental context area (49%), while countries focus the attention more on Process (50%). The outcome area is the second most representative for both sources (18% and 33%, respectively). The comparison of the common measures between the International Databases and the Countries led to the identification of 30 measures distributed across all five areas and representing 10 topics, such health expenditure, child care provider/workforce, prevention, specialist/hospital health care, health status, demographic, education, socio-economic and health-related behaviour.

Tracer Conditions

A report entitled Measures of Quality and Outcomes derived from large datasets (Liyanage et al., 2018) undertaken by MOCHA researchers from the University of Surrey have put forward an alternative approach to identifying indicators utilising information on tracer conditions collected from routinely collected datasets.

These tracer conditions cover the totality of care provided for children in primary care including ambulatory-sensitive conditions (such as diarrhoea and vomiting), chronic diseases (such as asthma), mental health and preventative

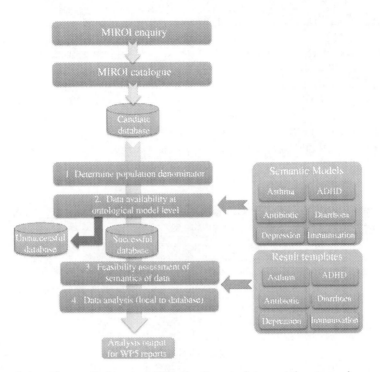

Figure 8.4.   Flow of the compilation of metadata catalogue and semantic models to harmonise case definitions and facilitate comparison from different data sources.

health. However, electronic medical databases and sources of routinely collected data relating to health care across the EU are heterogeneous. Thus, the researchers utilised a method that involved the compilation of a metadata catalogue and semantic models to harmonise case definitions and facilitate comparison from different data sources across the EU (Liyanage et al., 2016, 2017, 2018). This is summarised in Figure 8.4 and outlined in further detail in Liyanage et al. (2018).

Using indicators for these tracer conditions, the researchers found substantial, statistically significant and consistent variation in a number of health services and clinical quality indicators, especially of prescribing practices in primary child care systems based on the models of care adopted (Liyanage, Shinneman et al., 2018).

Conclusion

Chapter 7 has already shown the difficulty identified by the project's scientists of obtaining data about children, their health and the context in which services are trying to operate. This chapter then takes this further, by looking at approaches to health system quality and delivered service quality. Extensive work was undertaken by an expert group within the MOCHA project and reported separately in a detailed Deliverable, which not least captures an overview of activities in each of the 30 study countries. While this gives a rich analysis of a range of activities, it shows the comparatively early stages of this research in Europe and the opportunity for joint collaborative working at the conceptual and methodological levels, as well as at the data level mentioned in Chapter 7. In terms of the MOCHA project objective of appraising models of child primary health care, the results of this specific work show that the means of appraisal of system and service quality are not yet agreed or mature, as well as having inadequate data to fuel them.

References

Bos, E., & Batson, A. (2000). *Using immunization coverage for monitoring health sector performance: Measurement and interpretation issues.* Health and Nutrition Discussion Paper. The World Bank. Retrieved from http://documents.worldbank.org/curated/en/607721468763783070/Using-immunization-coverage-rates-for-monitoring-health-sector-performance-Measurement-and-Interpretation-Issues

Cattaneo, A., Cogoy, L., Macaluso, A., & Tamburlini, G. (2012). *Child health in the European Union.* Luxembourg: European Commission.

Chapple, S., & Richardson, D. (2009). *Doing better for children.* Paris: OECD Publishing.

Gini, C. (1936). On the measure of concentration with special reference to income and statistics, Colorado College Publication, General Series No. 208, 73–79.

Haverkate, M., D'Ancona, F., Giambi, C., Johansen, K., Lopalco, P. L., Cozza, V., ... VENICE project gatekeepers and contact points. (2012). *Mandatory and recommended vaccination in the EU, Iceland and Norway: Results of the VENICE 2010 survey on the ways of implementing national vaccination programmes.* Retrieved from https:\\doi.org\17.10.2807/ese.17.22.20183-en

Kavanagh, P. L., Adams, W. G., & Wang, C. J. (2009). Quality indicators and quality assessment in child health. *Archives of Disease in Childhood, 94*(6), 458–463.

Kendall, M. (1938). A new measure of rank correlation. *Biometrika, 30*(1–2), 81–89.

Liyanage, H., Hoang, U., Ferreira, F., Alexander, D., Rigby, M., Blair, M., & de Lusignan, S. (2017). Availability of computerised medical record system data to compare models of child health care in primary care across Europe. *Studies in Health Technology and Informatics, 244,* 8–12.

Liyanage, H., Hoang, U., Ferreira, F., & de Lusignan, S. (2018). *Report of measures of quality and outcomes derived from large datasets.* Retrieved from http://www.childhealthservicemodels.eu/wp-content/uploads/Deliverable-D14-5.2-Report-of-Measures-of-Quality-and-Outcomes-derived-from-large-data-sets.pdf

Liyanage, H., Luzi, D., De Lusignan, S., Pecoraro, F., McNulty, R., Tamburis, O., ... Blair, M. (2016). Accessible modelling of complexity in health (AMoCH) and associated data flows: Asthma as an exemplar. *Journal of Innovation in Health Informatics, 23*(1), 863. doi:10.14236/jhi.v23i1.863

Liyanage, H., Shinneman, S., Hoang, U., Ferreira, F., Alexander, D., Rigby, M., ... de Lusignan, S. (2018). Profiling databases to facilitate comparison of child health systems across Europe using standardised quality markers. *Studies in Health Technology and Informatics, 247*, 61–65.

Minicuci, N., Corso, B., Rocco, I., Luzi, D., Pecoraro, F., & Tamburis, O. (2017). *Innovative measures of outcome and quality of care in child primary care models.* Retrieved from http://www.childhealthservicemodels.eu/wp-content/uploads/2015/09/D7-Identification-and-Application-of-Innovative-Measures-of-Quality-and-Outcome-of-Models.pdf

Ortiz, I., Daniels, L. M., & Engilbertsdóttir, S. (Eds.). (2012). *Child poverty and inequality.* NewYork, NY: UNICEF.

Peoples-Sheps, M., Guild, P., Farel, A., Cassady, C. E., Kennelly, J., Potrzebowski, P. W., Waller, C. J. (1998). Model indicators for maternal and child health: An overview of process, product, and applications. *Maternal and Child Health Journal, 2*(4), 241–256.

Rigby, M. J., Köhler, L. I., Blair, M. E., & Mechtler, R. (2003). Child health indicators for Europe – A priority for a caring society. *European Journal of Public Health, 13*(3 Suppl), 38–46.

Simon, H. A. (1962). The architecture of complexity. *Proceedings of the American Philosophical Society, 106*, 467–482.

Simon, H. A. (1973). Structure of ill-structured problems. *Artificial Intelligence, 4*, 181–201.

Simon, H. A. (1996). *The sciences of the artificial.* Cambridge, MA: MIT Press.

Wolfe, I., Thompson, M., Gill, P., Tamburlini, G., Blair, M., Van Den Bruel, A., … McKee, M. (2013). Health services for children in Western Europe. *The Lancet, 381*(9873), 1224–1234. doi:10.1016/S0140-6736(12)62085-6

World Health Organization Regional Office for Europe. (2005a). *European strategy for child and adolescent health and development.* Copenhagen: WHO. Retrieved from http://apps.who.int/iris/handle/10665/107677

World Health Organization Regional Office for Europe. (2005b). *European strategy for child and adolescent health and development Information tool.* Copenhagen: WHO.

World Health Organization Regional Office for Europe. (2014). *Investing in children: The European child and adolescent health strategy 2015–2020.* Retrieved from http://www.euro.who.int/en/health-topics/Life-stages/child-and-adolescent-health/policy/investing-in-children-the-european-child-and-adolescent-health-strategy-20152020

Chapter 9

Measurement Conundrums: Explaining Child Health Population Outcomes in MOCHA Countries

Heather Gage and Ekelechi MacPepple

Abstract

The 30 MOCHA (Models of Child Health Appraised) countries are diverse socially, culturally and economically, and differences exist in their healthcare systems and in the scope and role of primary care. An economic analysis was undertaken that sought to explain differences in child health outcomes between countries. The conceptual framework was that of a production function for health, whereby health outputs (or outcomes) are assumed affected by several 'inputs'. In the case of health, inputs include personal (genes, health behaviours) and socio-economic (income, living standards) factors and the structure, organisation and workforce of the healthcare system. Random effects regression modelling was used, based on countries as the unit of analysis, with data from 2004 to 2016 from international sources and published categorisations of healthcare system. The chapter describes the data deficiencies and measurement conundrums faced, and how these were addressed. In the absence of consistent indicators of child health outcomes across countries, five mortality measures were used: neonatal, infant, under five years, diabetes (0–19 years) and epilepsy (0–19 years). Factors found associated with reductions in mortality were as follows: gross domestic product per capita growth (neonatal, infant, under five years), higher density of paediatricians (neonatal, infant, under five years), less out-of-pocket expenditure (neonatal, diabetes 0–19), state-based service provision (epilepsy 0–19) and lower proportions of children in the population, a proxy for family size (all outcomes). Findings should be interpreted with caution due to the ecological nature of the analysis and the limitations presented by the data and measures employed.

Keywords: Child health; primary care; European countries; regression modelling; mortality outcomes; Gross Domestic Product

Introduction

The Models of Child Health Appraised (MOCHA) countries (e.g. the 30 European Union and European Economic Area countries at the time of the study) are diverse socially, culturally and economically, and differences exist in their healthcare systems and in the scope and role of primary care (see Chapter 2). An economic analysis was undertaken that sought to explain differences in child health outcomes across the MOCHA countries.

Methods

The conceptual framework for the analysis was that of a production function for health, whereby health outputs (or outcomes) are assumed affected by several 'inputs' consistent with those reviewed in Chapter 2. Traditional production function approaches explain outputs of goods and services in terms of the resources that are used in their production, primarily natural resources, labour, capital and technology. In the case of health, those factors translate into the healthcare workforce (discussed further in Chapter 13), the capital equipment and technology that is used in the diagnosis and treatment of patients, and the drugs, devices and other consumables that are prescribed for managing medical conditions. Health, however, is also the product of other factors, including personal characteristics of the population (genes and health behaviours), socio-economic variables (such as income levels and living standards) and the structure and organisation of the healthcare system that delivers care.

The aim of the economic analysis was to explore the relationships between a range of health system variables, including the strength of primary care (a key variable of interest for the MOCHA project) and child health outcome indicators in the MOCHA countries, controlling for confounding country-level factors. The methodology was quantitative, namely, regression modelling to explore the relationship between explanatory factors and outcomes, based on countries as the unit of analysis. Data deficiencies, however, constrained the scope of the work. This chapter explains the measurement conundrums that were faced and how they were addressed. The results of the modelling are presented, but should be interpreted with caution due to the data-related compromises that were made.

Data and Methods

Child Health Outcome Indicators

The importance of population-level measures of child health for identifying progress, problems and priorities is well recognised, and proposals have been advanced for holistic national-level indicator sets that reflect quality in the care of specific conditions and more general indicators of health (Gill, O'Neill, Rose, Mant, & Harnden, 2014; Rigby, Köhler, Blair, & Metchler, 2003). The data to enable the use of such indicators in cross country analysis, however, are very limited, as discussed in Chapter 7. The range of outcome measures for children available from international health data sources are mostly focussed on a variety of vaccination and mortality rates. Information on other, more health-centred outcomes may be gathered in individual countries, but cross-national comparisons are only possible if sufficient numbers of countries can provide data, and there is agreement on the definitions that they use.

The outcome indicators used in this study are selected mortality rates that are reported across the MOCHA countries. Child mortality rates in Europe are generally low, but variability between countries does occur, providing an opportunity for investigating potential contributing factors. Being the inverse of health, the use of mortality indicators represents a compromise resulting from a lack of other data. Moreover, it is arguable that mortality is a poor indicator of quality of primary care. Vaccination rates were rejected as an alternative outcome for use in the analysis because they are delivered outside of primary care in some countries and are also influenced by legislation in some jurisdictions that requires parents (under threat of sanctions in some cases) to comply (Wells, 2017).

Five mortality measures were chosen for analysis: three relating to early years (neonatal, i.e. first 28 days; infant, i.e. first year; and under five years of age mortality per 1,000 live births) and two relating to mortality of children 19 years and younger per 100,000 population from two ambulatory care-sensitive conditions (diabetes and epilepsy). Emergency admissions to hospital by people with a range of ambulatory care-sensitive conditions are widely used as indicators of the quality of primary care (Tian, Dixon, & Gao, 2012). In the absence of hospitalisation data across MOCHA countries for children, mortality rates were used as a proxy.

Explanatory Variables

Two broad groups of factors were considered as potential influences on child mortality outcomes: socio-economic and socio-demographic characteristics of the countries, and healthcare system features. The choice of variables was constrained by data availability, and the variables available had limitations.

Three broad country-specific factors reported in international data sources were included in the analysis. First, gross domestic product (GDP) per capita was used as an indicator of income levels and economic strength of a country and hence its ability to spend on health care. This is the most widely used measure of a nation's living standards, although it has some significant limitations, including that it does not take account of the distribution of income in a country, which may be very inequitable (Amadeo, 2018). Secondly, the proportion of the population living in urban (rather than rural) areas was used to explore any potential influence this might have on the child mortality indicators. Lastly, the proportion of the country's population aged 19 years or less was included as a proxy for family size.

Among healthcare system factors that might affect health outcomes, health expenditure per capita is a likely key determinant. This, however, is represented by GDP per capita since these variables are highly correlated (see Chapter 13). Including both in the regression modelling would create statistical problems of multicollinearity. Other potential healthcare system influences on mortality that were sought for inclusion in the analysis related to access to health care, the healthcare workforce, the healthcare financing mechanism, how services are provided and the strength of primary care. Data reflecting each of these features were obtained, although some limitations applied.

Point-of-care charges might limit access to health care, and to proxy this, out-of-pocket (OOP) expenditure on health care as a proportion of total health care expenditure was incorporated. OOP expenditure data, however, have the drawback that they refer to a country's population as a whole, and not just to the use of health care by children. Information obtained from the MOCHA country agents (see Chapter 1) indicated complex systems of charging for children in many countries with exemptions in place depending on a variety of factors including age, family income, the nature of the condition and the type of medication. Only three countries (Norway, Sweden and United Kingdom) said there were no charges for children.

The workforce (size and composition) is a major component in the delivery of health care, and the number of general paediatricians (includes neonatologists, but excludes paediatric specialties such as psychiatry, cardiology, oncology, surgery etc.), general practitioners (GPs) and nurses per 100, 000 of the population are available in international datasets and were included as potential influences on activity levels and outcomes. In the context of an assessment of primary health care for children, however, these variables have drawbacks. In particular, the data are aggregated such that the work of GPs and nurses with children (rather than adults) cannot be isolated, and the allocation of nurses to the primary (rather than secondary) care sector is not provided.

Countries were classified according to (1) how their healthcare system was predominantly financed and (2) how care was predominantly provided. These classifications were based on the work of Böhm (Böhm, 2012; Böhm, Schmid, Götze, Landwehr, & Rothgang, 2013) which argues that financing and provision arrangements in a healthcare system create mechanisms and incentives that affect the way in which the actors (government, societal/non-governmental organisations and private individuals) in the system behave. For example, the service provision arrangements may affect the way in which doctors are paid (capitation vs fee-for-service or performance related) and this may affect their treatment decisions, with implications for the outcomes and experiences of patients (see Chapter 16; Wells, 2017). The financing dimension is broken down into state (raising money for health care through taxes or national insurance schemes), societal (social insurance) and private (private insurance or direct payments). Similarly, care is either provided by the public (state), non-governmental/societal organisations or the private sector. There are no examples of predominantly private financing or societal provision in the MOCHA countries (Table 9.1). The problem with these variables is that health systems are complex and financing

Table 9.1. Financing and service delivery classifications.

Country	Financing	Service Provision
Austria	Societal	Private
Belgium	Societal	Private
Bulgaria*	Societal	Private
Croatia*	Societal	Private
Cyprus*	State	State
Czech Rep.	Societal	Private
Denmark	State	State
Estonia	Societal	Private
Finland	State	State
France	Societal	Private
Germany	Societal	Private
Greece*	Societal	Private
Hungary	Societal	Private
Iceland	State	State
Ireland	State	private
Italy	State	Private
Latvia*	State	State
Lithuania*	State	Private
Luxembourg	Societal	Private
Malta*	State	State
Netherlands	Societal	Private
Norway	State	State
Poland	Societal	Private
Portugal	State	State
Romania		
Slovakia	Societal	Private
Slovenia	Societal	State
Spain	State	State
Sweden	State	State
UK	State	State

Source: Based on Böhm 2013, except countries marked *.
*Classified by Authors based on the European Observatory on Health Systems and Policies report (downloaded 2016).

and provision within countries is often through a blend of methods thus creating uncertainties in the categorisation, and in turn giving rise to issues for the interpretation of the results of any analysis.

A measure of the strength of primary care in each country was taken from the Primary Care Activity Monitor for Europe (PHAMEU) (Kringos, Boerma, van der Zee, & Groenewegen, 2013). The PHAMEU method scored primary care on seven dimensions, each being made up of a number of indicators. Three dimensions are related to structures (governance, economic conditions and workforce development) and four to processes (access, continuity, coordination and comprehensiveness). An overall primary care system strength was assigned by PHAMEU on the basis of the dimension scores (strong, medium and weak), and this measure was used as an explanatory variable in the regression modelling (Table 9.2). The limitation of this variable is that the dimensions, and underlying indicators, were defined with care of the general population in mind and different factors may be important in care of children. A full description of all variables included in the analysis is given in Table 9.3.

Analysis

The data for the quantitative variables were obtained for the 30 MOCHA countries for the 13-year period from 2004 to 2016 (maximum of 390 observations per variable, if there was no missing information) from the World Health Organization, World Bank and Eurostat. Summary descriptive statistics are provided in Table 9.4. The values of variables are shown by country for the last year for which data were available (Table 9.5). Categorical variables (primary care strength, financing and service provision) were fixed across all years (as in Tables 9.1 and 9.2).

A random effects model was estimated to examine the contribution of the primary care system, other healthcare system variables and country covariates to each mortality outcome measure. Random effects models are used in the analysis of hierarchical or panel data when it is assumed the variables are random, and there are no fixed on non-random factors. A Hausman test was performed to confirm the random effects estimator was consistent (Prob $> \chi^2 = 0.9028$). Missing data could not be regarded as randomly missing and were not imputed as they were greater than 25% of the data, reducing the number of countries included in the modelling. The model was re-run with GDP per capita, the proportion of the population in urban areas, OOP expenditure and workforce variables lagged by two years since changes in those factors may take time to have an effect on mortality. As is customary, GDP per capita was entered into the modelling in logarithmic form, making the coefficient equivalent to a growth rate.

Findings

Results of the random effects regression analyses are found in Table 9.6. They are presented separately for each outcome measure without any lagged variables and with a two-year time lag to capture the medium-term effects of changes in

Table 9.2. PHAMEU scoring system for the strength of the countries' primary care system (Kringos et al., 2013).

Country	The Structure of Primary Care			The Service-delivery Process of Primary Care				Overall Primary Care System Strength
	Primary Care Governance	Economic Conditions of Primary Care	Primary Care Workforce Development	Access to Primary Care	Continuity of Primary Care	Coordination of Primary Care	Comprehensiveness of Primary Care	
Austria	Medium	Medium	Weak	Medium	Weak	Weak	Weak	Weak
Belgium	Medium	Strong	Medium	Weak	Strong	Medium	Strong	Strong
Bulgaria	Medium	Weak	Weak	Weak	Medium	Weak	Strong	Weak
Croatia								
Cyprus	Weak	Weak	Weak	Weak	Medium	Weak	Weak	Weak
Czech Republic	Medium	Weak	Weak	Strong	Strong	Medium	Weak	Medium
Denmark	Strong	Medium	Strong	Strong	Strong	Strong	Medium	Strong
Estonia	Strong	Weak	Medium	Medium	Strong	Medium	Medium	Strong
Finland	Medium	Strong	Strong	Medium	Medium	Medium	Strong	Strong
France	Medium	Medium	Medium	Weak	Medium	Medium	Strong	Medium
Germany	Medium	Strong	Medium	Medium	Strong	Medium	Medium	Medium
Greece	Medium	Weak	Weak	Weak	Weak	Strong	Weak	Weak
Hungary	Weak	Medium	Medium	Strong	Medium	Weak	Weak	Weak
Iceland	Weak	Weak	Weak	Medium	Strong	Weak	Medium	Weak
Ireland	Weak	Weak	Strong	Weak	Strong	Weak	Medium	Weak
Italy	Strong	Strong	Medium	Medium	Weak	Medium	Weak	Medium
Latvia	Medium	Medium	Weak	Weak	Strong	Medium	Medium	Medium
Lithuania	Strong	Medium	Medium	Strong	Weak	Strong	Strong	Strong
Luxembourg	Weak	Weak	Weak	Weak	Weak	Medium	Medium	Weak

Table 9.2. (Continued)

Country	The Structure of Primary Care			The Service-delivery Process of Primary Care				Overall Primary Care System Strength
	Primary Care Governance	Economic Conditions of Primary Care	Primary Care Workforce Development	Access to Primary Care	Continuity of Primary Care	Coordination of Primary Care	Comprehensiveness of Primary Care	
Malta	Weak	Weak	Strong	Weak	Weak	Strong	Medium	Weak
Netherlands	Strong	Strong	Strong	Strong	Weak	Strong	Medium	Strong
Norway	Strong	Weak	Medium	Medium	Medium	Weak	Strong	Medium
Poland	Weak	Weak	Weak	Strong	Medium	Strong	Weak	Medium
Portugal	Strong	Medium	Strong	Strong	Medium	Medium	Strong	Strong
Romania	Strong	Strong	Medium	Medium	Medium	Weak	Weak	Medium
Slovak Rep.	Weak	Medium	Weak	Medium	Strong	Weak	Weak	Weak
Slovenia	Strong	Strong	Strong	Strong	Weak	Strong	Weak	Strong
Spain	Strong	Strong	Strong	Strong	Strong	Strong	Strong	Strong
Sweden	Medium	Medium	Medium	Medium	Weak	Strong	Strong	Medium
UK	Strong	Strong	Strong	Strong	Medium	Strong	Strong	Strong

Note: Indicators making up each dimension:

Governance of the primary care system: (1) health (care) goals, (2) policy on equity in access, (3) (de)centralisation of management and service development, (4) quality management infrastructure, (5) appropriate technology, (6) patient advocacy, (7) ownership of practices and (8) integration of primary care in the healthcare system.

Economic conditions of the primary care system: (1) healthcare expenditure, (2) primary care expenditures, (3) healthcare funding system, (4) employment status of primary care workforce, (5) remuneration system of primary care workforces and (6) income of primary care workforce.

Primary care workforce development: (1) profile of workforce, (2) recognition and responsibilities of disciplines, (3) education and retention, (4) professional associations, (5) academic status of primary care disciplines and (6) future development of workforce.

Access to primary care services: (1) availability of primary care services, (2) geographic access, (3) accommodation of accessibility (including physical access), (4) affordability, (5) acceptability, (6) utilisation and (7) equality in access.

Continuity of care: (1) longitudinal, (2) informational, (3) relational and (4) management.

Coordination of care: (1) gatekeeping system, (2) practice and team structure, (3) skill-mix in primary care, (4) integration of primary and secondary care and (5) integration of primary and public health.

Comprehensiveness of care: (1) medical equipment available, (2) first contact for common health problems, (3) treatment and follow-up of diseases, (4) medical technical procedures and preventive care, (5) mother/child/reproductive health care and (6) health promotion.

Table 9.3. Description of dependent and independent variables used in the analysis.

Variable	Description	Source	Years Available
Infant mortality	Number of deaths of children under one year of age per 1,000 live births	WHO global burden of disease	2004–2015
Neonatal mortality	Number of deaths of children within the first 28 days of life per 1,000 live births	WHO global burden of disease	2004–2015
Under-five years mortality	Number of deaths of children below the age of five per 1,000 live births	WHO global burden of disease	2004–2015
Diabetes mortality	Number of deaths from diabetes of children/young people below the age of 20 per 100,000 of population	WHO global burden of disease	2004–2016
Epilepsy mortality	Number of deaths from diabetes of children/young people below the age of 20 per 100,000 of population	WHO global burden of disease	2004–2016
GDP per capita, PPP	Gross domestic product per capita based on purchasing power parity (PPP). GDP is converted to international dollars using purchasing power parity rates. Data are in constant 2011 international dollars	World Health Organization's global health expenditure database	2004–2016
Out-of-pocket expenditure as % total health expenditure	Any direct outlay by households, including gratuities and in-kind payments, to health practitioners and suppliers of pharmaceuticals, therapeutic appliances, and other goods and services. It is a part of private health expenditure	World Health Organization's Global Health Expenditure database	2004–2016
% of total population living in urban areas	Proportion of people living in urban areas in a country in a given year, weighted average	The United Nations Population Division's World Urbanization Prospects	2004–2016

Table 9.3. (*Continued*)

Variable	Description	Source	Years Available
General paediatricians/100,000 of population	General paediatricians per 100,000 of the population. Inclusion – Paediatricians; Neonatologists; Medical interns or residents specialising in paediatrics. Exclusion- Paediatric specialties (e.g. child psychiatry, child/paediatric surgery, child/paediatric gynaecology, paediatric cardiology, paediatric oncology)	European health information gateway	2004–2014
General practitioners/100,000 of population	General practitioners per 100K population. Inclusion – General practitioners – District medical doctors – therapists – Family medical practitioners ('family doctors') – Medical interns or residents specialising in general practice. Exclusion – Paediatricians – Other generalist (non-specialist) medical practitioners	European health information gateway	2004–2015
Nurses/100, 000	Nurses per 100,000 population – Nursing professionals; nursing associate professionals and Midwives	European health information gateway	2004–2015
Population ages 0–19 as % of total population	Percentage of children and young people in population aged 19 years and under	Eurostat	2004–2016
Financing classification	Böhm classification of each country according to financing system; 0 = predominantly societal or social-based financing and 1 = predominantly state or tax financing	Böhm 2013	
Service provision classification	Böhm classification of each country according to service provision types; 0 = predominantly private service provision; 1 = predominantly state service provision	Böhm 2013	
Strength of primary care	Kringos classification of each country according to strength of primary care system (overall score): 0 = weak; 1 = strong; 2 = medium	Kringos 2013	

Table 9.4. Summary descriptive statistics of quantitative variables included in the analysis for the 30 MOCHA countries, 2004–2016 ($N = 390$ is complete data for all countries and all years).

Variables	N	Mean	Standard Deviation	Min	Max
Mortality rate/1,000 live births, neonatal	360	3.204	1.804	0.900	12.30
Mortality rate/1,000 live births, infant	360	4.629	2.730	1.500	19.50
Mortality rate/1,000 live births, under five years	360	5.519	3.098	1.900	22.40
Mortality rate <= 19 years/100,000 population, diabetes	390	0.0708	0.0474	0.0184	0.260
Mortality rate <= 19years/100,000 population, epilepsy	390	0.381	0.155	0.149	0.920
GDP per capita, $ PPP	390	35,096	15,243	11,736	97,864
% of population in urban areas	390	73.41	12.51	49.63	97.90
Population aged 0–19 years as % of total population	390	22.23	2.538	18.05	29.64
Out-of-pocket expenditure as % total health expenditure	330	20.44	9.769	5.221	49.70
General paediatricians/100,000 of population	265	14.28	6.236	3.900	30.09
General practitioners/100,000 of population	227	70.94	28.55	13.28	170.00
Nurses/100,000 of population	232	977.6	497.4	29	2,675

GDP growth per capita, out-of-pocket expenditure, urban living and the health-care workforce on child mortality.

Looking at the neonatal, infant and under-five years mortality, the significant negative coefficients indicate that GDP growth per capita is associated with reductions in mortality rates. For infant mortality, for example, the coefficient of the log of GDP (–2.02) represents a change in mortality associated with a 100% growth rate. Hence, a 1% increase in GDP growth per capita would be associated with a reduction of about 0.02 infant deaths per 1,000 live births, with this effect increasing slightly when a two-year lag is included. There is a similar, albeit smaller effect for neonatal mortality, and a larger effect for under-five years mortality. Hence, in a representative country with (say) 750,000 live births per annum, a 1% GDP growth rate would be associated with 0.02 × 750,000/1,000 = 15 fewer infant deaths per annum. Coefficients relate to

Table 9.5. Values of quantitative variables by country – last year for which data were available.

| Country | Outcome Measures: Mortality Rates | | | | | Explanatory Variables | | | | | | |
	/1,000 Live Births, Neonatal, 2015	/1,000 Live Births, Infant, 2015	/1,000 Live Births, Under Five Years, 2015	<=19 Years/100,000 Population, Diabetes, 2016	<=19 Years/100,000 Population, Epilepsy, 2016	GDP Per Capita, $ PPP, 2016	% of Population in Urban Areas, 2016	Population Aged 0–19 Years as % of Total Population, 2016	Out-of-pocket Expenditure as % Total Health Expenditure, 2014	Paediatricians/100,000 of Population, 2013	General Practitioners/100,000 of Population, 2013	Nurses/100,000 of Population, 2013
Austria	2.1	2.9	3.5	0.04	0.27	44,143.70	66.0	19.22	16.15	16.21	76.95	803.09
Belgium	2.2	3.3	4.1	0.03	0.37	41,945.69	97.9	22.57	17.81	12.65	111.67	–
Bulgaria	5.6	9.3	10.4	0.11	0.59	17,709.08	74.3	18.27	44.19	19.93	62.93	491.82
Croatia	2.6	3.6	4.3	0.02	0.56	21,408.55	59.3	20.28	11.21	18.52	53.72	658.48
Cyprus	1.5	2.5	2.7	0.12	0.19	31,195.51	66.8	23.44	48.71	–	–	512.92
Czech Republic	1.8	2.8	3.4	0.04	0.33	31,071.75	73.0	19.43	14.33	12.33	70.13	841.28
Denmark	2.5	2.9	3.5	0.05	0.26	45,686.48	87.8	22.83	13.36	7.02	–	1,685.66
Estonia	1.5	2.3	2.9	0.07	0.45	27,735.14	67.5	20.57	20.72	13.43	70.33	587.94
Finland	1.3	1.9	2.3	0.05	0.21	39,422.65	84.4	21.81	18.23	12.93	–	–
France	2.2	3.5	4.3	0.03	0.27	38,058.87	79.8	24.11	6.34	12.09	160.11	999.73
Germany	2.1	3.1	3.7	0.04	0.45	44,072.39	75.5	18.05	13.20	12.38	66.66	1,323.07
Greece	2.9	3.6	4.6	0.03	0.16	24,263.88	78.3	19.33	34.86	30.33	23.36	353.68
Hungary	3.5	5.3	5.9	0.04	0.41	25,381.29	71.7	19.48	26.59	–	–	659.65
Iceland	0.9	1.6	2	0.02	0.26	45,276.45	94.2	26.64	17.48	4.63	58.07	1,626.8
Ireland	2.3	3	3.6	0.04	0.34	62,828.34	63.5	27.57	17.66	9.86	73.17	–
Italy	2.1	2.9	3.5	0.05	0.17	34,620.13	69.1	18.31	21.19	29.01	75.05	634.19
Latvia	5.2	6.9	7.9	0.11	0.30	23,712.09	67.4	19.46	35.13	12.67	–	508.09

Lithuania	2.5	3.3	5.2	0.10	0.33	27,904.10	66.5	20.19	31.27	26.91	86.28	785.28
Luxembourg	0.9	1.5	1.9	0.02	0.33	97,018.66	90.4	22.40	10.60	14.91	85.95	1,230.12
Malta	4.4	5.1	6.4	0.07	0.22	35,694.04	95.5	19.83	28.86	13.93	80.30	744.16
Netherlands	2.4	3.2	3.8	0.04	0.40	47,128.31	91.0	22.53	5.22	9.54	78.50	–
Norway	1.5	2	2.6	0.08	0.34	63,810.79	80.7	24.06	13.61	13.92	78.05	1,720.93
Poland	3.1	4.5	5.2	0.03	0.26	26,003.01	60.5	19.90	23.46	13.17	21.75	587.46
Portugal	2	3	3.6	0.05	0.26	27,006.87	64.0	19.13	26.84	17.80	56.83	629.31
Romania	6.3	9.7	11.1	0.07	0.56	21,647.81	54.7	20.75	18.87	10.97	56.95	552.42
Slovak Rep.	4.2	5.8	7.3	0.05	0.47	29,156.09	53.5	20.44	22.54	–	–	607.81
Slovenia	1.4	2.1	2.6	0.02	0.15	29,803.45	49.6	19.33	12.07	26.22	49.78	838.08
Spain	2.8	3.5	4.1	0.03	0.21	33,261.08	79.8	19.34	23.99	25.53	75.15	532.40
Sweden	1.6	2.4	3	0.05	0.21	46,441.21	86.0	22.46	14.06	10.48	64.53	1,192.12
UK	2.4	3.5	4.2	0.05	0.47	38,901.05	82.8	23.30	9.73	15.10	79.57	867.61

Source: WHO global burden of disease (columns 2–6); WHO global health expenditure database (columns 7–10); European Health Information Gateway (columns 11–13).

Table 9.6. Results of regression modelling.

Variables	Neonatal Mortality/1,000 Live Births		Infant Mortality/1,000 Live Births		Under-five Years Mortality/1,000 Live Births		Mortality from Diabetes, Age 19 Years and Under/100,000 Population		Mortality from Epilepsy, Age 19 Years and Under/100,000 Population	
		Two-year lag		Two-year lag		Two-year lag		Two-year lag		Two-year lag
Log GDP per capita PPP	−1.255***	−1.565***	−2.012***	−2.441***	−2.388***	−2.848***	0.018	−0.026	0.091	−0.083
	[0.363]	[0.361]	[0.555]	[0.548]	[0.665]	[0.635]	[0.019]	[0.017]	[0.067]	[0.062]
Out-of-pocket as % total health expenditure	0.027**	0.036***	0.014	0.036*	0.023	0.058**	0.002**	0.002***	0.004	0.005*
	[0.014]	[0.014]	[0.021]	[0.021]	[0.025]	[0.025]	[0.001]	[0.001]	[0.003]	[0.003]
% of population in urban areas	−0.026*	−0.005	−0.033	0.008	−0.050*	−0.014	−0.001	−0.001	0.002	0.003
	[0.016]	[0.015]	[0.024]	[0.024]	[0.028]	[0.027]	[0.001]	[0.001]	[0.003]	[0.002]
Paediatricians/100,000 population	−0.017**	−0.019***	−0.032***	−0.035***	−0.037***	−0.039***	−0.000	−0.001*	−0.000	−0.002*
	[0.007]	[0.007]	[0.010]	[0.010]	[0.012]	[0.012]	[0.000]	[0.000]	[0.001]	[0.001]
GPs/100,000 population	−0.008*	−0.013***	−0.019***	−0.031***	−0.021***	−0.027***	−0.000**	−0.000	−0.002***	−0.002**
	[0.004]	[0.004]	[0.006]	[0.007]	[0.008]	[0.008]	[0.000]	[0.000]	[0.001]	[0.001]
Nurses/100,000 population	0.000	−0.000	0.000	0.000	0.000	0.000	−0.000	0.000	−0.000	−0.000
	[0.000]	[0.000]	[0.000]	[0.000]	[0.000]	[0.000]	[0.000]	[0.000]	[0.000]	[0.000]
Non-lagged variables										
% of population <= 19 years	0.421***	0.321***	0.651***	0.534***	0.763***	0.589***	0.013***	0.011***	0.033***	0.033***
	[0.031]	[0.033]	[0.047]	[0.051]	[0.056]	[0.058]	[0.002]	[0.002]	[0.006]	[0.006]

Financing (state=1 vs societal=0)	-0.008	0.060	0.149	0.120	0.084	0.078	-0.001	-0.004	-0.004	-0.031
	[0.660]	[0.602]	[1.030]	[0.953]	[1.147]	[1.020]	[0.021]	[0.017]	[0.090]	[0.077]
Service provision (state=1 vs private=0)	-1.072	-0.994	-2.075*	-2.007*	-2.254*	-1.994*	-0.022	-0.014	-0.215**	-0.164*
	[0.723]	[0.662]	[1.128]	[1.047]	[1.259]	[1.123]	[0.023]	[0.019]	[0.099]	[0.085]
Primary care overall score (strong=1 vs weak=0)	0.229	0.178	0.413	0.538	0.556	0.549	0.049**	0.037*	0.216**	0.176**
	[0.693]	[0.637]	[1.080]	[1.005]	[1.208]	[1.082]	[0.023]	[0.019]	[0.096]	[0.083]
Primary care overall score (medium=1 vs weak=0)	0.148	0.281	0.229	0.670	0.219	0.593	0.027	0.025	0.144	0.130
	[0.682]	[0.627]	[1.063]	[0.989]	[1.189]	[1.064]	[0.023]	[0.019]	[0.095]	[0.082]
Constant	9.194	13.131	15.295	19.474	18.966	24.404	-0.320	0.111	-1.414	0.271
	[4.402]	[4.379]	[6.742]	[6.692]	[8.002]	[7.658]	[0.222]	[0.197]	[0.780]	[0.717]
Observations	166	164	166	164	166	164	166	166	166	166
Number of countries	23	23	23	23	23	23	23	23	23	23

Note: Standard errors in brackets; ***$p < 0.01$. **$p < 0.05$. *$p < 0.10$.

marginal changes that only apply to the sample averages, with confidence intervals increasing away from the average.

The results also indicate that medical workforce density has a significant effect in reducing mortality rates. For neonatal mortality, for example, an increase in the number of general paediatricians (includes neonatologists) by 1 per 100,000 of the population is associated with, on average, a decrease in neonatal deaths of 0.017 per 1,000 live births. Likewise, an increase in the number of GPs by 1 per 100,000 population is associated with a decrease in neonatal deaths of 0.008 per 1,000 live births. Significant effects are also seen for infant and under-five years mortality; the effects are slightly larger with two-year lagged variables in the models. The average number of paediatricians in the MOCHA countries is about 14 per 100,000 of the population (Table 9.4). An increase in one paediatrician per 100,000 of the population in a country with 750,000 live births per annum would be associated with a reduction in neonatal deaths per 1,000 live births of 750,000/1,000*0.017 = 12.75 fewer deaths per annum. This calculation assumes no constraints on the availability of the technologies required for caring for newborns.

For ambulatory care-sensitive conditions in children and young people of 19 years or younger, however, growth in GDP per capita and density of general paediatricians show no significant effect on mortality rates. An increase in the number of GPs per 100,000 of the population has an effect on mortality, but it is very small, and not significant in the lagged diabetes model.

An increase in OOP expenditure as a percentage of total health expenditure is seen to significantly increase neonatal mortality rates and mortality from diabetes in children and young people aged 19 years and younger than 19 years. A 1% point increase in OOP payments as a percentage of total health expenditure, on average, is associated with an increase in diabetes deaths in the 0–19 age group by 0.002 deaths per 100,000 of the population, other things held constant; lower OOP expenditures are associated with lower mortality. This effect is also seen in neonatal and the under-five years mortality lagged model and marginally on mortality from epilepsy. In the neonatal model, a 1% point decrease in OOP expenditures as a percentage of total health expenditure is associated, on average, with a 0.027 fewer deaths per 1,000 live births.

Strength of primary care does not have a statistically significant effect on neonatal, infant and under-five years mortality. However, for diabetes and epilepsy mortality rates in children and young people aged 0–9 years, strong primary care systems, compared to weak systems, are associated with higher mortality rates. A country having a primary care system rated as strong is predicted to have higher mortality from diabetes of 0.049 per 100,000 of the population, compared to countries whose primary care system is rated as weak; the effect is 0.216 per 100,000 of the population in the epilepsy un-lagged model. When service provision is predominantly by the state rather than private enterprise, mortality rates from epilepsy ages 0–19 years are predicted to be lower by 0.215 per 100,000 of the population. Diabetes, neonatal, infant and under-five years mortality rates, however, are not affected by mode of service provision. The method of financing health care is unrelated to any mortality variable.

A higher proportion of a country's population in the 0−19 age group exerts a worsening effect on all types of mortality. For example, for infant mortality, a 1% point increase in the proportion of the population aged 0−19 years is associated, on average, with an increase in infant mortality by 0.651 per 1,000 live births. A 1% point increase in population of the population aged 0−19 is associated, on average, with an increase in deaths from diabetes in children and young people aged 0−19 years by 0.013 per 100,000 of the population.

Discussion

The results of the analysis suggest that mortality in the early years is lower in MOCHA countries where the GDP per capita is higher. GDP per capita is an indicator of average income levels and is closely correlated with expenditure on health care. Many other studies have consistently shown a significant positive effect of a country's GDP per capita and health expenditures on the health and well-being of the population (Swift, 2011) and on infant mortality in particular (Erdogan, Ener, & Arica, 2013; Nixon & Ulmann, 2006; Rad et al., 2013). Within MOCHA countries, lower mortality in early years is also associated with a larger medical workforce (GPs and general paediatricians) per 100,000 of the population. More GPs per 100,000 of the population is also a predictor of lower mortality among children and young people aged 0−19 years from epilepsy and diabetes.

Consistent across all mortality indicators was the independent effect of the number of children and young people in the population. As this increased, mortality rates rose, suggesting that larger family size is a risk factor. Higher OOP expenditure on health was associated with higher neonatal mortality and mortality from diabetes in the 0−19 age group, but not with other mortality indicators.

Healthcare system variables were mostly found to not significantly influence mortality. Countries with primary care systems that were classified as strong (compared to weak) were associated with higher mortality from diabetes and epilepsy in children and young people, although the strength of primary care was unrelated to mortality in the early years. State provision of health care rather than private was associated with lower epilepsy mortality, but no other mortality outcome. Financing mechanism was insignificant for all outcomes.

There are many drawbacks with the analysis that limit the inferences that can be drawn from it. As explained above, data deficiencies constrained the choice of both outcome measures and explanatory variables. The absence of consistent reporting of child *health* outcomes across countries necessitated the use of mortality indicators, which are inadequate measures of quality of primary care. Of the available explanatory variables, time series were incomplete, particularly with respect to workforce data, thereby reducing the number of countries included in the analysis and opening up the possibility of bias. Many quantitative and qualitative factors contribute to health outcomes, and the relationships are complex (Nixon & Ulmann, 2006). The model of health production that was used in this study is likely to have excluded many factors.

The key focus of the MOCHA project was on the quality of primary care for children, but available expenditure, workforce and outcome data are gathered for countries as a whole and information related to children and the primary care sector cannot be separated out. The use of the primary care quality indicator derived in the PHAMEU study (Kringos et al., 2013) in the analysis produced a counter-intuitive finding that stronger primary care systems are associated with higher mortality than in countries with systems classified as weaker. This may be because the criteria were selected for assessing primary care in general, and not specifically for evaluating the quality of primary care for children. In addition, the three-level overall score (strong, medium and weak) used in the analysis (an average of seven different dimensions) may have been insufficiently sensitive to reflect mortality differences. Other studies using a more disaggregated description of primary care have found associations with health outcomes (Macinko, Starfield, & Shi, 2003). Similarly, mortality rates were generally not affected by differences in healthcare system financing and service provision features between countries, possibly due to the breadth of the categories and within country variability.

Conclusion

This study presents one of the few cross-sectional, time series analyses that explores the association between healthcare system features, primary care quality and child mortality outcomes. Keeping in mind the ecological nature of the analysis, and the limitations presented by the data and measures employed, several tentative conclusions can be drawn. National health expenditure and the general medical workforce density appear to reduce mortality among infants and children and young people with conditions thought to be sensitive to primary care. OOP expenditure exerts pressure on the resources of families and worsens some indicators, while potentially deepening health inequalities.

References

Amadeo, K. (2018). *Standard of living*. Retrieved from http://www.thebalance.com/standard-of-living-3305758

Böhm, K. (2012). *Classifying OECD healthcare systems: A deductive approach*. Retrieved from http://www.socium.uni-bremen.de/f/4912881dfe.pdf

Böhm, K., Schmid, A., Götze, R., Landwehr, C., & Rothgang, H. (2013). Five types of OECD healthcare systems: Empirical results of a deductive classification. *Health Policy, 113*(3), 258−269. doi:10.1016/j.healthpol.2013.09.003

Budhdeo, S., Watkins, J., Atun, R., Williams, C., Zeltner, T., & Maruthappu, M. (2015). Changes in government spending on healthcare and population mortality in the European union, 1995−2010: A cross-sectional ecological study. *Journal of the Royal Society of Medicine, 108*(12), 490−498. doi:10.1177/0141076815600907

Erdogan, E., Ener, M., & Arica, F. (2013). The strategic role of infant mortality in the process of economic growth: An application for high income OECD countries. *Social and Behavioural Sciences, 99*, 19−25. doi:10.1016/j.sbspro.2013.10.467

Gill, P., O'Neill, B., Rose, P., Mant, D., & Harnden, A. (2014). Primary care quality indicators for children. *British Journal of General Practice, 64*(629), e752–e757. doi:10.3399/bjgp14X682813

Kringos, D. S., Boerma, W., van der Zee, J., & Groenewegen, P. (2013). Europe's strong primary care systems are linked to better population health but also to higher health spending. *Health affairs, 32*(4), 686–694. doi:10.1377/hlthaff.2012.1242

Macinko, J., Starfield, B., & Shi, L. (2003). The contribution of primary care systems to health outcomes within Organization for Economic Cooperation and Development (OECD) countries, 1970–1998. *Health Services Research, 38*(3), 831–865.

Nixon, J., & Ulmann, P. (2006). The relationship between health care expenditure and health outcomes. *The European Journal of Health Economics, 7*(1), 7–18. doi:10.1007/s10198-005-0336-8

Rad, E. H., Vahedi, S., Teimourizad, A., Esmaeilzadeh, F., Hadian, M., & Pour, A. T. (2013). Comparison of the effects of public and private health expenditures on the health status: A panel data analysis in eastern Mediterranean countries. *International Journal of Health Policy and Management, 1*(2), 163–167. doi:10.15171/ijhpm.2013.29

Rigby, M. J., Köhler, L. I., Blair, M. E., & Metchler, R. (2003). Child health indicators for Europe: A priority for a caring society. *European Journal of Public Health(Suppl), 13*(3), 38–46.

Swift, R. (2011). The relationship between health and GDP in OECD countries in the very long run. *Health Economics, 20*. doi:10.1002/hec.1590

Tian, Y., Dixon, A., & Gao, H. (2012). *Emergency hospital admissions for ambulatory care sensitive conditions.* Data briefing, The Kings Fund. Retrieved from https://www.kingsfund.org.uk/sites/default/files/field/field_publication_file/data-briefing-emergency-hospital-admissions-for-ambulatory-care-sensitive-conditions-apr-2012.pdf

Wells, H. (2017). Contribution to Blair, M., Rigby, M., Alexander, D. *Final report on current models of primary care for children* (Part I, Chapter 8). Retrieved from www.childhealthservicemodels.eu/wp-content/uploads/2017/07/MOCHA-WP1-Deliverable-WP1-D6-Feb-2017-1.pdf

Chapter 10

Services and Boundary Negotiations for Children with Complex Care Needs in Europe

Maria Brenner, Miriam O'Shea, Anne Clancy, Stine Lundstroem Kamionka, Philip Larkin, Sapfo Lignou, Daniela Luzi, Elena Montañana Olaso, Manna Alma, Fabrizio Pecoraro, Rose Satherley, Oscar Tamburis, Keishia Taylor, Austin Warters, Ingrid Wolfe, Jay Berry, Colman Noctor and Carol Hilliard

Abstract

Improvements in neonatal and paediatric care mean that many children with complex care needs (CCNs) now survive into adulthood. This cohort of children places great challenges on health and social care delivery in the community: they require dynamic and responsive health and social care over a long period of time; they require organisational and delivery coordination functions; and health issues such as minor illnesses, normally presented to primary care, must be addressed in the context of the complex health issues. Their clinical presentation may challenge local care management. The project explored the interface between primary care and specialised health services and found that it is not easily navigated by children with CCNs and their families across the European Union and the European Economic Area countries. We described the referral-discharge interface, the management of a child with CCNs at the acute–community interface, social care, nursing preparedness for practice and the experiences of the child and family in all Models of Child Health Appraised countries. We investigated data integration and the presence of validated standards of care, including governance and co-creation of care. A separate enquiry was conducted into how care is accessed for children with enduring mental health disorders. This included the level of parental involvement and the presence of multidisciplinary teams in their care. For all children with CCNs, we found wide variation in access to, and governance of, care. Effective communication between the child, family and health services remains challenging, often with fragmentation of care delivery across the health and social care sector and limited service availability.

Keywords: Acute-community interface; access to care; complex care needs; complex mental health care needs; integrated care; child

Introduction

Every child has a right to the highest attainable standard of health care, including those with complex care needs (CCNs) (see Chapters 4 and 16), which is a cohort of children often neglected in policy and research priorities in primary care. Improvements in neonatal and paediatric care mean that more children with CCNs are surviving into adulthood, but by their very nature, children with CCNs, and their families, place great challenges on healthcare delivery in the community. Although the provision of care closer to home for such children is a policy objective internationally, in most countries, the necessary integration of health services is insufficient, and there is wide variation in systems of care for these children. As a result, the interface between primary care and more specialised services is not easily navigated by children and families across the European Union (EU) and European Economic Area (EEA) countries. To identify the particular challenges faced by children with CCNs and their families, we explored the referral-discharge interface, the management of the child with CCNs at the acute–community interface, the social care interface, nursing preparedness for practice and the experiences of the child and family (Brenner, O'Shea, & Larkin, 2017; Clancy, Montañana-Olaso, & Larkin, 2017; Keilthy, Warters, Brenner, & McHugh, 2017; Wolfe, Lignou, & Satherley, 2017) by means of an extensive set of questionnaires to the MOCHA country agents (CAs) (see Chapters 1 and 2).

Data Integration

Collectively, we focused on two key areas in the integration of data to identify the issues that emerged pertaining to the optimum care for children with CCNs at the acute–community interface: to demonstrate how each area was linked and to identify how there would be meaningful integration of the various data gathered. We used business process analysis to reconstruct the child's care pathway through the identification of the actors and the activities performed to address a child's CCNs. This often complex care process was described in the project by using Unified Modelling Language (UML) methodology (Luzi, Pecoraro, & Tamburis, 2016). In addition to this, the experiences of children and young people living with long-term conditions were sought by MOCHA project partners, DIPEx International (see Chapter 3). This group of qualitative interviewers conducted interviews with young people and their parents to provide insight into the experiences of children and parents in terms of primary health care for children and the primary/secondary care interface. It was not possible nor methodologically appropriate to conduct these interviews in all MOCHA countries, so qualitative researchers from five representative countries worked collaboratively to explore patients' experiences in Czech Republic, Germany, The Netherlands, Spain and United Kingdom.

We identified key themes from each area of work and the core facilitators of optimum integration of care at the acute–community interface. Due to the complexity of this subject, we verified the findings of our integration of the data to ensure the findings were supported by exemplars of good practice, provided through self-report of the CAs in the participating countries. This occurred in two ways, the CAs read through our draft reports and commented on the representation of their data and the research team returned to the raw data to verify each standard which emerged in our collective analysis (see also Chapters 1 and 2).

Validated Principles and Standards of Care for Children Living with Complex Care Needs

We grouped our data into three principles and standards of care: access to care, co-creation of care and effective integrated governance. For each of these principles and standards, CAs in 30 countries were asked questions about the experiences of children with three tracer conditions needing complex care input. These three tracer conditions were chosen and presented to the CAs by means of a short vignette. This process allowed the exploration of a child's experience and the wider family experience of caring for a child with considerable needs. The tracer conditions also allowed us to cover a wide variety of ages from infant to 18 years of age (for a full explanation and analysis, see Brenner et al., 2017, Brenner et al., 2018a, b). The three tracer conditions were as follows:

(1) traumatic brain injury (TBI) (15-year-old boy, previously healthy who suffered a head injury in a skateboard accident) – responses from 26 out of 30 MOCHA countries;
(2) long-term ventilation (LTV) (18-month-old boy, with chronic lung disease due to bronchopulmonary dysplasia; and ventilator dependent since birth) – responses from 27 out of 30 MOCHA countries; and
(3) intractable epilepsy (seven-year-old girl with intractable epilepsy, suffering from multiple seizures daily, she comes from a non-EU migrant family, her father only speaks his native language, and her mother has basic knowledge of the official language of their host country) – responses from 27 out of 30 MOCHA countries.

Access to Care

We explored the access to care experienced by a child with CCNs, in terms of appropriateness of care, as well as availability of services and geographical, linguistic and cultural access to care. Our findings for the three tracer conditions, including the key issues are described in Table 10.1.

Co-creation of Care

This principle encompasses a number of key features of managing the health and care of a child with complex needs, including coordinating the services required, engagement and empowerment of the family (and child if able) to manage care at home where possible, support and advocacy where needed and an overall plan for long-term care. Our main findings are shown in Table 10.2, and more detailed results and analysis can be found in Brenner et al. (2017a, b), Brenner et al. (2018a, b).

Effective Integrated Governance

This is an aspect of care that ensures good quality of care and also encompasses the mechanisms by which a family can access and obtain help to co-ordinate the care they need in the community. This is a principle that many EU and EEA countries struggle to uphold, and concerns were raised about inequity of service provision (see also Chapter 5). Examples of our findings are shown in Table 10.3. For more detailed analysis and data, see Brenner et al. (2017a, b), Brenner et al. (2018a, b).

Services and Boundary Negotiations for Children with Complex Mental Health Needs in Europe

Children with complex mental care needs are defined as those with substantial care needs resulting from one or more conditions, which require access to multiple health and social support services. These needs can be best fulfilled when their care is integrated so that children and their families receive a continuum of preventive and curative services according to their needs over time and across different levels of the health system. Thus, in addition to describing the approach to managing the care of children with enduring complex mental health care needs, the aim of this study was also to identify facilitators and barriers to achieving a continuum of care at the interface of primary care (Brenner et al., 2017a; Kamionka & Taylor, 2017).

Methods

In addition to an extensive survey of the MOCHA CAs, this study incorporates a qualitative exploration of patient and family experiences (through DIPEx International, see Chapter 3), business process models of actors involved in

Table 10.1. Access to care for children with complex care needs.

Principles and Standards of Care	Supporting Data of Optimum Practice Identified from MOCHA and Identified Deficits
Principle 1: Access to care	
1.1 Children have access to age-specific and developmentally appropriate care	Data from Portugal highlights the benefits from an adolescent perspective: *When this is the case, care is much more adjusted and adolescents get much more integrated care across several areas: developmental/puberty; mental health, oral health, vision health, hearing assessment, sexual health nutrition and counselling.* (Portugal)
1.2 There is a pathway in place to access non-urgent specialist care in the community 24/7	Several countries provided examples of good practice regarding access to urgent care in the community, including having 24/7 access to a physician to seek clinical care advice
1.3 Where possible children are cared for by the same doctor and nurse on each consultation	Several countries identified a need for a comprehensive system of care for children with disabilities, which can provide consistent care to children and their families
1.4 Community complex care centres are established where the population and specialist expertise exists to support the child with CCNs and their family	*Centres for complex care [...] to support of the families of children with disabilities and chronic diseases [...] treatment and medical and psychosocial rehabilitation; long-term treatment and rehabilitation [...] education of parents for home-care [...].* (Bulgaria)
1.5 There is technical support in the community to assist parents caring for a child living with CCNs in the home	*The parents together with the transitional care person of the hospital and the social worker discuss and organise all the technical equipment, social support which is needed.* (Austria)

Table 10.1. (*Continued*)

Principles and Standards of Care	Supporting Data of Optimum Practice Identified from MOCHA and Identified Deficits
1.6 Electronic health records are used to support communication and continuity of care across the acute–community interface	*All health care providers should use digital records […] where the next care providers and parents can get an overview of services performed in the past as well as a plan for the future.* (Estonia)
1.7 Children and families have access to community pharmacists	*A community-based pharmacy system exists whereby the pharmacist is part of the primary care team, aware of the child's background and illness.* (Estonia and Portugal)
1.8 A child living with CCNs receives ongoing preventative care screening and developmental checks	61.4% of countries responding have mechanisms in place to support the preventative screening, assessment and referral of children living with CCNs
1.9 The results of all screening are disseminated to all health services caring for the child and communicated to the child's parent(s)/guardian(s)	Half of all countries responding have mechanisms in place to disseminate the results of health screening to providers engaged in the care of children with intractable epilepsy
	Half of all countries responding have mechanisms in place to disseminate the results of all screening to the parent(s)/guardian(s) of children with intractable epilepsy
1.10 Families have access to a transportation service that can enable the child, and their assisted technology devices, to attend daily activities and health and social care visits	Parent(s)/guardian(s) receive assistance from the State and healthcare providers with the daily transport requirements of their children in approximately a quarter of all countries responding
1.11 All information provided to families of children living with CCNs is linguistically appropriate	Over one-third of all countries responding have mechanisms in place to support the provision of linguistically appropriate information material to the families of children living with CCNs

1.12 All information provided to families of children living with CCNs is culturally appropriate

Over one-third of all countries responding have mechanisms in place to support the provision of culturally appropriate information material to the families of children assisted with LTV or with intractable epilepsy

1.13 When a child living with CCNs has a medical crisis there is direct access to, and discharge from, a Paediatric ED and/or a Paediatric Intensive Care Unit

Nearly two-thirds of all countries responding have a process in place which facilitates direct access to/from a Paediatric Intensive Care Unit for children assisted with LTV

1.14 Children have timely assessment for, and access to, rehabilitation services

An excerpt from data highlights some challenges in relation to the provision of rehabilitation services for adolescents following a TBI:

[...] accessibility varies a lot. In several local rehabilitation centres, the staff have very little knowledge about the need for intensive training after a TBI. (Sweden)

1.15 Paediatric palliative care services are available to the child and family when required.

Nearly two-thirds of countries responding have paediatric palliative care services available when required for children assisted with LTV

1.16 Children have timely access to respite care services

The absence of respite care services for children living with CCNs was repeatedly documented as a major concern

1.17 Children have access to diagnostic tests in primary care that enable prevention and early detection of health concerns

More than half of countries responding have mechanisms which support and facilitate preventative screening and developmental assessments for children with intractable epilepsy

Table 10.2. Co-creation of care for children with complex care needs.

Principles and Standards of Care	Supporting Data of Optimum Practice Identified from MOCHA and Identified Deficits
Principle 2: Co-creation of care	
2.1 A discharge planning coordinator is available to the child and family when transitioning from the acute to the community setting	Nearly two-thirds of countries responding have a discharge planning coordinator in place for the transition of an adolescent with a TBI from the acute hospital environment to the community-based setting
2.2 There is a standardised system to identify the clinical support needs for the child transitioning to home	*Parents will be trained in the ICU in tracheostomy care, equipment, medicines etc. by the physicians and nurses in charge prior to their discharge to home.* (Austria)
2.3 Parents are supported to be clinically ready to care for their child at home, in an incremental manner	*[…] the child comes to a step down unit, where the parents share a greater part of care themselves, but know they can always call someone for support […] Only when the parents feel safe and do well, and agree, the child will be discharged to home.* (Austria)
2.4 There is a written personalised plan of care for the child, developed in consultation with the child's parent(s)/guardian(s) and members of the healthcare team	The majority of countries responding develop a written personalised care plan for a child assisted with LTV in consultation with members of the health care teams
2.5 A named care coordinator is appointed to the child living with CCNs and their family to support multidisciplinary engagement and care in the community	A number of countries provided good examples highlighting the importance of the care coordinator role in supporting integration at the acute–community interface
2.6 Family advocacy groups are involved in making recommendations to home and community-based services	Over one-third of all countries responding have input from a family advocacy groups for children following a TBI or children assisted with LTV

2.7 There is a standardised assessment of sibling support needs	*For siblings of children and/or adolescents with TBI there are 'Siblings-days' [...] they get information about TBI and they can share their experiences.* (Netherlands)
2.8 The child, their parent(s)/guardians(s) and siblings have access to psychological support	The majority of countries responding indicated access to psychological support for families from professionals with paediatric expertise
2.9 Children are included in national quality improvement initiatives for their care	Over one-third of all countries responding include the views of children in national quality improvement initiatives
2.10 Data are collected on the child's experience of care	Only one-sixth of all countries responding collect data from adolescents with TBI (where cognition allows)
2.11 Data are collected on the experience of care from the perspectives of parents(s), guardians(s) and siblings	Over one-third of all countries responding collect data on experience of care from the perspective of parent(s)/guardian(s) of children living with CCNs
2.12 A plan of care is prepared with adult healthcare services before an adolescent is transferred from paediatric services	One-third of all responding countries have a plan of care prepared with the adult healthcare service providers prior to the transfer to adult services
2.13 Data are collected on the experience of transitioning from paediatric to adult services from the perspective of the adolescent	No country reported that they collect data on the transition of care of adolescents with a TBI
2.14 Data are collected on the experience of transitioning from paediatric to adult services from the perspective of the parent(s)/guardians(s)	One country reported that they collect data on the experience of transitioning from paediatric to adult services from the perspective of parent(s)/guardian(s) of adolescents with a TBI

Table 10.3. Effective integrated governance for children with complex care needs.

Principle 3: Effective Integrated Governance	
3.1 Primary care providers have access to specialist support when caring for a child living with CCNs	The majority of responding countries indicated that primary care providers routinely have access to specialist support when caring for a child living with CCNs
3.2 Specialist advanced nurse practice roles are developed in the community for the care of children living with CCNs	*Recent developments have included the development of Advance Nurse Practitioner posts in Children's Epilepsy which respondents unanimously agreed was a significant positive move to enhance access to services.* (Ireland)
3.3 There are standardised systems in place for the assessment of the child living with CCNs in the community, including the deteriorating child	This was repeatedly identified as an issue of potential inequity in access to, and delivery of, care to these children and their families
3.4 There are standardised processes for the clinical handover of the child living with CCNs to and from acute care services	Very few countries indicated any evidence of a strategic and systemic network to co-ordinate care. Where reported, this seemed dependent on personal and professional relationships
3.5 There is systematic identification of all health and social care providers who care for a child living with CCNs	Over one-third of all countries responding have a system in place that can identify all of the healthcare providers caring for children living with CCNs
3.6 There is systematic identification of all voluntary agencies who care for children living with CCNs	The role of the voluntary sector in providing primary care services was widely viewed as an increasing ad hoc network, requiring governance to ensure quality of care delivery
3.7 There is a system in place to govern all care delivery to the child living with CCNs in the home	The majority of countries responding reported challenges in governance of care in the home and suggested that a national strategy on the management of children on LTV would begin to address many of the issues raised

3.8 There is specialist training in the care of children with CCNs for primary care providers caring for these children and their families	Inadequate education of nursing staff to provide care was repeatedly reported as a significant challenge to the provision of optimum care
3.9 There is appropriate education for all social care staff caring for children living with CCNs	Inadequate training of social care staff was repeatedly reported as a significant challenge to the provision of optimum care
3.10 There is a retention policy for skilled healthcare staff who care for children living with CCNs	Training and retention of skilled healthcare staff was identified as a key facilitator for the integration of care across all exemplar complex conditions
3.11 There is a national data base of children living with CCNs	National databases of children living with CCNs were repeatedly identified as necessary to support optimum integration of care for children living with CCNs
3.12 Quality assurance mechanisms are in place for service providers caring for children living with CCNs	Over one-third of all countries responding indicated that they have mechanisms in place to support quality assurance
3.13 There are cross-border initiatives in place where no specialist centre exists nationally for children living with CCNs	Given the variance in the specialist care, the needs of children living with CCNs across the EU/EEA cross-border specialist healthcare initiatives were identified as a critical part of the healthcare infrastructure to support access to care, particularly for island nations
3.14 There are national integrated care programmes in place to support care delivery at the acute–community interface	The establishment of integrated care programmes was one of the most significant changes to occur during the last five years in relation to integration of care for all exemplar complex conditions
3.15 There is a school health system to support the child living with CCNs	The absence of a structured school health system was identified as a barrier to equitable access to education for children living with CCNs across the EU/EEA

Table 10.3. (*Continued*)

Principle 3: Effective Integrated Governance	
3.16 There is appropriate training for school teachers and education support staff when a child is living with CCNs	The introduction of specialised training for school teachers was identified as a significant and positive trend across the EU/EEA
3.17 There is special reference to promoting the welfare of children with disabilities within wider child protection legislation	In some countries, the welfare of children with disabilities is promoted within the wider child protection legislation; other countries aspire to this to support the care of children living with CCNs
3.18 There is safeguarding training for children with communication difficulties for all health and social care staff	Training for professionals to communicate with individuals with disabilities that impact on their communication, as well as online peer-support for professionals, is available in a small number of countries

complex care (using UML) and a mixed-methods study conducted by Murdoch Children's Research Institute in Australia, which was conducted in collaboration with the MOCHA project. The range of methods and perspectives used adds to the understanding of the complex and multi-faceted topic of care for complex mental health conditions.

Autism spectrum disorder (ASD) and attention deficit hyperactivity disorder (ADHD) were selected as tracer mental health conditions, as they are charac-terised by their persistent care needs across the specialised and general psychi-atric, medical and social services (Lai, Lombardo, & Baron-Cohen, 2013; Thapar & Cooper, 2015). The main part of our investigation consisted of a mixed-methods study of 30 European countries to collect survey data and quali-tative commentary from key informants in each country (see Chapter 1). The questionnaire was composed of patient vignettes and the adapted from the Standards for Systems of Care for Children and Youth with Special Health Care Needs and Complex Care European Survey of Change (Association of Maternal and Child Health Programs and Lucile Packard Foundation for Children's Health, 2014). The analysis of the qualitative responses from the MOCHA CAs was conducted to identify basic, organising and global themes that influence the interface of primary care. The methodology adopted in studying the manage-ment of children and adolescents with complex mental healthcare conditions is described in full in Kamionka and Taylor (2017).

Key Themes Influencing Care for Children with Enduring Mental Health Needs at the Primary Care Interface

The results from this study fall into two main domains: firstly, relating to coord-ination within multidisciplinary structures, and secondly, relating to attitudes and awareness within the wider societal context. The public and political context provides the framework within which organisations, practitioners and parents must operate when providing and supporting services, communicating with each other and advocating for a child's care (see also Chapters 16 and 17). Access to appropriate care, parental involvement and multidisciplinary expertise were identified as the key interrelated factors facilitating and being facilitated by coordination. This is illustrated in Figure 10.1.

We developed a business process model (UML) to illustrate some of the key processes and complexity involved in the care of children with ADHD and ASD, highlighting the actors and level of collaboration involved both in provid-ing health and social care preventive screening and developmental checks, and in the development and implementation of a written personalised plan. Our ana-lysis suggests that collaboration is more developed for the care of children on the autistic spectrum than for children with ADHD and for health care more than for social care. This is illustrated in Figure 10.2.

Key principles in providing care for children with complex mental health needs from multiple perspectives were derived under three main principles; access to care, parental involvement and multidisciplinary.

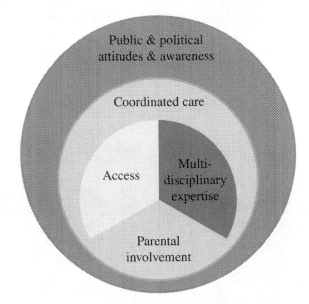

Figure 10.1. Model of key themes influencing the care of children with enduring mental health needs at the primary care interface.

Access to Care

Children with complex mental healthcare issues are in need of multi-faceted care services, and this premise was acknowledged across all of the EU/EEA countries. Thus, the term access to care covers the area of availability of specialist at a knowledge-based and a structural level. Access to care includes equity of access to normal primary care and other services for children with an identified mental health condition. This proved to be a strong theme as services for both ADHD and ASD suffered from a shortage of specialist care at different points during the care continuum.

- *Ongoing screening and developmental checks should be provided regardless of detected mental health conditions.* Several countries responded that these children are not necessarily are being offered ongoing screening and developmental checks. Many reported that elements regarding developmental health were incorporated into the personalised written plan of care but there was no consensus on which elements of development health should be included.
- *Care provision should be accessible regardless of the geographic location of the child and family.* The vast majority of the countries described geographic differences where clustering of services and expertise in some regions leave other regions with less coverage.
- *Care services to supporting children with mental health conditions should be in place in primary, secondary and social care.* Across the EU/EEA countries, it was widely recognised that the care services should exist across all the care

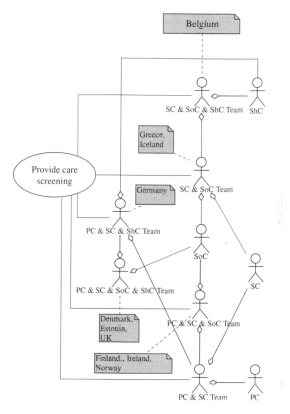

Figure 10.2. An Example of UML use of case diagram: provision of screening services for children with autism. *Notes*: PC = primary care professionals; SC = secondary care; SoC = social care; ShC = school care.

sectors. 'More community-based services are needed in order to provide suitable care for children with autism. Additionally, healthcare providers with specific knowledge under the spectrum of autism are required for the optimal care of children with autism'. (Cyprus, ASD).

- *Access to care should follow a stepped care approach.* Most countries reported following a stepped care approach in providing care which places primary care in a central role.
- *Consideration should be given to the regional differences of young people and their families.* A range of feedback highlighted the need to incorporate the differences in culture and structure of families and local communities. [...] *Family centred services should be an important part of the organisation and development of all services. However, as yet there is limited formal implementation of family centred services in the country* (Iceland, ASD).
- *Care pathways should be put in place to support care delivery at the interface between services.* Most countries noted the difficulties in providing care across sectors. Three countries reported to have specific care pathways for children

with either ADHD or ASD. The rest had only partially developed pathways or no pathways at all. Of those who care pathways, few had clearly described roles for the different care providers.

- *There should be a review of fee-based care, which can act as a barrier to accessing care for low-income families.* Several countries reported to have fee-based care systems, especially in secondary and tertiary care. This was not noted in the Scandinavian countries.
- *Transparent referral procedures support continuity of care.* This is necessary to support safe care given the number of people involved in care provision.
- *Attention to transition between services and/or lifespan changes are a part of the personal care plan of every child with mental health conditions.* The vast majority reported not to have policies or procedures to ensure continuity of care when transitioning to adult services. Many countries identified lack of knowledge about the persistent nature of ADHD as a barrier to continuity of care in this transition period.
- *Political awareness and collaboration is necessary to facilitate access to different services.* Nearly all of the EU/EEA countries reported that there is a long-standing problem of disinterest and a lack of political awareness of ASD and ADHD which was identified as a barrier in ensuring care services. Nonetheless several countries state that public and political awareness has increased within the last five years.

Parental Involvement

As part of co-creation of care, it is important that parents, and where possible, the child, are involved in any care plan and supported to carry out that plan in a practical manner. We asked about particular means by which this can be achieved.

- *Parents should be included as partners in their child's care.* Parental involvement was consistently identified as key to insuring, facilitating and coordinating care.
- *Parents should receive information about their child's care in a linguistically and culturally appropriate manner.* It was widely agreed across EU/EEA countries that this linguistic or culturally appropriate information was not prioritised. However, parents/guardians of children with ASD were in general more involved in reviewing materials than parents/guardians of children with ADHD.
- *The families of children with mental health conditions should be provided with psychosocial support.* There was consensus about the need for parents and sibling of children with ASD and ADHD to receive psychosocial support.
- *Parents and parent advocacy groups should be invited to participate in the development of policies and procedures affecting their child.* The specialist knowledge of parent and parent advocacy groups about the children's care needs was broadly recognised between the countries as facilitator in ensuring better care services and increase awareness.

- *Parents should be provided with an overview of the skill set of the caregiver caring for their child, and of their specific professional role.* An overview of caregivers was identified as supporting the care plan.
- *Parents should be provided with an overview of all possible accessible care services.* Parents/guardians were identified as the main help seeker and care facilitator.
- *Parents should have a voice in quality assurance at regional and national level.* Parents were identified as crucial in assessing quality. It was found that parents, and parent advocacy groups, of children with ASD positively influenced a focus on quality assurance.

Multidisciplinary Teams

The care provided to children with ASD or ADHD involves many different healthcare and social care professionals located in several different settings. This study identified considerable evidence that good communication between multidisciplinary teams improves outcomes for the child and facilitates better working conditions for the service providers. In the context of CCNs for those with long-term mental health conditions, we identified a number of key facilitating factors.

- *There needs to be a level of knowledge regarding childhood mental health conditions which should be insured, both with regard to the health and social care aspects of treatment.* The basis for multidisciplinary teams' collaboration was a commonly shared knowledge and there was a clear tendency among the EU/EEA countries that the level of knowledge was lacking, particular in social services. Gaps in knowledge of mental health conditions was identified across the EU/EEA for health and social care professionals.
- *Responsibilities between caregivers should be clearly communicated and coordinated.* Many countries stated difficulties in insuring continuity of care across sectors because of a lack of or undefined cross-sectoral communication and coordination.
- *A personalised care plan should be accessible for all professionals who are involved in the child's care, across both sectors and services.* Due to the multifaceted care needs, every country in the study had identified several care providers. The written care plan was the main shared document which could facilitate communication and coordination between professionals.
- *The results of screening and assessments should be accessible for all caregivers.* Many countries reported that their healthcare professionals corresponded on assessments, however few countries reported that reports were shared with social care services.
- *Professionals across sectors should be included as partners in regional and national quality assurance initiatives.* In general, the healthcare sector was more influential at national level than social care.
- *A standard for the multidisciplinary approach in care provision for children with mental health conditions should be encouraged as it would heighten the degree of coordination between healthcare and social care services.* Despite the different structures across the EU/EEA countries, all aimed at incorporating a

multidisciplinary approach in the care provision. (The different organisations can be seen in the UML diagram.)

- *Primary care providers should have specialised training in the care and treatment of children with mental health conditions.* Nearly every country had primary care — mainly the GPs — as gatekeepers to care. *Mostly family physicians/GPs or primary care paediatricians [are responsible for providing general health care to these children] (but most of them have very little knowledge about the treatment of such kids)*, Lithuania, ADHD.
- *Social care providers should also have specialised training in the care and treatment of children with mental health conditions.* Many countries identified a gap in specialist knowlege in social care.
- *All personnel involved in the treatment of children with mental health conditions should have training in the coordination of care packages.*
- *School health systems should provide specialised training and need to be able to support and educate the child with a mental health condition.* Many countries identified schools as a central scene for both identification of the child's mental health needs and the place for providing community-based care. Many countries identified specialised trained professionals in schools as a scarce yet highly important resource.

Summary

Children with CCNs and their families place great challenges on health and social care delivery for many reasons: they require dynamic and responsive health and social care over a long period of time; they require organisational and delivery coordination functions; health issues such as minor illnesses, which are normally presented to primary care and must be addressed in the context of the complex health issues; and finally. Our collective findings in MOCHA are that the existing integration of health and social care services is generally found to be insufficient, with wide variation in access to, and governance of, care for these children. It is acknowledged that some initiatives are beginning in this area across the EU; however, there remain extensive challenges. These include communication of a child and family's needs at the acute—community interface, confusion over points of accessing care and no defined system of documenting care needs and care delivery in a manner that can be accessible for the family and the multidisciplinary team when families cross between acute and community care services. There is a small window of opportunity in a child's life to address key issues of care that can have a positive or negative influence on subsequent adaptation and coping by a child living with CCNs and their family. This need for timeliness in care transcends the principles and standards developed, cognisant of the initial need for a timely transition to home when a child has CCNs, the ongoing importance of timely assessment of needs, the timely identification of any deterioration and the timely management of care to support transitions to end-of-life care.

Similarly, children with complex mental health conditions face challenges due to the fragmentation of the continuum of care delivery across primary /

secondary care and across the health and social care sector. In most European countries, the structure of care is moving towards more specialisation in both the health and social care systems, which have increased needs for a comprehensive coordination of services and a higher demand for specialists in mental health care. In addition, the gaps in the continuum of care also stem from the limited availability of services for children and young people with mental health problems. Thus, the barriers to care delivery are not only rooted in clinical complexities, but also rooted in complexity at the meso-level of service design. A general lack of public and political awareness of mental health disorders can hinder the development of optimal cross-sectoral care pathways. Fundamental to the discussion regarding optimal care integration for children with complex mental health needs are issues specific to the exemplar conditions, as described, but further, these are also indicative of issues relating to mental health in general, in contrast with physical health. The care of children with mental health conditions depends on the discipline and perspective of clinicians, who are reliant on less demonstrable, externally measurable symptoms, resulting in a wider variety of possible treatment pathways. Care pathways in mental health are therefore very different from in physical health, where tangible symptoms can be measured. The multiple subjective perspectives as to the causal factors of childhood mental health problems and the subsequent impact of these perspectives in the preferred treatment options make uniformity in mental health service coordination problematic. However, the core principles of involvement of families in treatment, coherent transitions, multi-agency working and specialist training for professionals involved in the care of children will all benefit the improvement of care coordination and ultimately benefit the experience of children and their families.

References

Association of Maternal and Child Health Programs and Lucile Packard Foundation for Children's Health. (2014). *Standards for systems of care for children and youth with special health care needs.* Washington: Association of Maternal and Child Health Programs. Washington. Retrieved from https://www.lpfch.org/publication/standards-systems-care-children-and-youth-special-health-care-needs

Brenner, M., Alma, M., Clancy, A., Larkin, P., Lignou, S., Luzi, D., ... Blair, M. (2017a). *Report on needs and future visions for care of children with complex conditions.* Retrieved from http://www.childhealthservicemodels.eu/wpcontent/uploads/20171130_Deliverable-D11-2.4-Report-on-needs-andfuture-visions-for-care-of-children-with-complex-conditions.pdf

Brenner, M., O'Shea, M., & Larkin, P. (2017b). *Final report on the current approach to managing the care of children with complex care needs.* Brussels: EU Commission. Retrieved from http://www.childhealthservicemodels.eu/publications/deliverables/. Accessed on September 5, 2018.

Brenner, M., O'Shea, M. P., Larkin, P., Luzi, D., Pecoraro, F., Tamburis, O., ... Blair, M. (2018a). Management and integration of care for children living with complex care needs at the acute—community interface in Europe. *Lancet Child and Adolescent Health, 2*(E11), 822—831. doi:10.1016/S2352-4642(18)30272-4

Brenner, M., O'Shea, M. P., McHugh, R., Clancy, A., Larkin, P., Luzi, D., … Blair, M. (2018b). Principles for provision of integrated complex care for children across the acute—community interface in Europe. *Lancet Child and Adolescent Health, 2*(11), 832—838. doi:10.1016/S2352-4642(18)30270-0

Clancy, A., Montañana-Olaso, E., & Larkin, P. (2017). Nursing preparedness for practice. In M. Brenner, M. Alma, A. Clancy, P. Larkin, S. Lignou, D. Luzi, … M. Blair (Eds.), *Report on needs and future visions for care of children with complex conditions*. Brussels: EU Commission. Retrieved from http://www.child-healthservicemodels.eu/wp-content/uploads/20171130_Deliverable-D11-2.4-Report-on-needs-and-future-visions-for-care-ofchildren-with-complex-conditions.pdf

Kamionka, S. L., & Taylor, K. (2017). *Report on requirements and models for supporting children with complex mental health needs and the primary care interface.* Retrieved from http://www.childhealthservicemodels.eu/wp-content/uploads/2017/07/20171130_Deliverable-D10-2.3-Report-on-requirements-and-models-for-supporting-children-with-complex-mental-health-needs-and-the-primary-care-interface.pdf

Keilthy, P., Warters, A., Brenner, M., & McHugh, R. (2017). *Final report on models of children's social care support across the EU and the relationship with primary health care.* Retrieved from http://www.childhealthservicemodels.eu/wpcontent/uploads/2017/07/20170728_Deliverable-D9-2.2-Final-report-onmodels-of-hildren%E2%80%99s-social-care-support-across-the-EU-and-the-relationship-with-primary-health-care.pdf

Lai, M., Lombardo, M. V., & Baron-Cohen, S. (2013). Autism. *Lancet, 383*(9920), 896—910. doi:10.1016/S0140-6736(13)61539-1

Luzi, D., Pecoraro, F., & Tamburis, O. (2017). Appraising Healthcare Delivery Provision: A Framework to Model Business Processes. *Studies in health technology and informatics* 235, 511—515.

Thapar, A., & Cooper, M. (2015). Attention deficit hyperactivity disorder. *Lancet, 387*(10024), 1240—1250. doi:10.1016/S0140-6736(15)00238-X

Wolfe, I., Lignou, S., & Satherley, R. M. (2017). Referral—discharge interface. InM. Brenner, M. Alma, A. Clancy, P. Larkin, S. Lignou, D. Luzi, … M. Blair (Eds.), *Report on needs and future visions for care of children with complex conditions.* Retrieved from http://www.childhealthservicemodels.eu/wpcontent/uploads/20171130_Deliverable-D11-2.4-Report-on-needsand-future-visions-for-care-of-children-with-complex-conditions.pdf

Chapter 11

School Health Services

Danielle Jansen, Johanna P. M. Vervoort, Annemieke Visser,
Sijmen A. Reijneveld, Paul Kocken, Gaby de Lijster and
Pierre-André Michaud

Abstract

Models of Child Health Appraised (MOCHA) defines school health services (SHSs) as those that exist due to a formal arrangement between educational institutions and primary health care. SHSs are unique in that they are designed exclusively to address the needs of children and adolescents in this age group and setting.

We investigated SHSs have been provided to schools and how they contribute to primary healthcare services for school children. We did this by mapping the national school health systems against the standards of the World Health Organization, and against a framework measuring the strength of primary care, adapting this from an existing, adult-focused framework.

We found that all but two countries in the European Union and European Economic Area have SHSs. There, however, remains a need for much greater investment in the professional workforce to run the services, including training to ensure appropriateness and acceptability to young people. Greater collaboration between SHSs and primary care services would lead to better coordination and the potential for better health (and educational) outcomes. Involving young people and families in the design of SHSs and as participants in its outputs would also improve school health.

Keywords: School health services; children; adolescents; primary care; Europe, organization, content

Introduction

School Health Service (SHS) is an important aspect of primary care for children. We define SHS as health services provided to enrolled pupils by healthcare professionals and/or allied professionals, such as social workers, health visitors, counsellors, psychologists and dental hygienists, irrespective of the site of service provision. The services should be mandated by a formal arrangement between the educational institution and the provider healthcare organisation (Baltag & Saewyc, 2017). SHS generally focuses on promoting and protecting health and well-being, early diagnosis, preventing and controlling of diseases of pupils. SHS can be school-based, community-based or integrated in primary care. There are two countries that do not have SHS. This does however not mean that these two countries do not have health services for school age children at all. These two countries have only organized the health services for children in a different way; for example via other healthcare providers or healthcare organizations in primary care, that are often closely linked to the school system. Because valuing health services for school age children not provided by SHS professionals is not the aim of this part of the study, we are not able to provide an evaluation of this kind of care.

SHSs play a number of different roles:

- SHSs have the opportunity to reach a large group of pupils and influence their health behaviour during different stages of life (Baltag, Pachyna, & Hall, 2015; Bersamin, Garbers, Gaarde, & Santelli, 2016).
- Evidence exists that when SHSs are available, pupils are more likely to access health care and thus eliminate barriers to access to care (Anderson & Lowen, 2010; Bains & Diallo, 2016; Bersamin et al., 2016).
- High-quality SHS is related to positive health and educational outcomes in disadvantaged pupils (Bersamin et al., 2016; Knopf et al., 2016).
- SHS may have an important role in supporting children with chronic illnesses, such as diabetes. Integrating care needs of these children may help pupils to stay at school and prevent missing school (Leroy, Wallin, & Lee, 2017). SHS might also reduce the use of other healthcare services such as emergency care or hospitalisation (Bersamin et al., 2016).

In this chapter, we present the comparison of MOCHA findings on SHS with the WHO quality standards in SHS and competence for SHS professionals (Hoppenbrouwers et al., 2014).

Methods

Data on SHS were collected in 30 European countries from the MOCHA country agents. These data describe the organisational structure and process of functioning of health systems. Data collection comprised a number of steps. We first adapted the Primary Health Care Activity Monitor for Europe (PHAMEU) framework for primary care for adults to SHS for children and adolescents (Jansen et al., 2018). The original PHAMEU framework focuses on primary care for the general population, whereas the framework applicable for the MOCHA project has to focus especially on primary care for children and adolescents. In accordance with the PHAMEU framework, the organisational structure of SHS is divided into three structure dimensions: governance, economic conditions and workforce development and in four process delivery dimensions: access, continuity, coordination and comprehensiveness. Each dimension is detailed in features that are in turn specified into indicators.

In order to adapt the structure and process dimensions of the PHAMEU framework into a framework applicable for exploring health systems for children and adolescents, we undertook two steps: (1) we reviewed the literature on structure and process dimensions for SHS and (2) we discussed the results of step 1 with experts and asked them which dimensions, features or indicators to add to or remove from the PHAMEU-framework in order to make it more applicable for children and adolescents. This resulted in the adjusted PHAMEU framework applicable for children and adolescents.

Based on this adjusted PHAMEU framework, we collected data on the dimensions across 30 European countries via the MOCHA country agents and from existing databases. We analysed the data in order to describe the organisational structure in the 30 countries. In the final step, we compared our data with that of the WHO for quality standards in SHS and competence for SHS professionals (Hoppenbrouwers et al., 2014). The framework consists of standards that are assumed to be beneficial for the health of school-aged children and adolescents.

The main quality standards are as follows:

- *Standard 1*: an intersectoral national or regional normative framework involving the ministries of health and education and based on children's rights is in place to advice on the content and conditions of service delivery of SHS.
- *Standard 2*: SHSs respect the principles, characteristics and quality dimensions of child- and adolescent-friendly health services and apply them in a manner that is appropriate to children and adolescents at all developmental stages and in all age groups. Principles of accessibility, equity and acceptability also apply to the way in which SHSs engage with parents.
- *Standard 3*: SHS facilities, equipment, staffing and data management systems are sufficient to enable SHS to achieve their objectives.
- *Standard 4*: collaboration between SHS, teachers, school administration, parents and children, and local community actors (including healthcare providers) is established and respective responsibilities are clearly defined.
- *Standard 5*: SHS staff have clearly defined job descriptions, adequate competences and a commitment to achieving SHS quality standards.
- *Standard 6*: a package of SHS services based on priority public health concerns is defined, supported by evidence-informed protocols and guidelines. The service package encompasses population-based approaches, including health promotion in the school setting, and services developed on an approach based on individual needs.

- *Standard 7*: a data management system that facilitates the safe storage and retrieval of individual health records, monitoring of health trends, assessment of SHS quality (structure and activities) and research is in place. Additional specifications are listed below, where appropriate.

We collected data on the most essential features and indicators of SHSs by means of two questionnaires, which were sent at two different time points (July 2016 and April 2017). The aim of the two questionnaires was to develop a good understanding of the most essential features and indicators of the MOCHA-adapted PHAMEU framework regarding SHS.

The first questionnaire was a replication of a previously conducted European-wide survey, which was carried out by the World Health Organization in 2009 (Baltag & Levi, 2013; World Health Organization, 2010a). The aim of the replication study was to understand how SHS is organised in 2016 and the differences in the two time points.

A second questionnaire was sent to the country agents, which asked additional questions that were not part of the first questionnaire. The second questionnaire asked about issues such as governance, organisation and service delivery models, staffing, content of the SHS and main challenges each country faced in the organisation and delivery of SHS.

Results

Functions of School Health Services

Of the 30 EU/EEA countries, all have SHS, except for Spain and Czech Republic. In terms of health priorities, all countries' SHSs considered lifestyle-related issues to be a priority for pupils. These included subjects such as physical activity, healthy eating and tackling substance abuse. SHSs are involved in the development and implementation of specific programmes to improve children's health and discuss these issues. In the following text, we present the comparison of the MOCHA findings with the WHO framework for SHS (Hoppenbrouwers et al., 2014).

How School Health Services Are Governed and Organised

In the majority of the countries, the development of what is described by the WHO Framework as the 'content and scope', 'workforce' and 'funding' of SHS is a shared responsibility of national and local, and health and education authorities (Standard 1). The involvement of both sectors and both levels (national and local) is important for successful SHSs. National health and educational authorities may provide political and financial support and facilitate the development and implementation of SHS. The regional or local health and educational authorities can tailor the service to the needs of the local population and thereby increase responsiveness. Involvement of both levels may therefore take the best of both, but needs also coordination and good dialogue between authorities (World Health Organization, 2010b). In addition, almost half of the countries had a policy to ensure that SHS facilities, equipment, staffing and data management systems are sufficient to enable SHS to achieve their objectives.

Equity and Access
In the countries that have SHS, theoretically we can assume that most pupils have access to health services in schools. In the majority of the participating countries, there were no great variations in SHS between regions and there are often national regulations for SHS, which means that if followed, equity of access is increased. We also asked the MOCHA country agents to identify the policies on school dropouts and on vulnerable pupils in their country. Half of the countries had a comprehensive policy: in most cases, this existed as inter-professional meetings to discuss school absenteeism and dropout, guidelines for schools to improve integration and education of pupils and opportunity for vulnerable pupils or pupils who drop out to see a doctor.

The accessibility of SHS may be influenced by the way it is organised: SHS can be school-based, a distinct structure in the health system, or offered by providers in primary care. In most countries SHS provision is a mixture of types or organisation. For example, school based mixed with primary care involvement in countries like Estonia, Finland and Poland or a distinct structure mixed with primary care involvement in countries like Germany, Ireland and Portugal. Baltag and Levi (2013) hypothesised that the proximity of SHS to the children (school-based SHS) may increase accessibility of SHS. Table 11.1 shows the indicators of access to SHSs.

Quality Assurance
Quality management infrastructure contains a number of mechanisms that need to be in place to assure adequate quality of care. In more than half of the countries, quality management infrastructure is safeguarded by working with clinical recommendations, regulation and/or standard sets, as reflected in the WHO framework Standard 2 principle effectiveness. In most of these countries, the quality recommendations or standards were performed by SHS themselves or by external inspection. It was less common for the results of the quality assessments to be published. A limitation of the MOCHA investigation was that we could only ask about the presence or absence of standards, but not the type or aim of the existing standards and therefore have no information on the quality of the standards.

Collaboration
SHS tasks are very complex and comprehensive, and for them to work effectively, it requires good collaboration between professionals, for example with other primary healthcare professionals. The WHO Standard 4 (Hoppenbrouwers et al., 2014) aims to encourage and highlight collaboration between SHS professionals, teachers, school administration, parents and children and local community actors (including other healthcare providers). The MOCHA study focused on cooperation between SHS and other forms of primary care services, for which in about

Table 11.1. Essential indicators of access of SHS.

Country	National Availability of SHS					Geographic Access	
	Healthcare Providers[a]	Time SHS Providers Spent in School	Possibility of Individual Contact from School Entry to Graduation	Organisation of SHS Provision[b]	Room Available for Use by School Health Personnel	Shortage of SHS Staff	
Austria	Doctor	Half time bigger schools/regularly to once a year	Once a year	Distinct	Partly	some
	Other	Once a year				
Belgium-F	Nurse/other	Once/twice a week	As often as needed/	Distinct	Yes and no	Some
	Doctor	On demand	3–9 times			
Belgium-W	Nurse	Once/twice a week	As often as needed/	Distinct	Yes and no	Some
	Doctor/other	On demand	3–9 times			
Bulgaria	Nurse	Once/twice a week	As often as needed	School based/ PC	Yes	Some
	Doctor	Depends on no pupils				
Croatia	Nurse/doctor	Once/twice a week	As often as needed	Distinct	No	Some
Cyprus	Nurse/doctor/ other	Once/twice a week	3–9 times	Distinct	Yes	Some
Czech Republic	Not applicable	Not applicable	Not applicable	Not applicable	Not applicable	Some

Denmark	Nurse/doctor/ other	Depends on no pupils	As often as needed/ 3–9 times	School based	Yes	Some
Estonia	Nurse	Depends on no pupils	Once a year	School based/ PC	No	Some
Finland	Nurse/doctor Other	Part time	As often as needed/ once a year	School based/ PC	Yes	Some
France	Nurse Other	–	As often as needed/ three times or less	School based/ distinct	No	Some
Germany	Doctor Other	Part time	3–9 times	Distinct/PC	Yes	Some
Greece	Other	–	3–9 times	PC	No	–
Hungary	Nurse/doctor	Once/twice a week	3–9 times	School based/ PC	Yes	Some
Iceland	Nurse Doctor	Depends on no pupils (> 800) Once a year	As often as needed	School based	Yes	Some
Ireland	Nurse/doctor	Once/twice a month	3–9 times	Distinct/PC	Yes	Some
Italy	Doctor/other	–	3–9 times	Distinct/PC	No	Some
Latvia	Nurse/other Doctor	Fulltime Part time	As often as needed	School based/ PC	Yes	Some
Lithuania	Nurse	Depends on no pupils	As often as needed	School based/ PC	Yes	Some

Table 11.1. (*Continued*)

Country	National Availability of SHS					Geographic Access
	Healthcare Providers[a]	Time SHS Providers Spent in School	Possibility of Individual Contact from School Entry to Graduation	Organisation of SHS Provision[b]	Room Available for Use by School Health Personnel	Shortage of SHS Staff
Luxembourg	Nurse/medical doctor/social worker	–	As often as needed/ 3–9 times	Distinct/PC	Yes	Severe
Malta	Nurse/doctor/ other	Once/twice a month	3–9 times	Distinct/PC	Yes	Severe
Netherlands	Nurse, Doctor Other	Time spent differ	As often as needed	Distinct	No	Some
Norway	Nurse/doctor Other	Part time	3–9 times	School based	Yes	Severe
Poland	Nurse Other	Fulltime (>800), part time (>400), once/twice a week (<400)	As often as needed/ 3–9 times	School based/ PC	Yes	Some
Portugal	Nurse Doctor/other	Once/twice a week Once/twice a month	As often as needed/ at least five times/ year	Distinct/PC	Yes	Some

	Nurse/doctor/some dentist	Full/part time depends on no pupils	As often as needed	School based/PC	Yes	Some (severe in rural and small cities)
Romania	Nurse/doctor/some dentist	Full/part time depends on no pupils	As often as needed	School based/PC	Yes	Some (severe in rural and small cities)
Slovakia	Doctor/other	Full or part time/on demand	As often as needed	PC	No	Severe
Slovenia	Doctor/other	Periodically	As often as needed	Distinct	Yes	Severe
Spain*	Not applicable	Not applicable	Not applicable	Not applicable	Not applicable	—
Sweden	Nurse/doctor/other	Depends on no pupils	As often as needed	School based	Yes	Some
UK ENG	NA	—	As often as needed	School based/distinct/PC	Yes	Adequate
UK NI	—	—	—	—	—	—

[a]**Nurse** School nurse, **Doctor** School doctor, **Other** Other health care providers, such as health care assistant

[b]**School based** SHS is based in schools, **Distinct** SHS is a distinct structure, SHS personnel not based in schools, **PC** SHS offered by primary health care providers

*Spain: Health care for school-aged children in Spain (curative, preventive and health promotion issues) is integrated into primary care services and coordinated with the school system, although it is not formally a School Health System

half of the countries, formal national recommendations were formulated. Some countries have regulations for the exchange of information between SHS and other healthcare professionals, and some countries have formal agreements on cooperation and division of tasks between the different services. Half of the countries do have formal recommendations that support inter-professional working within SHS.

Tasks, Roles and Competence of SHS Staff

Standard 5 of the WHO framework states the need for SHS professionals to have job descriptions, competences and a commitment to achieve SHS quality standards. In MOCHA, this standard was operationalised by paying attention to composition of the SHS team, existence of job descriptions, knowledge and skills of SHS providers and the ratio of SHS provider-to-pupil.

In the vast majority of the participating countries, SHS is provided by a multidisciplinary team of health professionals, consisting most often of at least a school nurse and a school doctor. In almost half of the countries, this team is supplemented by other types of health professionals. We found no norms in the literature regarding the composition of the most effective SHS teams, but we did so regarding the important role of the school nurse (Council on School Health, 2008).

SHS providers have a clearly defined and written job description in more than half of the countries. We do not know whether this description distinguishes only task and roles of SHS providers or also describes their contact and communication with primary care services, which is – according to the WHO (2010b) – also an important aspect of a good functioning SHS. Table 11.2 shows the essential indicators of the school health workforce (see also Chapter 13).

Baltag and Levi (2013) hypothesised the importance of dedicated school health personnel, referring to experienced and trained healthcare providers who are also perceived by children and adolescents as familiar and accessible. The knowledge and skills of SHS providers are acknowledged as important factors to enable the SHS to function optimally (Hoppenbrouwers et al., 2014). SHS providers in only one-third of the countries were reported to be adequately trained, and specialisation in SHS is required for employment in only half of the countries. SHS providers in one-third of the countries have access to supervision and feedback on their performance.

In most countries, information on the ratio of SHS provider-to-pupil was not available or depended on the size of school. This variable was therefore not easy to translate to a national level. All countries indicated that there is a shortage of SHS personnel, in some cases, severe. The American Academy of Paediatricians recommends a full-time school nurse in every school, a ratio of one school nurse per 750 students and a strong partnership among school nurses, school physicians, other school health personnel and paediatricians (Council on School Health, 2008), something that does not seem to be often achieved in Europe.

Table 11.2. Essential indicators of workforce in school health services.

Country	Type of SHS Providers		Tasks and Role of SHS Providers in Medical Care and as Liaison			Professional Status	Trained and Competent Staff			
	SHS providers[1]	Working in a team	Tasks in medical care[2]	Availability of mental health emergencies[3]	Liaison role is clearly defined[4]	Clearly defined jobs	Adequate, somewhat or not trained	Training in emergency care[5]	Specialisation SHS is needed for employment	Access to supervision and feedback on performance
Austria	B/C/D/E/H	No	Acute/chronic	B/C/D	t/p/c	Partly	Somewhat	1/2/3/4	No	No
Belgium-F	A/B/C/D	Yes	Chronic	No	t/p	–	Somewhat	–	Yes[6]	–
Belgium-W	A/B/C/D	Yes	Chronic	–	t/p	–	Somewhat	–	Yes[6]	–
Bulgaria	A/B	Yes	Acute	Onsite help	No	Yes	Somewhat	–	No	Yes
Croatia	A/B/D	Yes	Chronic	No	t/p/h/c	Yes	Adequate	1/2/3	Yes	Yes
Cyprus	A/B/D	Yes	No	C	No	Yes	Adequate	1/3	Yes[7]	No
Czech R	Not applicable	Not applicable	Not applicable	Not applicable	Not applicable	Not applicable	Not applicable	Not applicable	Not applicable	Not applicable
Denmark	A/B/C/E/F	No	No	–	p	No	Adequate	NA	Yes	No
Estonia	A	No	Chronic	Onsite help	h	No	Somewhat	1/2/3	No	No
Finland	A/B/D	Yes	All tasks	B	t/p/h/c	Yes	Somewhat	1/2/3	Yes	Yes
France	A/B/G	Yes	Med/chronic	–	t/p/h/c	Yes	Adequate	NA	Yes	Yes
Germany	E/H	No	No	No	No	No	Somewhat	–	No	No
Greece	H	–	No	C	–	Yes	–	1/2/3	No	No
Hungary	A/B/E	NA	Acute/chronic	No	h	Yes	Somewhat	1/2/3	Yes	No

Table 11.2. (Continued)

Country	Type of SHS Providers		Tasks and Role of SHS Providers in Medical Care and as Liaison			Professional Status		Trained and Competent Staff		
	SHS providers[1]	Working in a team	Tasks in medical care[2]	Availability of mental health emergencies[3]	Liaison role is clearly defined[4]	Clearly defined jobs	Adequate, somewhat or not trained	Training in emergency care[5]	Specialisation SHS is needed for employment	Access to supervision and feedback on performance
Iceland	A/B	No	All tasks	No	t/p/h	Yes	Somewhat	1/2/3	No	Yes
Ireland	A/B/E	Yes	Acute (only dentist)	No	t/p/h	Yes	Somewhat	3	No	Yes
Italy	H	Yes	No	C/D	t/p/h/c	No	Adequate	3	No	No
Latvia	A/B	No	All tasks	No	No	No	Somewhat	1/2/3/4	Yes	Differs
Lithuania	A/H	Yes	Acute/chronic	No	t/h/c	No	Somewhat	1/2/3	No	No
Luxembourg	A/B/D/E	NA	Chronic	Onsite help	p/h	Yes	Somewhat	Yes	No	No
Malta	A/B/H	Yes	All tasks	No	t/p/h	Yes	Not	1/2/3	No	Yes
Netherlands	A/B/G	Yes	No	No	t/p/h/c	Yes	Adequate	NA	Yes	Yes
Norway	A/B/C/F	No	No	No	t/p/h/c	Yes	Adequate	1/2/3	Yes	Differs
Poland	A/E/H	Yes	All tasks	No	t/p/h/c	Yes	Adequate	1/2/3	Yes[7]	Yes
Portugal	NA	Yes	Chronic	Onsite help	t/p/h/c	Yes	Somewhat	1/2/3	No	Yes
Romania	A/B/E	No	All tasks	No	p/h	Yes	Somewhat	1/2/3	Yes	No
Slovakia	H	NA	Med/acute	No	No	No	Not	4/5	No	No

Slovenia	A/B/C/D/E	Yes	All tasks	C	t/p/h/c	Yes	Adequate	No	Yes	Yes
Spain*	Not applicable	Not applicable	Not applicable	Not applicable	Not applicable	Not applicable	No	Not applicable	Not applicable	Not applicable
Sweden	A/B/C/D	No	All tasks	–	t	Yes	Adequate	1/2/3	Yes[7]	No
UK ENG	–	Yes	Chronic	No	–	Yes	Adequate	3	Yes	Yes
UK NI	–	–	–	–	–	Yes	–	3	Yes	Yes

Notes: [1]*A* – School nurse, *B* – School doctor, *C* – Psychologist, *D* – Social worker, *E* – Dentist, *F* – Physical therapist, *G* – Healthcare assistant and *H* – Other.
[2]*Med* – Administration of medication, *Acute* – Provision of care in case of injury or acute illnesses, *Chronic* – Management of pupils with chronic illnesses, *All* – Task in all mentioned options and *No* – SHS is not involved in direct medical care.
[3]*Onsite help* – There is onsite help in schools, with immediate referral from the school nurse, *B* – There is specialist help available onsite the school, via the school nurse, *C* – Help is available within a few hours and *No* – Not equipped.
[4]*t* – Liaises with teachers, *p* – Liaises with parents, *h* – Liaises with other health services, *c* – Liaises with other community health services and *No* – No clearly defined roles.
[5]*1* – Benign injuries, *2* – Loss of consciousness, *3* – Emergency care, *4* – Other and *NA* – SHS doesn't provide emergency care.
[6]Only for school doctors.
[7]Only for school nurse.
*Spain: Health care for school-aged children in Spain (curative, preventive and health promotion issues) is integrated into primary care services and coordinated with the school system, although not formally a School Health System

Data Management

Early access to up-to-date information for providers of SHSs is essential to deliver high-quality care, and this is defined as a criterion in Standard 7 of the WHO framework. Eighteen of the 28 responding countries have a policy for schools to keep and update information concerning the health of children, and about one-third have a policy to ensure ease of access to this information.

Stakeholders' Involvement

A policy aimed at the involvement of stakeholders is a topic included in several WHO standards. We found that stakeholders' involvement is, in general, only weakly developed, especially as regarding the involvement of medical insurers and parents. Medical providers and children were more often, directly or indirectly involved, for example through identifying the needs of children by means of epidemiological data. A more active involvement of families, informal caretakers and teachers in SHSs was described to be a challenge by most country agents. MOCHA has described the importance of involving children and young people in services that address them (see Chapter 3), and the added value of involving stakeholders is increasingly recognised in the literature on school health (Baltag et al., 2015; World Health Organization, 2010b), in particular the benefits of involving children and adolescents (Anderson & Lowen, 2010; Jourdan et al., 2016).

Services Provided by School Health Services

SHSs provide a wide range of services in MOCHA countries that have a SHS. In the majority of countries, the providers are involved in medical care, particularly in the management of pupils with chronic illness and care in the case of injury or acute illness. Almost all countries' SHS took an active role in preventive care, in the form of screening, disease prevention and promoting good mental health. Differences exist, however. In the types of screenings which are undertaken in schools, visual acuity and weight/height/hearing screenings were performed by most countries, and STI screening was less often performed. Almost all responding countries performed disease prevention activities, such as vaccinations, referrals for health conditions, infection control, surveillance of school's hygiene conditions and emergencies handling. In addition, in more than two-thirds of the MOCHA countries, schools have a national policy on health-promoting schools, indicating that in many countries, a healthy setting for living, learning and working is seen as important (World Health Organization, 2018).

Another important part of the WHO framework is the respect for the principles, characteristics and quality dimensions of child- and adolescent-friendly health services and apply them in a manner that is appropriate to children and adolescents at all developmental stages and in all age groups, which is discussed in Chapter 12.

Discussion and Implications Regarding SHS

One of our most important findings is that of the 30 countries, all except two have a SHS. We compared our findings with the 'gold standard' of SHS, the WHO-framework for quality standards in SHS and competence for SHS professionals (Hoppenbrouwers et al., 2014). The majority of countries perform well against the framework in terms of having a shared responsibility between national and local governance, and health and education authorities for the development of the content and scope, workforce and funding of SHS. More than half of the countries also stand up well against the framework regarding quality management infrastructure, multidisciplinary team working and the establishment of a policy for schools to keep and update information concerning the health of children and having policy on easy access to this information. Encouragingly, also in more than two-thirds of MOCHA countries, schools have a national policy on being a health-promoting school (World Health Organization, 2018).

Nevertheless, there are two major concerns for European SHS when comparing with the WHO standards. A first major concern is a lack of policies to ensure that SHS facilities, equipment, staffing and data management systems are sufficient to enable SHS to achieve their objectives in most of the countries. Our country agents also expressed this concern in their feedback, specifically that

- There is some or a severe shortage of SHS professionals.
- SHS providers are not adequately trained.
- In only half of the countries, specialisation in SHS is needed for SHS professionals.

A second major concern regards the ease of collaboration between SHS professionals, teachers, school administration, parents and children and local community actors (including other healthcare providers). Only about half of the countries who responded as part of the MOCHA project have formal recommendations on effective collaboration between SHS and other forms of primary care or on interdisciplinary working within SHS. In addition, in only half of the responding countries, the multidisciplinary team – often consisting of a school nurse and a school doctor – is supplemented by other types of health professionals. Finally, involvement of families, informal caretakers and teachers in providing SHS is lacking or difficult to achieve in most of the countries.

Implications and Recommendations

This project has resulted in a valuable overview of the different features and indicators of which SHS in different countries exist. This provides many options for countries regarding alternatives for their current system. With this overview, it is possible for countries, to see how other countries have organised parts of the SHS and which options are preferred by most of the countries.

Recommendation 1

European countries should not only invest in more SHS professionals but also in adequately trained SHS professionals to robustly address the specific needs of school-aged children and adolescents (Ambresin, Bennett, Patton, Sanci, & Sawyer, 2013; Committee on Adolescence, 2008; Farre et al., 2015; Michaud & Baltag, 2015; Michaud, Weber, Namazova-Baranova, & Ambresin, 2018).

Recommendation 2

European countries should invest in collaboration between SHS and other primary care professionals. It might be hypothesised that particularly in the case of children with chronic disorders or multimorbidity, effective collaboration between SHS and primary and secondary care, but also with teachers, may offer a breadth of experience and optimise treatment, and thereby improve educational and health outcomes (Baltag & Levi, 2013; Hunt, Barrios, Telljohann, & Mazyck, 2015; Kamionka & Taylor, 2017; Kringos et al., 2013). Collaboration between SHS and the public health sector (and also with parents and adolescents, see recommendation 5) may lead to more integrated and coordinated care, which can result in more accessible and responsive care (Anderson & Lowen, 2010; Kamionka & Taylor, 2017).

Recommendation 3

More involvement of families (both parents and children/adolescents) in SHS policy is needed. Active involvement of parents and children/adolescents in the design, planning, implementation and evaluation of services is of great importance for an efficient and effective SHS (Anderson & Lowen, 2010; Brenner et al., 2017; Ingram & Salmon, 2010). A participatory approach involving children and adolescents focusing on the necessary conditions to reduce risk factors and enhance young people's health is seen as a useful way of optimally matching the policy to the needs and possibilities of children and adolescents (Brenner et al., 2017; Jourdan et al., 2016).

References

Ambresin, A. E., Bennett, K., Patton, G. C., Sanci, L. A., & Sawyer, S. M. (2013). Assessment of youth-friendly health care: A systematic review of indicators drawn from young people's perspectives. *Journal of Adolescent Health, 52*(6), 670–681. doi:10.1016/j.jadohealth.2012.12.014

Anderson, J. E., & Lowen, C. A. (2010). Connecting youth with health services: Systematic review. *Canadian Family Physician, 56*(8), 778–784.

Bains, R. M., & Diallo, A. F. (2016). Mental health services in school-based health centers: Systematic review. *The Journal of School Nursing, 32*(1), 8–19.

Baltag, V., & Levi, M. (2013). Organisational models of school health services in the WHO European Region. *Journal of Health Organisation and Management, 27*(6), 733–746. doi:10.1108/JHOM-08-2011-0084

Baltag, V., Pachyna, A., & Hall, J. (2015). Global overview of school health services: Data from 102 countries. *Health Behavior and Policy Review, 2*(4), 268–283. doi:10.14485/HBPR.2.4.4

Baltag, V., & Saewyc, E. (2017). Pairing children with health services: The changing role of school health services in the twenty-first century. In A. Cherry, V. Baltag, & M. Dillon (Eds.), *International handbook on adolescent health and development* (pp. 463–477). Cham: Springer.

Bersamin, M., Garbers, S., Gaarde, J., & Santelli, J. (2016). Assessing the impact of school-based health centers on academic achievement and college preparation efforts: Using propensity score matching to assess school-level data in California. *The Journal of School Nursing, 32*(4), 241–245.

Brenner, M., Alma, M., Clancy, A., Larkin, P., Lignou, S., Luzi, D., ... Blair, M. (2017). *Report on needs and future visions for care of children with complex conditions.* Retrieved from http://www.childhealthservicemodels.eu/wpcontent/uploads/20171130_Deliverable-D11-2.4-Report-on-needs-andfuture-visions-for-care-of-children-with-complex-conditions.pdf

Committee on Adolescence. (2008). Achieving quality health services for adolescents. *Pediatrics, 121*(6), 1263–1270.

Council on School Health. (2008). The role of the school nurse in providing school health services. *The Journal of School Nursing, 24*(5), 269–274.

Farre, A., Wood, V., Rapley, T., Parr, J. R., Reape, D., & McDonagh, J. E. (2015). Developmentally appropriate healthcare for young people: A scoping study. *Archives of Disease in Childhood, 100*(2), 144–151.

Hoppenbrouwers, K., Baltag, V., Michaud, P., Stronski, S., Pattison, D., Vesna, J., Edelsten, M., Juricic, M., Kuzman, M., Lahti, I., & Schammert-Prenzler A. (2014). *European framework for quality standards in school health services and competences for school health professionals.* Copenhagen: World Health Organization. Retrieved from http://www.euro.who.int/__data/assets/pdf_file/0003/246981/European-framework-for-quality-standards-in-school-health-services-and-competences-for-school-health-professionals.pdf?ua=1

Hunt, P., Barrios, L., Telljohann, S. K., & Mazyck, D. (2015). A whole school approach: Collaborative development of school health policies, processes, and practices. *Journal of School Health, 85*, 802. doi:10.1111/josh.12305

Ingram, J., & Salmon, D. (2010). Young people's use and views of a school-based sexual health drop-in service in areas of high deprivation. *Health Education Journal, 69*(3), 227–235.

Jansen, D. E. M. C., Visser, A., Vervoort, J. P. M., van der Pol, S., Kocken, P., Reijneveld, S. A., & Michaud, P. (2018). *School and adolescent health services in 30 European countries: A description of structure and functioning, and of health outcomes and costs.* Retrieved from http://www.childhealthservicemodels.eu/wp-content/uploads/Deliverable-173.1_Final-report-on-the-description-of-the-various-models-of-school-health-services-and-adolescent-health-services.pdf

Jourdan, D., Christensen, J. H., Darlington, E., Bonde, A. H., Bloch, P., Jensen, B. B., Bentsen, P. (2016). The involvement of young people in school- and community-based noncommunicable disease prevention interventions: A scoping review of designs and outcomes. *BMC Public Health, 16*(1), 1123. doi:10.1186/s12889-016-3779-1

Kamionka, S. L., & Taylor, K. (2017). *Report on requirements and models for supporting children with complex mental health needs and the primary care interface.* Retrieved from http://www.childhealthservicemodels.eu/wp-content/uploads/2017/07/20171130_Deliverable-D10-2.3-Report-on-requirements-and-models-for-supporting-children-with-complex-mental-health-needs-and-the-primary-care-interface.pdf

Knopf, J. A., Finnie, R. K., Peng, Y., Hahn, R. A., Truman, B. I., Vernon-Smiley, M., et al. (2016). School-based health centers to advance health equity: A community guide systematic review. *American Journal of Preventive Medicine, 51*(1), 114–126. doi:10.1016/j.amepre.2016.01.009

Kringos, D., Boerma, W., Bourgueil, Y., Cartier, T., Dedeu, T., Hasvold, T. ... Groenewegen, P. (2013). The strength of primary care in Europe: An international comparative study. *British Journal of General Practice, 63*(616), e742–50. doi:10.3399/bjgp13X674422

Leroy, Z. C., Wallin, R., & Lee, S. (2017). The role of school health services in addressing the needs of students with chronic health conditions: A systematic review. *The Journal of School Nursing, 33*(1), 64–72. doi:10.1177/1059840516678909

Michaud, P., & Baltag, V. (2015). *Core competencies in adolescent health and development for primary care providers: Secondary core competencies in adolescent health and development for primary care providers* (p. 49). Geneva: World Health Organization. Retrieved from http://apps.who.int/iris/bitstream/handle/10665/148354/9789241508315_eng.pdf;jsessionid=93E92FABAC0C4597630456D02BC4D55B?sequence=1

Michaud, P., Weber, M., Namazova-Baranova, & Ambresin, A. (2018). Improving the quality of care delivered to adolescents in Europe: A time to invest. *Archives of Disease in Childhood.* doi:10.1136/archdischild-2017-314429

World Health Organization. (2010a). *Pairing children with health services – The results of a survey on school health services in the WHO European region.* Retrieved from http://www.euro.who.int/__data/assets/pdf_file/0006/112389/E93576.pdf

World Health Organization. (2010b). *Monitoring the building blocks of health systems: A handbook of indicators and their measurement strategies.* Retrieved from http://www.who.int/workforcealliance/knowledge/toolkit/26.pdf

World Health Organization. (2018). *What is a health promoting school?* Retrieved from http://www.who.int/school_youth_health/gshi/hps/en/

Chapter 12

Primary Care for Adolescents

Pierre-André Michaud, Johanna P. M. Vervoort and Danielle Jansen

Abstract

Adolescence is a time when a young person develops his or her identity, acquires greater autonomy and independence, experiments and takes risks and grows mentally and physically. To successfully navigate these changes, an accessible and health system when needed is essential.

We assessed the structure and content of national primary care services against these standards in the field of adolescent health services. The main criteria identified by adolescents as important for primary care are as follows: accessibility, staff attitude, communication in all its forms, staff competency and skills, confidential and continuous care, age appropriate environment, involvement in health care, equity and respect and a strong link with the community.

We found that although half of the Models of Child Health Appraised countries have adopted adolescent-specific policies or guidelines, many countries do not meet the current standards of quality health care for adolescents. For example, the ability to provide emergency mental health care or respond to life-threatening behaviour is limited. Many countries provide good access to contraception, but specialised care for a pregnant adolescent may be hard to find.

Access needs to be improved for vulnerable adolescents; greater advocacy should be given to adolescent health and the promotion of good health habits. Adolescent health services should be well publicised, and adolescents need to feel empowered to access them.

Keywords: Adolescents; health care; preventive care; primary care services; mental health; sexual and reproductive health

Introduction

Adolescents (defined in this survey as individuals aged 10–19 years) have specific needs compared with younger children. They are in the process of developing their identity and acquiring autonomy, their bodies and minds are growing, and it is a time of experimenting and risk-taking, and increasing independence (Jansen et al., 2018; Michaud, Blum, & Ferron, 1998; WHO, 2014b). Adolescents need to feel confident in their ability to access primary care services, in the form of advice, prevention and treatment services – independently of their parents or guardians if appropriate (Michaud et al., 2010). Models of Child Health Appraised (MOCHA) has identified young people as an important group in terms of their health and also in terms of children's rights (United Nations General Assembly, 1990). Adolescents should be respected and involved as much as possible in all decisions regarding their life and their health. To provide optimal services, the primary healthcare system and the health professionals providing services need to recognise the needs of adolescents and adapt policies accordingly (Sawyer et al., 2014).

The health of an adolescent depends on many factors that lie beyond the healthcare system, such as the economic situation of the country, the climate and the culture, the organisation of the educational system, the presence or absence of preventive activities and so on (see Chapter 17; Patton et al., 2012; Patton et al., 2016; World Health Organization, 2014b; World Health Organization, 2017; WHO, 2014a). MOCHA investigated the extent to which the current health systems of European countries met the healthcare needs of adolescents aged 10 – 18, as being the upper age of childhood as defined by the Convention on the Rights of the Child (CRC) (United Nations, 1989).

There are models of quality health care available for adolescents (Michaud & Baltag, 2015; Michaud, Weber, Namazova-Baranova, & Ambresin, 2018; World Health Organization, 2014; World Health Organization, 2015a; World Health Organization, 2015b; World Health Organization, 2015c), most of which refer to the concept of adolescent/youth-friendly health services and care jointly developed by the World Health Organization (WHO), United Nations Children's Fund (UNICEF) and United Nations Population Fund (UNFPA). These models have also been validated by young people themselves (Ambresin, Bennett, Patton, Sanci, & Sawyer, 2013), as a result of surveys about the main ingredients of fair and high-quality health services and care. The main criteria mentioned by young people in this survey are as follows:

- accessibility (flexible schedule, possibility to drop in), location (public transportation), affordability (financial coverage) and equity;
- staff attitude: respectful, supportive, empathetic, trustworthy and honest;
- communication: developmentally appropriate, understandable, active listening and provision of information;
- staff competency and skills, both technical and medical (health care), and comprehensive and holistic approach (multi professional: e.g. providing

curative and preventive services in the broad area of adolescent health, including mental health, substance use, sexual & reproductive health) (see Chapter 13);

- guideline-driven care: confidentiality, autonomy, privacy and continuity of care;
- age appropriate environment: clean and teen-oriented physical space, health information, access to internet, pamphlets and leaflets;
- involvement in health care, participation, shared decision-making approach and continuity of care;
- equity and respect of adolescents' rights (CRC); and
- link with the community, networking approach and community support;

These comments align closely with MOCHA findings from young people about their experiences of primary care (see Chapter 3), and MOCHA sought to address whether the experience of primary healthcare services met these standards.

This report complements the survey on school health services, as described in Chapter 11, and assesses the extent to which the structure and content of primary care services comply with available standards in the field of adolescent health care.

Methods

We created a questionnaire on adolescent primary care services to be sent to the MOCHA country agents (see Chapter 1). The questionnaire was divided into three sections and contained 43 questions on structural and content issues that are specific to adolescent care. Each section began with a typical clinical vignette to assist the Country Agent in understanding what information was expected. These included the existence of guidelines or policies regarding adolescent-friendly health services and care, the respect of adolescent rights, access of adolescents to appropriate health care as well as the continuity of care. The two last sections of the questionnaire focussed on two major healthcare areas during adolescence: mental health and self-harm, and sexual and reproductive health. Complete data from all thirty countries were available for analysis.

Results

Adolescent Primary Care Services

We assessed the country agent answers against the existing adolescent-friendly health services and care (AFHSC) guidelines. Thirteen out of the 30 countries surveyed indicated that they were aware of and follow the AFHSC guidelines, and a document to this end is available nationally. However, it was impossible to ascertain whether the documents are applied and to what extent. One of the questions tackled the existence of specialised services for adolescents. More than half the countries (16/30) have set up such specialised centres to deliver adolescent health care, although these are likely to be in selected cities and not in all regions of a country. Some units address specific issues (such as sexual

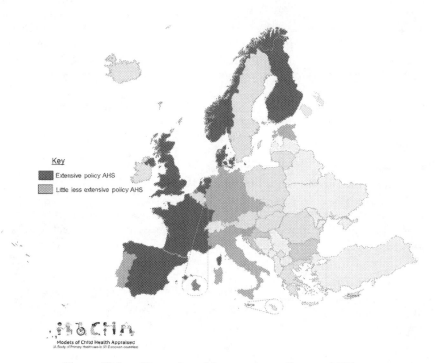

Figure 12.1.   Countries with extensive policy on AHS.

and reproductive life or mental health), and some are more broadly oriented. Many, if not most, are run by multidisciplinary team ($N = 16$), and in eleven countries, the country agents claim that professionals in charge have received formal training in adolescent health (see Chapter 13). Figure 12.1 shows the countries that have an extensive policy on adolescent health services as recommended currently (Kokotailo et al., 2018). For more information, see Jansen et al. (2018).

Adolescents' Rights and Ethical Issues

The respect of confidentiality and privacy is, according to young people, of utmost importance, and this applies to all countries of the world (see Chapter 3; Baltag & Mathison, 2010; Bell, Breland, & Ott, 2013; Committee on Adolescence, 2016; National Research Council and Institute of Medicine, 2009; World Health Organization, 2016; Michaud et al., 2010). Indeed, when it comes to discussing sensitive issues such as sexual conduct or contraception, risk-taking, problematic eating patterns or substance use, young people need to be confident that the healthcare professional will not disclose information unless the situation is life threatening or unless the adolescent feels comfortable to disclose. However, the right to confidentiality is linked with the young person's decision-making capacity (competence), and healthcare providers are not necessarily well equipped to assess such a capacity (Michaud, Blum, Benaroyo,

Zermatten, & Baltag, 2015). In 13 out of the thirty countries surveyed, the existence of a formal legislation or policy tackling the issue of confidentiality was confirmed by country agents. Five countries also have policies but restricted by an age range. In only nine countries, guidelines are available about how to assess a young person's competence. Another important aspect of confidentiality is the right of a young person to access health care without the knowledge of parents. In 20 countries, adolescents have the right to consult a doctor without parents (or any substitute) knowing, and in around the same proportion of countries, adolescents have the right to choose their doctor themselves ($N = 17$). Finally, shared decision-making, for example the right to refuse a treatment or choosing another alternative than the one chosen by the parents, is a right that should be given to competent young patients. In around half of the countries ($N = 9$), a policy exists to guarantee such a right.

Access to Health Care
Access to health care is an important issue for adolescents. Blair, Rigby, and Alexander (2017) stated that most European countries provide some kind of sustainable insurance system that covers the healthcare expenditures of children and young people. The potentially limiting factors to access of adolescents to health care is thus more likely linked to a lack of knowledge of what exists and where to be able to consult freely and expect high-quality health care. In addition to this, it is sometimes difficult to access services because of a lack of availability, due to under-resourcing or a shortage of health professionals skilled in adolescent health care. This is particularly pertinent to so-called vulnerable adolescents, such as migrants and adolescents from deprived socio-economic background or 'drop-out' adolescents who are homeless or in temporary accommodation. Globally, around 50% of countries have developed policies or strategies that aim to improve access to care for adolescents facing situations of vulnerability. In around half of the countries ($N = 16$), it is possible for adolescents in such situations to consult primary care spontaneously. Half of the countries are able to offer translators if needed, at least in some regions, and/or to provide professionals who have an expertise in cross-cultural issues. Moreover, just about two thirds of the countries ($N = 20$) have policies which encourage an inter-professional approach to disruptive behaviour adolescents having left or being about to leave the mainstream educational system (see Chapter 11).

Access to Mental Health Care and Sexual and Reproductive Health Care
Issues such as conduct disorders, violence, depression and self-harm/suicide are increasingly recognised as important threats to adolescents' mental health (Nair et al., 2015; Patton et al., 2012; Potrebny, Wiium, & Lundegard, 2017; Steinberg et al., 2017). The majority of countries ($N = 25$) have some kind of suicide prevention programme, and a similar number are able to provide same-day referral appointments for suicide or mental health breakdown, but only half ($N = 14$) of the surveyed countries provide guidelines to primary care physicians as how to screen for mental health problems and disorders in adolescents, and only

Table 12.1. Indicators of quality management for mental health services and sexual and reproductive health care for adolescents.

Country	Quality Management Infrastructure	
	Guidelines PC Screening Young People on Mental Health Issues	Guidelines/Standards for PC Professionals about Adolescent Pregnancy
Austria	No	No
Belgium-F	Unclear	No
Bulgaria	Yes	No
Croatia	Yes	No
Cyprus	No	No
Czech Republic	Yes	No
Denmark	No	Yes
Estonia	Yes	Yes
Finland	Yes	Yes
France	Unclear	Yes
Germany	Yes	No
Greece	Yes	No
Hungary	No	–
Iceland	No	No
Ireland	Yes	Yes
Italy	Yes	No
Latvia	No	No
Lithuania	Unclear	No
Luxembourg	No	No
Malta	No	No
Netherlands	Yes	No
Norway	No	No
Poland	No	Yes
Portugal	Yes	No
Romania	No	No
Slovakia	No	No
Slovenia	Yes	No
Spain	Yes	Yes
Sweden	No	No
UK ENG	Yes	Yes

fourteen provide recommendations as how to screen for adolescent mental health problems (Table 12.1).

In all the countries who replied to the questionnaire ($n = 30$), it is possible for a young person to obtain emergency contraception. In about half of the countries ($n = 24$), there are multiple options where a young person can obtain emergency contraception, such as in a pharmacy, a health clinic, the emergency department of a hospital or via a primary care practitioner. 25 countries have multiple options to obtain pregnancy tests, and in most countries ($n = 24$), condoms are easily available. Only eleven countries, however, provide oral contraception free of charge, although, on the whole, adolescents can obtain such contraception easily in most countries, but in only 16 countries, it is possible for the adolescents to visit a doctor without their parents knowing. More than half of the surveyed countries ($N = 16$) have centres which provide counselling and care in sexual and reproductive health (although some centres address all ages, not specifically adolescents). In terms of primary care, however, only eight countries have specific guidelines or policies about how to address adolescent pregnancy.

Summary

Although around half of the MOCHA countries have adopted policies or guidelines that aim to secure equal access to primary care for most adolescents, including the most vulnerable, many countries of the EU and EEA lag far behind the current standards of quality health care for adolescents. The situation seems not to have improved since ten years (Ercan et al., 2009) Only a minority of countries are equipped to identify and respond to mental health emergencies and life-threatening behaviour. Access to contraception is good in most countries, but very few have developed guidelines for practitioners to help care for a pregnant adolescent. In addition, while many countries support the concept of confidential health care, only a small number provide guidelines to professionals as how to address adolescents' competence. This situation is all the more problematic as evidence suggests that the quality of primary care services has a positive effect on the health of young people (Carai, Bivol, & Chandra-Mouli, 2015; Kalamar, Bayer, & Hindin, 2016; Sanci et al., 2015). Addressing the need for specific training of health professionals is of prime importance to improve the delivery of adolescent-focused health care (see Chapter 12), and successfully addressing the complex, changing needs of adolescents (World Health Organization, 2015c).

In summary, there is a need for *all* European countries to endorse policies and strategies regarding adolescent-friendly primary care in order to improve access and quality of care for young people. The creation of specific youth clinics and addressing other important primary care services, such as public or private consultation offices and hospitals, will help to achieve these aims. No country comprehensively responds to the many facets of quality adolescent care: some have strong policies but do not secure easy access while others are in the opposite situation. Thus, all European countries, and especially those that have a weak corpus of policies, recommendations or specific healthcare strategies (Cyprus, Hungary, Iceland, Latvia, Lithuania, Malta, Poland, Romania and Slovakia) can begin improvement in different ways.

- Physicians, especially those involved in scientific organisations or in public health activities should advocate for adolescent health, sensitising colleagues and policy-makers to the importance of this cohort. Adoption of good life-styles during this period of life will profoundly affect their health for the rest of their life (see Chapter 2).
- Addressing health-compromising behaviour, supporting healthy habits is the responsibility of adolescents' primary care providers (Patton et al., 2014, 2016; World Health Organization, 2017). European countries must develop policies and strategies which improve access to adolescents facing situations of vulnerability; particularly in the area of mental health and sexual and reproductive health. Schools, ambulatory settings and hospitals should offer easily identified, low-threshold comprehensive health care and a culturally appropriate approach, given the number of migrant adolescents being hosted in most European countries (see Chapter 11).
- Also, services to adolescents, even if they follow the evidence-based standards, will not be effective if young people themselves are inadequately informed or able to access them. It is the task of both the education and the healthcare systems to assist young people to understand their rights and responsibility for their health, and how and where to access to adequate care.
- One of the best ways to improve the quality of care delivered to adolescents is to improve the training of healthcare providers (Michaud et al., 2017). This is addressed in Chapter 13.

References

Ambresin, A. E., Bennett, K., Patton, G. C., Sanci, L. A., & Sawyer, S. M. (2013). Assessment of youth-friendly health care: A systematic review of indicators drawn from young people's perspectives. *Journal of Adolescent Health, 52,* 670–681. doi:10.1016/j.jadohealth.2012.12.014

Baltag, V., & Mathison, A. (2010). *Youth-friendly health policies and services in the European region: Sharing experiences* (p. 267). Copenhagen: World Health Organization.

Bell, D. L., Breland, D. J., & Ott, M. A. (2013). Adolescent and young adult male health: A review. *Pediatrics, 132*(3), 535–546.

Blair, M., Rigby, M., & Alexander, D. (2017). *Final report on current models of primary care for children.* Retrieved from www.childhealthservicemodels.eu/wp-content/uploads/2017/07/MOCHA-WP1-Deliverable-WP1-D6-Feb-2017-1.pdf

Carai, S., Bivol, S., & Chandra-Mouli, V. (2015). Assessing youth-friendly-health-services and supporting planning in the Republic of Moldova. *Reproductive Health, 12,* 98.

Committee on Adolescence. (2016). Achieving quality health services for adolescents. *Pediatrics, 138*(2).

Ercan, O., Alikasifoglu, M., Erginoz, E., Janda, J., Kabicek, P., Rubino, A., ... Vural, M. (2009). Demography of adolescent health care delivery and training in Europe. *European Journal of Pediatrics, 168*(4), 417–426.

Jansen, D. E. M. C., Visser, A., Vervoort, J. P. M., van der Pol, S., Kocken, P., Reijneveld, S. A., & Michaud, P. (2018). *School and adolescent health services in 30 European countries: A description of structure and functioning, and of health outcomes and costs.* Retrieved from http://www.childhealthservicemodels.eu/wp-content/uploads/Deliverable-173.1_Final-report-on-the-description-of-the-various-models-of-school-health-services-and-adolescent-health-services.pdf

Kalamar, A. M., Bayer, A. M., & Hindin, M. J. (2016). Interventions to prevent sexually transmitted infections, including HIV, among young people in low- and middle-income countries: A systematic review of the published and gray literature. *Journal of Adolescent Health, 59*(3 Suppl), S22–31.

Kokotailo, P. K., Baltag, V., & Sawyer, S. M. (2018). Educating and training the future adolescent health workforce. *Journal of Adolescent Health, 62*(5), 511–524.

Michaud, P. A., Berg-Kelly, K., Macfarlane, A., & Benaroyo, L. (2010). Ethics and adolescent care: An international perspective. *Current Opinion in Pediatrics, 22*(4), 418–422.

Michaud, P. A., Blum, R. W., Benaroyo, L., Zermatten, J., & Baltag, V. (2015). Assessing an adolescent's capacity for autonomous decision-making in clinical care. *Journal of Adolescent Health, 57*, 361–366. doi:10.1016/j.jadohealth.2015.06.012

Michaud, P. A., Schrier, L., Ross-Russel, R., van der Heijden, L., Dossche, L., Copley, S., ... Ambresin, A. E. (2017). Paediatric departments need to improve residents' training in adolescent medicine and health: A position paper of the European Academy of Paediatrics. *European Journal of Pediatrics, 177*(4), 479–487. doi:10.1007/s00431-017-3061-2

Michaud, P., & Baltag, V. (2015). *Core competencies in adolescent health and development for primary care providers* (p. 49). Geneva: World Health Organization.

Michaud, P., Blum, R., & Ferron, C. (1998). "Bet you I will!" Risk or experimental behavior during adolescence? *Archives of Pediatrics & Adolescent Medicine, 152*, 224–226.

Michaud, P., Weber, M., Namazova-Baranova, L., & Ambresin, A. (2018). Improving the quality of care delivered to adolescents in Europe: A time to invest. *Archives of Disease in Childhood, 104*(3), 214–216.

Nair, M., Baltag, V., Bose, K., Boschi-Pinto, C., Lambrechts, T., & Mathai, M. (2015). Improving the quality of health care services for adolescents, globally: A standards-driven approach. *Journal of Adolescent Health, 57*(3), 288–298.

National Research Council and Institute of Medicine. (2009). *Adolescent health services.* Washington, DC: National Academic Press.

Patton, G. C., Coffey, C., Cappa, C., Currie, D., Riley, L., Gore, F., ... Ferguson, J. (2012). Health of the world's adolescents: A synthesis of internationally comparable data. *Lancet, 379*(9826), 1665–1675.

Patton, G. C., Ross, D. A., Santelli, J. S., Sawyer, S. M., Viner, R. M., & Kleinert, S. (2014). Next steps for adolescent health: A Lancet commission. *Lancet, 383*(9915), 385–386.

Patton, G. C., Sawyer, S. M., Santelli, J. S., Ross, D. A., Afifi, R., Allen, N. B., ... Viner, R. M.. (2016). Our future: A Lancet commission on adolescent health and wellbeing. *Lancet, 387*(10036), 2423–2478.

Potrebny, T., Wiium, N., & Lundegard, M. M. (2017). Temporal trends in adolescents' self-reported psychosomatic health complaints from 1980-2016: A systematic review and meta-analysis. *PLoS One, 12*(11), e0188374.

Sanci, L., Chondros, P., Sawyer, S., Pirkis, J., Ozer, E., Hegarty, K., ... Patton, G. (2015). Responding to young people's health risks in primary care: A cluster randomised trial of training clinicians in screening and motivational interviewing. *PLoS One, 10*(9), e0137581.

Sawyer, S. M., Ambresin, A. E., Bennett, K. E., & Patton, G. C. (2014). A measurement framework for quality health care for adolescents in hospital. *Journal of Adolescent Health, 55*(4), 484–490.

Steinberg, L., Icenogle, G., Shulman, E. P., Breiner, K., Chein, J., Bacchini, D., ... Takash, H. M. (2017). Around the world, adolescence is a time of heightened sensation seeking and immature self-regulation. *Developmental Science, 21*(2), e12532.

United Nation General Assembly. (1990). *United nation convention on the rights of the child.* New York, NY: UN General Assembly.

United Nations. (1989). *Convention on the rights of the child, UNICEF.*

World Health Organization. (2014). *Health for the world's adolescents: A second chance in the second decade.* Geneva: World Health Organization. Retrieved from https://www.who.int/maternal_child_adolescent/documents/second-decade/en/

World Health Organization. (2014a). *European framework for quality standards in school health services and competences for school health professionals* (Vol. 1, p. 11). Copenhagen: World Health Organization Regional Office for Europe.

World Health Organization. (2014b). *Health for the world's adolescents: A second chance in the second decade.* Geneva: World Health Organization.

World Health Organization. (2015a). *Children's rights in primary health care. Assessment and improvement Tool for Children and Adolescents aged 12-18* (Vol. 3, p. 50). Copenhagen: World Health Organization.

World Health Organization. (2015b). *Core competencies in adolescent health and development for primary care providers: Including a tool to assess the adolescent health and development component in pre-service education of health-care providers* (p. 58). Geneva: World Health Organization.

World Health Organization. (2015c). *Global standards for quality health-care services for adolescents: A guide to implement a standards-driven approach to improve the quality of health care services for adolescents.* Volume 1: Standards and criteria. Geneva: World Health Organization.

World Health Organization. (2016). *Improving the quality of care for reproductive, maternal, neonatal, child and adolescent health in the WHO European region* (p. 50). Copenhagen: World Health Organization.

World Health Organization. (2017). *Global accelerated action for the health of adolescents (AA-HA!): Guidance to support country implementation.* Geneva: World Health Organization.

Chapter 13

Workforce and Professional Education

Mitch Blair, Heather Gage, Ekelechi MacPepple,
Pierre-André Michaud, Carol Hilliard, Anne Clancy,
Eleanor Hollywood, Maria Brenner, Amina Al-Yassin and
Catharina Nitsche

Abstract

Given that the workforce constitutes a principal resource of primary care, appraisal of models of care requires thorough investigation of the health workforce in all Models of Child Health Appraised (MOCHA) countries. This chapter explores this in terms of workforce composition, remuneration, qualifications and training in relation to the needs of children and young people. We have focused on two principal disciplines of primary care; medicine and nursing, with a specific focus on training and skills to care for children in primary care, particularly those with complex care needs, adolescents and vulnerable groups. We found significant disparities in workforce provision and remuneration, in training curricula and in resultant skills of physicians and nurses in European Union and European Economic Area Countries. A lack of overarching standards and recognition of some of the specific needs of children reflected in training of physicians and nurses may lead to sub-optimal care for children. There are, of course, many other professions that also contribute to primary care services for children, some of which are discussed in Chapter 15, but we have not had resources to study these to the same detail.

Keywords: Workforce; medical education; nursing education; adolescent medicine; primary care; child health; human resource; training

Introduction

Physicians and nurses provide preventive care, education and guidance as well as diagnostic, curative care and management of the mental and physical disorders of childhood. Analysis within Models of Child Health Appraised (MOCHA) countries has shown that the size of the primary care workforce affects outcomes for children (Chapter 5). The ability to communicate with children in an inclusive, non-threatening but nevertheless informative and authoritative manner is essential (Alma, Mahtani, Palant, Klůzová Kráčmarová, & Prinjha, 2017). The MOCHA project has investigated the acquisition of these skills by means of analysis of medical and nursing training curricula.

The Primary Care Workforce

In most countries, the healthcare workforce is comprised of multiple professional groups with diverse skills and roles. In addition to including front-line personnel of all types and levels whose roles are in the direct delivery of care, healthcare systems are run on a daily basis by significant numbers of managers, administrators and support staff whose roles are not patient facing. Establishing overall expenditure on the human resource contribution to the production of healthcare additionally needs to incorporate resources committed to training. Workforce data that are available from MOCHA countries are limited and relate only to broad groups of professionals such as general practitioners (GPs), nurses and paediatricians (including community paediatricians and neonatologists, but excluding paediatric specialties such as child psychiatry, oncology, cardiology and surgery). The distribution of the workforce between primary and secondary care is not reported, although it would usually be assumed that GPs and community paediatricians work in primary care. The available data are not routinely captured, with information related to 2013 being the most recent at the time of writing (2018), as shown in Table 13.1.

On a national level, gross domestic product (GDP) per capita (a recognised indicator of a country's standard of living) is highly correlated with health expenditure per capita (Pearson correlation: 0.92, 2016 from Table 13.1). Hence, among the MOCHA countries, those with the highest GDP per capita have the highest health expenditure (e.g. Luxembourg and Norway) and vice versa (e.g. Romania and Latvia). There is also a direct relationship between the size of the workforce and health expenditure, although at a disaggregated level, this is affected by healthcare system features. A primary care-based system, for example, will tend to result in a higher ratio of GPs and community paediatricians to specialist doctors. In MOCHA countries, the total number of nurses correlates strongly with health expenditure per capita, but the association is less strong for GPs (Pearson correlation coefficients nurses 0.688, GPs 0.362). Cross-tabulating the MOCHA typology of models for child health care (GP led, paediatrician led, mixed) with the number of paediatricians per 100,000 of the population confirms the lower proportions of non-specialist paediatricians in GP led systems (see Table 13.2). The tendency for paediatrician-led countries to

Table 13.1. Healthcare expenditure and workforce data for the MOCHA countries.

Countries	GDP Per Capita: PPP, US$ (2016)[a]	Health Expenditure Per Capita, PPP: Constant 2011 International US$ (2014)[b]	Population Total (2016)	% of Population, 19 Years and under (2016)	Physicians, Paediatric Per 100,000 Population (2013)[b]	General Practitioners, Per 100,000 Population (2013)[b]	Nurses Per 100,000 Population (2013)[b]
Austria	44,143.70	5,038.88	8,712.137	19.22	16.21	76.95	803.09
Belgium	41,945.69	4,391.60	11,358.379	22.57	12.65	111.67	–
Bulgaria	17,709.08	1,398.88	7,131.494	18.27	19.93	62.93	491.82
Croatia	21,408.55	1,652.12	4,213.265	20.28	18.52	53.72	658.48
Cyprus	31,195.51	2,062.37	1,170.125	23.44	–	–	512.92
Czech Republic	31,071.75	2,146.32	10,610.947	19.43	12.33	70.13	841.28
Denmark	45,686.48	4,782.06	5,711.870	22.83	7.02	–	1,685.66
Estonia	27,735.14	1,668.31	1,312.442	20.57	13.43	70.33	587.94
Finland	39,422.65	3,701.14	5,503.132	21.81	12.93	–	–
France	38,058.87	4,508.13	64,720.690	24.11	12.09	160.11	999.73
Germany	44,072.39	5,182.11	81,914.672	18.05	12.38	66.66	1,323.07
Greece	24,263.88	2,098.05	11,183.716	19.33	30.33	23.36	353.68
Hungary	25,381.29	1,826.68	9,753.281	19.48	–	–	659.65
Iceland	45,276.45	3,881.70	332.474	26.64	4.63	58.07	1,626.8
Ireland	62,828.34	3,801.06	4,726.078	27.57	9.86	73.17	–
Italy	34,620.13	3,238.89	59,429.938	18.31	29.01	75.05	634.19
Latvia	23,712.09	940.30	1,970.530	19.46	12.67	–	508.09

Table 13.1. (*Continued*)

Countries	GDP Per Capita, PPP, US$ (2016)[a]	Health Expenditure Per Capita, PPP: Constant 2011 International US$ (2014)[b]	Population Total (2016)	% of Population, 19 Years and under (2016)	Physicians, Paediatric Per 100,000 Population (2013)[b]	General Practitioners, Per 100,000 Population (2013)[b]	Nurses Per 100,000 Population (2013)[b]
Lithuania	27,904.10	1,718.02	2,908.249	20.19	26.91	86.28	785.28
Luxembourg	97,018.66	6,812.08	575.747	22.40	14.91	85.95	1,230.12
Malta	35,694.04	3,071.63	429.362	19.83	13.93	80.3	744.16
Netherlands	47,128.31	5,201.70	16,987.330	22.53	9.54	78.5	–
Norway	63,810.79	6,346.62	5,254.694	24.06	13.92	78.05	1,720.93
Poland	26,003.01	1,570.45	38,224.410	19.90	13.17	21.75	587.46
Portugal	27,006.87	2,689.94	10,371.627	19.13	17.8	56.83	629.31
Romania	21,647.81	1,079.26	19,778.083	20.75	10.97	56.95	552.42
Slovakia	29,156.09	2,179.05	5,444.218	20.44	–	–	607.81
Slovenia	29,803.45	2,697.67	2,077.862	19.33	26.22	49.78	838.08
Spain	33,261.08	2,965.82	46,347.576	19.34	25.53	75.15	532.4
Sweden	46,441.21	5,218.86	9,837.533	22.46	10.48	64.53	1,192.12
United kingdom	38,901.05	3,376.87	65,788.574	23.30	15.1	79.57	867.61

Notes: [a]World Bank, International Comparison Program database. [b]World Health Organization Global Health Expenditure database. [c]United Nations, Department of Economic and Social Affairs, Population Division (2017). World Population Prospects. GDP, gross domestic product; PPP, purchasing power parity.

Table 13.2. Density of paediatricians by MOCHA typology of primary care for children.

MOCHA Typology of Primary Care for Children	More Than 20 Paediatricians per 100k Population	Less Than 20 Paediatricians per 100k Population
GP led		Bulgaria, Denmark, Estonia, Finland, Ireland, Malta, Netherlands, Norway Portugal, Romania and UK
Paediatrician led	Greece, Italy, Slovenia	Croatia, Czech Rep., Germany
Mixed	Lithuania, Spain	Austria, Belgium, Iceland, France, Latvia, Luxembourg, Poland, Sweden

have lower GDPs (except Germany) accounts for the negative correlation between health expenditure per capita and the density of paediatricians (Pearson correlation −0.208).

There are many drawbacks with the data that are available which restrict the conclusions that can be drawn. Despite attempts by the international organisations that assemble the data to ensure uniformity of definitions across countries, local practices may affect the compilation of the statistics. Also, data are only available after a lag and situations and systems are often undergoing reform.

Training in Primary Care

International variability in healthcare expenditures may extend to differences in professional training and methods of care delivery. To gain further understanding of such features, a series of questions were asked of the MOCHA country agents, as outlined in Table 13.3. Responses are summarised in Tables 13.4 and 13.5. Training is discussed later in the chapter.

With the exception of Slovakia, where children in primary care are treated by single practitioners (paediatricians), responses indicated that the health professionals worked in a multidisciplinary team either in a community practice or a group practice. This was regardless of GDP level or model type (GP or paediatrician led, or mixed). Policies around case load sizes varied, as did whether health promotion and prevention functions were conducted within primary care. About one half of countries reported national salary scales; just over one half reported data available on the primary care workforce (Table 13.4).

In terms of training of healthcare professionals (Table 13.5), it was clear from the 28 responses that in all countries, paediatricians had mostly six years of

Table 13.3. Questions on workforce sent to Country Agents.

Category	Question
Found in Table 13.4	
On organisation of care	What type of primary care system is available? Q1
	Is there a regulatory upper limit (maximum number) of children that a primary care paediatrician or GP can have in their list? Q2
	Within your primary care system, how is the healthcare workforce organised to provide services? Options: single practitioner, multidisciplinary team, paediatric group practice, GP group practice, other model Q3
On health promotion and health promotion/curative care services	Are universal prevention and health promotion services (e.g. immunisation, routine developmental examinations) provided in the primary care setting described above, or by a separate preventive health service? Q4
	Are there suggested caseloads for staff numbers who provide universal prevention and health promotion services? Q5
	Is the case load of Q5 based on population size, geographical area/transport conditions, socio-economic factors, other? Q6
	Are there suggested case loads for staff numbers who provide curative care within the primary care setting? Based on population size, geographical area/transport conditions, socio-economic factors, other? Q7
On salary and national datasets	Does your country have a national salary scale for the members of the primary care system? Q8
	Does your country have a dataset for the number of staff (by group) in the primary care system? Q9
Found on Table 13.5	
On training of paediatricians	On average, how many years mandatory training at college/university level does a paediatrician working in primary health care have? (If possible and appropriate, split into general medical education (medical faculty) and paediatric-specific education (postgraduate)). Q10

Table 13.3. (*Continued*)

Category	Question
	• What type of (if any) postgraduate specialisation does the paediatrician have? Q10a
	• In what type of setting does the postgraduate training take place? (e.g. in hospital, or in community-based clinics under the supervision of a primary care paediatrician). Q10b
On training of GPs	On average, how many years mandatory training at college/university level does a GP working in primary health care have? Q11
	• What type of (if any) postgraduate specialisation does the GP have? (If possible and appropriate, split into general medical education, and general practice-specific education). Q11a
	• In what type of setting does the postgraduate training take place? (e.g. in hospital paediatric ward, or emergency department, or in community-based clinics or GP offices under the supervision of a primary care/public health physician). Q11b
On training of nurses	On average, how many years mandatory basic training at college/university level does a registered nurse need to undertake this additional qualification/work in universal prevention and health promotion services nursing service for all children (e.g. public health nurse, health visitor, other)? Are these postgraduate qualifications? Q12
	In your country, what type of (if any) postgraduate specialisation does a nurse need to work in universal prevention and health promotion services nursing service for all children (e.g. paediatrics, public health, community health, other), Q12a and what is the duration of that training? Q12b

Table 13.4. Primary care (PC) workforce configuration, summary of Country Agent responses.

Country	Type of PC System for Children (Q1)	Regulatory Maximum Number of Children on Doctor List (Q2)	How Workforce Organised to Provide Services (Q3)					Prevention/ Promotion in Primary Care or Separate? (Q4)	Suggested Caseloads Prevention/ Promotion? (Q5)	What is Suggested Case Load Based on? (Q6)	Suggested Caseloads Curative? (Q7)	National Salary Scale Primary Care? (Q8)	Available Datasets Primary Care Staff? (Q9)
			1	MDT	PN	GPN	5						
Austria	Combined	N		x				N	N		N	N	N
Belgium	Combined	N		x	x	x	x	N	Y & N		N	N	Y & N
Bulgaria	GP led	Y (2,500~)	x					N	N		N	N	N
Croatia	Combined	Y (1,000)		x	x	x	x	Y	Y	Pop; other	Y	Y	Y
Cyprus	Paediatrician led	Y (30)	x					N	N		N	N	N
Czech rep.	GP led	N	x				x	N	N		Y	N	N
Denmark	Combined	Y (1,600)	x	x	x	x		Y	Y	–	Y & N	Y	Y
Estonia	GP led	N	x			x		N	Y	Pop; geog	Y	N	Y
Finland	Combined	N		x				N	Y	Pop; geog	N	N	Y
Germany	Paediatrician led	N	x	x	x	x		Y	Y	–	Y	Y	Y
Greece	Combined	N	x	x				Y	N		N	Y	N
Hungary	Combined	N	x		x			Y	Y		Y	Y	Y
Iceland	Combined	N		x		x		Y	Y	Pop; geog	N	Y	Y
Ireland	Combined	N		x				Y	Y	Pop	Y	Y	Y
Italy	Combined	Y (1,000)	x		x			Y	N	Pop; geog	Y	Y	N
Latvia	Combined	Y (800)			x	x		Y	Y	Pop; geog	Y	Y	Y

Lithuania	Combined	Y (varies)	x	x			x		N	N	Pop	Y	N N
Malta	Combined	N	x	x					Y	Y		N	Y Y
Netherlands	Other	N				x			Y	Y		N	Y Y
Norway	Combined	N	x	x	x	x			N	N		N	N N
Poland	Combined	Y (2,950~)			x				N	N		N	N Y
Portugal	Combined	N		x					Y	Y	Pop	N	Y Y
Romania	GP led	N	x	x			x	x	N	N	Pop; geog; other	Y	Y Y
Slovakia	Paediatrician led	Y (1,000)	x						N	N	Pop	Y	N Y
Slovenia	Combined	N	x	x					Y	Y	Pop	Y	Y N
Spain	Paediatrician led	Y (2,000)	x	x					Y	Y	Pop; geog; soc-ec	Y	Y Y
Sweden	*	*		x					*	*	*	*	* *
UK	GP led	N	x	x		x			N	Y		Y	N Y

Notes: Missing data: France, Luxembourg, Sweden. *Clarification needed/missing data; ~ people not children; N = No, Y = Yes; Pop – Population; Geog – Geography/Transport; Soc-ec – Socio-economic factors.

How primary care workforce organised. 1, Single practitioner; MDT, multidisciplinary team in community practice; PN, paediatric group with nursing staff; 4 GPN, group with nursing staff; 5, Other.

Table 13.5. Country Agent responses to questions on training of workforce for children in primary care.

Country	Paediatrician			GP			Nursing		
	Mandatory Training, Years (Q10)	Postgraduate Specialisation, Years (Q10a)	Type of Postgraduate Specialisation (Q10b)	Mandatory Training, Years (Q11)	Postgraduate Specialisation, Years (Q11a)	Type of Postgraduate Specialisation (Q11b)	Mandatory Basic Training Prevention/ Promotion, Years (Q12)	Postgraduate Specialisation, Years (Q12a)	Type of Postgraduate Specialisation (Q12b)
Austria	3	27 Months	Hospital	3	Generic	Hospital, GP office, practice	3, Paediatric school for nurses.	Certified paediatric nurse – no additional specialisation	N
Belgium	5	5	Hospital	3	6m, Paediatrics	GP office, hospital	4, general	Community health, paediatrics	N
Bulgaria	6	4	Paediatrics	3	3	General medicine	4, General	None	N
Croatia	6.25	5	Paediatrics	6.25	4	Paediatric-specific	3, General	Optional	N
Cyprus	6	4	Paediatrics	6	4	Postgraduate training	*, General	Public health or Community	N
Czech Rep.	5	5	*	No GPs	*		3, General	Professional module	
Denmark	6	5	Hospital	5–5.5	4.5	Hospital depts	3.5	1.5, health visitor	N
Estonia	6	4	Paediatrics	6	5, residency	Family medicine	4, General	Community care	N

Finland	6	Paediatrics. Other	6	6	General practice, other	4, Public health	None	3.5, General
Germany	5	Hospital	6.25	5	Specialist medical training	—	None	Y
Greece	4	Paediatrics. Other	6	4	General medicine	4, General nurse	Optional, paediatric	N
Hungary	*	Paediatrics. Other	3	2.2	Paediatric	4, Midwifery	None*	N
Iceland	4–5	Paediatrics	*	*	None	4, General	Optional; primary care	N
Ireland	*	Minimum requirements	5–6	4	*	4, General	Public health	N
Italy	5	Paediatrics	3	*	General medicine	3, General	Optional; masters	N
Latvia	4	Paediatrics. Other	6	3	Family medicine	4, University; 2, College	Ambulatory/ child care	1 Year
Lithuania	5	Paediatric surgery. Other	6	3	Family medicine	3.5, General nurse	Optional; community	N
Malta	5	Paediatrics	5	3	General practice	4, General; 3, Diploma	Optional; public health	N
Netherlands	2	Preventive	3	*	Postgraduate	4, General	Optional; children	N
Norway	5	Paediatrics	6	Generic	None	3, General	Public health	N
Poland	5	Paediatrics	6	*	Family medicine.	3, General	*	N

Table 13.5. (*Continued*)

Country	Paediatrician			GP				Nursing	
	Mandatory Training, Years (Q10)	Postgraduate Specialisation, Years (Q10a)	Type of Postgraduate Specialisation (Q10b)	Mandatory Training, Years (Q11)	Postgraduate Specialisation, Years (Q11a)	Type of Postgraduate Specialisation (Q11b)	Mandatory Basic Training Prevention/ Promotion, Years (Q12)	Postgraduate Specialisation, Years (Q12a)	Type of Postgraduate Specialisation (Q12b)
Portugal	6	5	Paediatrics	6	4	Paediatrics, internal / General/ family	4, General	Optional; paediatrics	N
Romania	6	5	Paediatrics	6	3	Family medicine	3/4, General	*	N
Slovakia	6	5	Paediatrics	6	3	Core specialisations	4, General	Optional; public health	N
Slovenia	6	5	Paediatrics	6	4	Hospital/ clinic/GP off	4, Secondary; 3, college		N
Spain	6	4	Paediatrics	6	4	General medicine	4, General	Paediatrics	N
Sweden	5	5.5	*	5	*	*	3, General	Optional; Paediatric/ district	N
UK	8	*	Paediatrics	5	3	General practice	3/4, General	Optional; Children's/ health visiting	N

Notes: Missing data: France, Luxembourg.

mandatory training. The Czech Republic, Malta and Sweden offer a minimum of five years. On average, almost all countries offered four to five years' post-graduate specialisation. This is in line with the European Academy of Paediatrics (EAP) recommendations (European Academy of Paediatrics, EAP, 2018). GP training, however, had more variability (EAP, 2018). All countries had a minimum of three years mandatory training with more than half of the country responses offering six years mandatory medical training and most requiring further specialisation in general practice/family medicine after the mandatory training. Paediatric specialisation was mentioned by three countries: Croatia, Hungary and Poland.

Looking at training requirements for nurses in 28 countries (Table 13.5), there was a minimum of three years mandatory basic training requirement for general nurses with optional specialisations in most countries. Eight countries specifically mention paediatric/children postgraduate/specialist training; others refer to community nursing and primary care. Hungary identified midwifery as a mandatory basic training. Midwifery in Hungarian context refers to Visiting Nurses.

Undergraduate (Basic) Medical Training

Healthcare professionals in primary care support the individual child to achieve optimal health within the context of the family and wider community. Undergraduate medical training, therefore, addresses the huge variety of requirements a physician needs to care for children, over and above their basic education on human physiology, illness, diagnostics and therapies. These include the following:

- checks on children's development (in the form of 'well child reviews'), early identification of any impairments or conditions that require treatment or management and the support of children living in vulnerable circumstances, for instance those experiencing abuse, those already in the care system (see Chapter 5), and those with a long-term, possibly complex, physical or mental condition (see Chapter 10);
- identification of children at risk of poor physical or mental health, such as those vulnerable to discrimination, poverty, traumatic experiences and migrant status and where possible assist in preventive activities;
- adaptation to the child's changing needs as they age and to the current situation of the child. This requires competencies to be attained in topics such as nutrition, parenting, children's rights and understanding of the (child) health system in the country;
- communication skills and the management of a consultation with two parties (the child and the parents) and an empathic style of interaction (see training in adolescent health); and
- training and experience in multi and inter disciplinary work with professionals such as social workers or the justice system (Završnik et al., 2018).

Table 13.6. A whole population approach: patient segments in child health.

Population Group 'Segments'	Examples of Activities/Conditions
Healthy child	Advice, health protection and promotion, immunisation, mental health and wellbeing, nutrition, child development and growth
Child with social needs	Complex family and schooling issues, children in care of the State, self-harm and substance misuse
Child with complex health needs	Severe neurodisability, Down syndrome, long-term ventilation, intractable epilepsy, ADHD and autism
Child with single long-term condition	Asthma, eczema, allergy, diabetes, coeliac disease and continence issues
Acutely mild-moderately unwell child	Common cold, flu, rash, ear infection and urinary tract infection
Acutely severely unwell child	Sepsis, meningitis, traumatic brain injury, acute appendicitis or other surgical emergency

Source: Klaber and Watson (2015).

These requirements provide many training challenges, which are addressed by European Union (EU) and European Economic Area (EEA) countries in subtly different ways. Table 13.6 illustrates a framework for describing the child health population in primary care settings. This has the advantage of classifying clinical groups of children and some of their typical health needs and is useful for appraising the curricula against and reflects our selected tracer conditions in MOCHA. The full framework has both time and equity dimensions in recognition of the changing needs of the developing child and young person as well as the need to ensure coverage of all children in a population.

Curriculum recommendations by a number of European paediatric associations exist, but national decisions have to be made regarding the content of medical school curricula; thus, there is a variety of extent and type of training undertaken by medical students in the EU and EEA countries, in general, and then specifically regarding children.

As one of the special groupings we were interested in, the basic requirements of training to work with vulnerable children in particular are outlined in Figure 13.1.

In Figure 13.1, the smaller circle represents basic medical (undergraduate) training. These qualifications and knowledge are required for all practitioners as a basis of medical studies. The larger circle represents specialist (postgraduate) training, which includes the qualifications and knowledge required for health professionals specialising in child health and treatment.

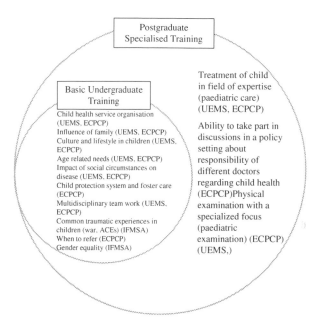

Figure 13.1.   Skills and qualifications required to adequately treat and monitor vulnerable children.

Figure 13.1 is based on the recommendations by European Union Medical Specialties (UEMS 2015), European Confederation of Primary Care Paediatricians (ECPCP 2018) and International Federation of Medical Student Associations (IFMSA 2017) for undergraduate and postgraduate training.

Time and cost restraints in the MOCHA project meant that in order to explore the content of medical training in the EU and EEA countries, we identified three representative countries (Bulgaria, Germany and Iceland) based on the levels of GDP, child poverty and Gini coefficient, in which we identified how the current training programme prepares paediatricians and GPs to work with different vulnerable groups of children including specific knowledge, attitudes and skills. We asked the MOCHA country agents to provide us with medical curricula of their country, either a national curriculum, if it existed, or that of the largest medical school in their country as a representative example of training of physicians in primary care. We then reviewed the medical curricula against the standards recommended by the European bodies for medical education in terms of the physician model of care, Gini-coefficient and the levels of child poverty. The three representative countries are shown in Table 13.7 and Table 13.8 (see Chapter 12).

We reviewed the undergraduate study programmes identified by the MOCHA country agents of the three countries to see whether the curriculum

Table 13.7. Three representative countries.

	Lead Medical Practitioner	Number of Children 0–19 Years	Gini Co-efficient (Source: OECD/ Eurostat)	Child Poverty (%)*
Bulgaria	GP	1,335,049	0.37	41.3%
Germany	Primary care paediatrician	14,550,756	0.29	20.0%
Iceland	Mixed service	89,316	0.25	13.0%

Notes: *http://www.oecd.org/social/income-distribution-database.htm.

Table 13.8. Characteristics of the European medical schools' curricula analysed by MOCHA.

Country Medical School	Type of Reference/Data*	Number of Medical Students (Per Institution)	Duration of Undergraduate Training (Years)
Bulgaria *Sofia*	List of mandatory courses including European Credit Transfer System (ECTS)**	4,000 in total	6
Germany *Munich*	List of mandatory courses	500/year	6
Iceland *Reykjavik*	List of learning goals	50/year	3 + 3*

Notes: *Bsc + Msc degree. http://www.oecd.org/social/income-distribution-database.htm.
**ECTS, https://ec.europa.eu/info/education/study-or-teach-abroad/selecting-university-or-other-institution/higher-education-system_en.

listed or covered the following topics related to health management of vulnerable children in the three identified countries:

- paediatric chronic conditions;
- development of a child;
- mental health of a child;
- disability and complex medical conditions;
- children in palliative care;
- trauma (such as accidents);
- child protection (including Adverse Childhood Experiences (ACEs));
- looked-after children (LAC);
- cultural challenges and immigration;

- refugees;
- poverty, homelessness (socio-economic status (SES)); and
- discrimination (including gender equality).

The coverage of the curricula of these topics is described in Table 13.9.

Preparing Students for Management of Vulnerable Children in Undergraduate Programmes in Bulgaria, Germany and Iceland

We found that that the various topics related to vulnerable children were not well described in the undergraduate medical training programmes. This may represent a suboptimal minimum knowledge and skills in this regard. Our findings are shown in Table 13.10.

Mandatory Undergraduate Courses Related to Health Care of Vulnerable Children

All three countries covered the topics *Development*, *Mental Health* and *Trauma (other than ACEs)* in their courses in paediatrics. However, further details as to the content of these courses were not provided. It is possible that the mandatory course on psychiatry may cover additional aspects of *Development*, *Mental Health* and *Trauma (other than ACEs)* in children. Subgroups of vulnerable children including children subject to child protection plans, children affected by cultural challenges and immigration, refugees and children in poverty or who are homeless were not identified in the curricula, so it is impossible to establish if the needs of these cohorts are specifically addressed. Germany was the only country that listed palliative care in the training programme, but not with a focus on children.

Training in Personal and Interpersonal Skills

Communication skills and knowledge about the national health system, multidisciplinary work and representation of the medical point of view (for instance in a court of law) were not overtly covered in any of the curricula, except in Iceland. Organisation and time management were not covered in any of the curricula.

Qualifications of a Doctor to Deal with Cases in a Paediatric and Social Setting

We investigated how undergraduate training prepares future doctors to cope with emotionally challenging situations. Iceland covered the skills *Talk about difficult cases, coping strategies* and *Knowledge about their own limits as a doctor* (in terms of own knowledge and when to seek other advice) in their curricula. Bulgaria listed *Sports for students in year 1* which might contribute to encourage the students to learn about work—life balance, but this was the only country of the three that did so. In Germany, a mentor programme is available and may include discussion of difficult cases. We found no data from students giving feedback on the training programme in any of the three countries. None of the countries addressed the importance of social determinants of health and how these

Table 13.9. Mandatory courses related to health care of subgroups of vulnerable children in Bulgaria, Germany and Iceland.

Country Medical School	Bulgaria Sofia	Germany Munich	Iceland Reykjavik
Paediatric chronic condition	Paediatrics	Paediatrics	Paediatrics
Development	Paediatrics	Paediatrics	Paediatrics
Mental health	Psychiatry^Paediatrics	Psychiatry^Paediatrics	Psychiatry^Paediatrics
Disability; complex medical condition	Physiotherapy^Rehabilitation^	Rehabilitation^	Rehabilitation^
Children in palliative care	Not listed	Palliative medicine^	Not listed
Trauma (other than ACEs*)	Psychiatry^Paediatrics	Psychiatry^Paediatrics	Psychiatry^Paediatrics
Child protection including ACEs*	Not listed	Not listed	Not listed
LAC	Not listed	Not listed	Not listed
Cultural challenges and immigration	Not listed	Not listed	Not listed
Refugees	Not listed	Not listed	Not listed
Poverty, homelessness (SES#)	Not listed	Not listed	Not listed
Discrimination	Not listed	Not listed	Not listed

Notes: ^not only focused on vulnerable children; not listed: not listed in outline of undergraduate study programme. * Adverse Childhood Experiences

Table 13.10. Skills and qualifications to overcome challenges in adequate treatment of vulnerable children.

Country Medical School	Bulgaria Sofia	Germany Munich	Iceland Reykjavik
Communication	Not listed	Not listed	Covered^
Organisation and time management	Not listed	Not listed	Not listed
Child health in the context of the society	Social medicine^	Social medicine^	Social medicine^
Children's rights, ethics, impact of SES	Ethics^; Other not listed	Ethics^; Other not listed	Ethics^; Other not listed
Knowledge to give preventative advice (nutrition, parenting, risk factors like environment and hygiene, projects, UNICEF, WHO)	Environment^Other not listed	Environment^Other not listed	Environment^Other not listed
Knowledge about the national health system to provide information for support and to enable access for the patient to different health services (e.g. referral)	Not listed	Not listed	Covered^
Multidisciplinary team work	Not listed	Not listed	Covered^
Giving evidence in court/coroner	Not listed	Not listed	Covered^

Notes: ^Not only focused on vulnerable children; not listed: not listed in outline of undergraduate study programme.

Table 13.11. A child health provider's required qualifications.

Country Medical School	Bulgaria Sofia	Germany Munich	Iceland Reykjavik
Talk about difficult cases, coping strategies	Not listed	Mentor programme	Covered
Knowledge about own limit (exceeded personal skills, exceeded medical treatment)	Not listed	Not listed	Covered
Work−life balance	Sports for the student in year 1	Not listed	Not listed
Possibilities to give feedback on the training	No data	No data	No data

Note: Not listed: not listed in outline of undergraduate study programme.

affect child health outcomes − even in countries with a high level of poverty and inequality (represented by Bulgaria in our examples). Table 13.11 summarises our findings in the three exemplar countries.

Training in Adolescent Health Medicine

Adolescent medicine involves acquiring specific competences and skills to develop a mutually respectful relationship between the physician and the adolescent. These include the following:

- respecting adolescents' rights and confidentiality (Kokotailo, Baltag, & Sawyer, 2018; Michaud, Berg-Kelly, Macfarlane, & Lazar, 2010; Michaud, Blum, Benaroyo, Zermatten, & Baltag, 2015; United Nations, 1989);
- developing appropriate screening and counselling approaches to review an adolescent's lifestyle;
- navigating family conflicts or addressing situations that may pose ethical dilemmas; and
- acquiring the capacity to deal with health issues such as exploratory and risk behaviours, mental health and sexual and reproductive health (Baltag & Mathison, 2010; Michaud et al., 2018, 2010; World Health Organization, 2014; World Health Organization, 2015a).

For effective outcomes, medical and nursing students should be trained to deal concretely with clinical situations by means of interactive participative sessions, bedside teaching and observation, discussions of videos or testing their skills with simulated patients (Hardoff, S. Benita, & Ziv, 2008).

Several documents have recently outlined how high-quality health care can be achieved for adolescents (Ambresin, Bennett, Patton, Sanci, & Sawyer, 2013; Michaud, Weber, Namazova-Baranova, & Ambresin, 2018; Nair et al., 2015; Sawyer, Ambresin, Bennett, & Patton, 2014; World Health Organization, 2016), and a recent publication of the World Health Organization suggests that there are several core elements of quality care pertaining specifically to adolescents, in which the healthcare providers' competencies play a pivotal role (World Health Organization, 2015b; Michaud & Baltag, 2015).

In MOCHA, we surveyed the country agents as to the extent of training in adolescent medicine and care in 30 countries. We sought to evaluate the number of European countries providing under- and postgraduate training curricula specifically focusing on the field of adolescent medicine and health, either as a stand-alone topic or as sessions embedded in the programme of other disciplines. In addition to the country agents, the questionnaire was sent to members of the European Association of Paediatrics (EAP) and the 'young EAP' group whose members extend beyond the 30 MOCHA countries. Further details about the survey can be found in the study by Jansen et al. (2018).

Results

Status of Adolescent Medicine and Health within European Countries

Only 10 countries from the MOCHA project (Croatia, Finland, France, Greece, Italy, Portugal, Slovenia, Spain, Sweden and the UK) and three from outside the EU (Moldova, Switzerland and Turkey) have some units where paediatric residents can train in specialised wards with tutors specifically trained in adolescent medicine, but it is likely that these are situated only in selected parts of the country. Sixteen countries (Austria, Bulgaria, Croatia, Czech Republic, Denmark, Finland, France, Greece, Italy, Malta, Norway, Portugal, Slovenia, Spain, Sweden and the UK) and three from outside the EU or EEA (Israel, Switzerland and Turkey) have set up a national association for adolescent health. Finally, four MOCHA countries (Bulgaria, Czech Republic, Finland and Spain (pending)) and two non-MOCHA countries (Armenia and Ukraine) have a formal title for physicians specialising in adolescent medicine and health in each country.

Under- and Postgraduate Training in the Field of Adolescent Medicine and Health

Stand-alone sessions encourage learners to look at adolescents as patients with specific health needs (World Health Organization, 2015). We asked if these were present or whether the teaching of adolescent health issues is embedded in the mainstream curriculum tackling issues such as mental health or reproduction in general. Table 13.12 gives an overview of the answers received from all participating countries: the dark grey colour indicates good training coverage, the light grey indicates some coverage, and the white colour indicates no or little coverage among various professions and disciplines.

Table 13.12. Training in adolescent health delivered within various disciplines and important topics in primary care, across all participating countries.

	Cat	Student SA	I Paed SA	II Paed SA	GPs SA	Gyn SA	Psych SA	School SA	Nurse SA	Topics Stud	Topics Paed	Topics GPs	Ward	CME	Spec	Assoc
Armenia		No	Mandatory	Mandatory	Optional	Optional	Mandatory	Not appl	Not that I know	All	Most	Few	No	All	Yes	No
Austria		Opt	Mand	Opt	Opt	Opt	Opt	Mand	No		All	Few	No	All	No	Yes
Belgium		No	Not SA	Not SA	Not SA	Not SA	Mand	Mand	No	All	All	Few	No	Ment h	No	No
Bosnia Herzeg		No	Not SA	Not SA	Opt	Opt	Opt	Not applic	No	Most	Ethics	None	No	Most	No	No
Bulgaria		Opt SA	Not appl	Opt	Opt	Opt	Opt	Mand	Yes SA	None	None	None	No	All	Yes?	±
Croatia		Mand SA	Not SA	Mand	Not SA	Mand	Mand	Mand	No	All	All	All	±	All	No	Yes
Cyprus	C	No	Not SA	Not SA	Not appl	Not appl	Not appl	Not SA	No	Most	None	None	No	Some	No	No
Czech Republic		Mand SA	Mand SA	Mand SA	Not SA	Not SA	Not SA	Not appl	No	All	All	None	No	Some	Yes	Yes
Denmark	Λ	No	Not appl	Not SA	Not SA	Not SA	Not SA	Not appl	No	None	Some	None	No	None	No	Yes
Estonia	Λ	No	Not SA	Not SA	Not SA	Not SA	Not SA	Not SA	No	Most	Most	All	No	SRH	No	No
Denmark	Λ	No	Not appl	Mand SA	Not SA	Not SA	Not SA	Not appl	No	None	Some	None	No	None	No	Yes
Estonia	Λ	No	Not SA	Not SA	Not SA	Not SA	Not SA	Not SA	No	Most	Most	All	No	SRH	No	No

Finland	A	Opt SA	Mand SA	Mand SA	Opt SA	Opt SA	Opt SA	Mand SA	Spec SA	All	All	All	Partly	All	Yes	Yes
France		No	Opt SA	Opt SA	Not SA	Not SA	Opt SA	Not SA	No	Most	Most	Few	Partly	All	No	Yes
Germany	A	No	Mand SA	Mand SA	Opt SA	Opt SA	Mand SA	Not appl	No	Some	Several	Few	No	Several	No	No
Greece		Opt SA	Mand SA	Opt SA	Opt SA	Mand SA	Mand SA	Not appl	No	Few	None	None	Yes	Several	Yes	Yes
Hungary		No SA	Not SA	Not SA	Not SA	Not SA	Mand SA	Mand SA	No	Some	Few	Few	No	Several	No	No
Iceland	C	No	Not SA	Not SA	Not SA	Not SA	Not SA	Not SA	No	Most	All	All	No	Some	No	No
Ireland		No	Not SA	Mand SA	Mand SA	Opt SA	Opt SA	Not SA	No	Few	Few	Few	No	Few	No	No
Israel		No	Not SA	Not SA	Not SA	Not SA	Not SA	Not SA	No	Few	Several	Few	No	Few	No	No
Italy		No	Mand SA	Mand SA	Opt SA	Opt SA	Opt SA	Not appl	Spec SA	Few	All	No	Yes	Several	No	Yes
Latvia	C	No	Not SA	Not SA	Not SA	Opt SA	Mand SA	Not appl	No	All	Few	Few	No	None	No	No
Lithuania	C	No	Not SA	Not SA	Not SA	Not SA	Not SA	Not appl	Spec SA	Some	All	All	No	All	No	Yes
Malta	C	No	Mand SA	Mand SA	Mand SA	Mand SA	Mand SA	Not appl	Spec SA	All	All	Some	No	Several	No	No
Moldova		Opt SA	Mand SA	Opt SA	Opt SA	Opt SA	Opt SA	Mand SA	Spec SA	All	All	All	Yes	Most	No	Yes
Netherlands	A	No	Not appl									All	No	None	No	No

Table 13.12. (Continued)

Norway		Yes stand SA	Opt SA	Opt SA	Opt SA	Opt SA	Opt SA	Opt SA	Spec SA	All	All	All	All	No	Few	No	Yes
Poland	C	No	Mand SA	Not SA	Not SA	Not SA	Not SA	Not SA	Spec SA	All	All	All	Some	No	None	No	No
Portugal		Opt SA	Opt SA	Opt SA	Opt SA	Not appl	Not appl	Not appl	Spec SA	All	All	All	Few	Yes	Several	No	Yes
Romania	C	No	Opt SA	Opt SA	Not appl	Opt SA	Opt SA	Mand SA	No	Few	Few	Few	Few	No	All	No	No
Serbia		No	No SA	Opt SA	No SA	Opt SA	Mand SA	Not SA	No	None	Several	Several	Some	No	Several	No	No
Slovenia	C	Mand SA	Mand SA	Mand SA	Opt SA	Mand SA	Mand SA	Mand SA	Spec SA	All	All	All	All	Yes	All	No	Yes
Spain	A	Opt SA	Mand SA	Mand SA	Mand SA	Not appl	Not appl	Not appl	Yes SA	Several	All	Few	Few	Yes	All	Pending	Yes
Sweden		No	Mand SA	Mand SA	Mand SA	Opt SA	Opt SA	Mand SA	Spec SA	Several	All	All	All	Yes	All	No	Yes
Switzerland		Mand SA	Opt SA	Not SA	Not SA	Not SA	Not SA	Not SA	Some	All	All	All	All	Yes	All	No	Yes
Turkey		Mand SA	Opt SA	Opt SA	Opt SA	Not SA	Opt SA	Not SA	No	All	All	All	All	Yes	Most	No	Yes
Ukraine		Mand SA	Not SA	Not SA	Not SA	Not SA	Not SA	Not SA	No	Few	Few	Few	Few	No	None	Yes	No
United Kingdom	A	No	Not appl	Opt SA	Opt not SA	Opt not SA	Opt not SA	Opt not SA	No	Most	All	Most	Most	Yes	Few	No	Yes

Notes: SA, stand-alone sessions; stud, medical students; Paed I, primary care paediatricians; Paed II, secondary care paed; GPs, general practitioners; school doctors; topics: in dark shade = all or most topics covered; ward: in dark shade: possibility to train in specialised adol. wards and specialisation in adol health and country-based association in adol health.

Undergraduate Curricula

Seven countries reported that some stand-alone teaching is available and mandatory for medical students, and another seven countries report optional stand-alone teaching. In terms of content, a number of countries provide sessions tackling specific adolescent health issues, either as stand-alone sessions or as part of the programme of larger disciplines (paediatrics, psychiatry and gynaecology): for instance, communication skills are taught in some form in 17 countries, ethical issues in 18 countries, how to assess lifestyles in 19 countries, the area of sexual and reproductive health in 22 countries and the field of mental health in 22 countries. Interestingly, countries that propose mandatory stand-alone training for medical students cover all the five areas considered as critical. In terms of nursing education, very few countries propose sessions specifically dedicated to adolescent health, only Bulgaria and Spain do so. Ten countries have implemented such courses as part of a specialisation process, but 24 countries do not provide any stand-alone training.

Postgraduate Curricula

Only four MOCHA countries, (Italy, Slovenia, Spain and Sweden), and Armenia and Moldova from outside the EU and EEA, provide stand-alone training sessions to residents in paediatrics and in family practice (overall primary care doctors). In other words, the majority of countries provide some specific sessions dealing with adolescent health, to primary and secondary care paediatricians, but in most cases, these are optional and embedded in sessions dealing with other topics. The content of training provided to future paediatricians varies, depending on the issue: Communication skills as well as topics related to sexual and reproductive health are taught in around 20 countries, while screening of lifestyles, ethics, and mental health seem better covered (respectively, in 25, 28 and 29 countries).

The coverage among family physicians, gynaecologists and psychiatrists is much lower, as can be seen in Table 13.12. Only two MOCHA countries, Ireland and Spain, plus Moldova from the non-EU countries offer mandatory sessions to GPs or gynaecologists. Ten countries provide sessions dealing with adolescent health to psychiatrists, but tend to tackle only mental health. The educational opportunities covering important topics in adolescent health are optional in 15 countries. The session content to junior GPs varies little and includes communication skills, ethics, screening of lifestyles and issues related to sexual and reproductive life; these are covered in only 16–18 countries and the area of mental health in 23 countries.

Continuing Medical Education (CME)

Table 13.12 shows that the percentage of countries organising CME training sessions is similar to that of postgraduate training in adolescent health. It is largely the same countries who provide training at postgraduate level that do so within CME curricula. Only nine countries offer CME sessions in all areas considered as important to adolescent health and in nine countries, there are no sessions on adolescent health and medicine.

Quality of Adolescent Primary Care and Amount and Content of Training
The MOCHA project attempted to identify three clusters of countries with different levels of standards of adolescent care. Countries belonging to the first group are Denmark, Finland, the Netherlands, Spain and the UK (England) and to a lesser extent are Croatia, Czech Republic, Estonia, Germany, Italy, Portugal and Slovenia. These countries have implemented policies and strategies which guarantee good access to health care for adolescents, as well as a respect of confidentiality and other aspects of 'adolescent friendly' care (Ambresin et al., 2013; Baltag & Mathison, 2010; Tylee, Haller, Graham, Churchill, & Sanci, 2007). The second group includes Austria, Belgium (French-speaking), Bulgaria, Greece, Ireland, Luxembourg, Norway and Sweden, which have developed only basic policies in adolescent health training, and the third group of Cyprus, Hungary Iceland, Latvia, Lithuania, Malta, Poland, Romania and Slovakia does not meet most standards.

While there is some consistency between the quality of adolescent health care and the amount and content of training delivered in countries such as Finland, Germany, the Netherlands, Spain and the UK, it is puzzling that Denmark and Estonia were classified high in terms of quality of care despite not offering adequate training in the field.

The Nursing Workforce

Nurses are the largest single profession within the European health workforce with over six million nurses in the region (World Health Organization, 2018). They play a critical role in public health, working across the breadth of primary and community care services, such as GP or primary care paediatrician-led practices, health centres, preventative health services, school health services (SHS), home care and residential services. A skilled and competent nursing workforce can influence not only people's health outcomes but also the practices and policies needed to achieve change (World Health Organization, 2013).

The MOCHA project has described the nursing workforce and has proposed key components for inclusion in education and training programmes for nurses in primary care for children (See Hilliard, Clancy, Hollywood, & Brenner, 2018). There is considerable variation in the distribution and scope of the nursing role across Europe. In some countries, nursing may be the first point of contact for children and families with a medical issue, and some nurses have advanced practice roles with varying degrees of diagnostic, prescriptive and referral authority (Blair, Rigby, & Alexander, 2017; Maier & Aiken, 2016). The various primary care configurations manifest themselves in differing models of nursing services, such as working exclusively with a health promotion and prevention remit, having a specific paediatric caseload, or working within a 'cradle to grave' model. The MOCHA examination of SHS (see Chapter 11) similarly identified variations in nurses' roles across the MOCHA countries, ranging from administering immunisations and preventative screening to managing minor illnesses or injuries to assessing the educational and participation needs of children with chronic healthcare needs (Jansen et al., 2018).

This variation in the role and configuration of the nursing workforce within primary care, and the multiplicity of other variables which influence primary care outcomes, creates a challenge when attempting to evaluate the contribution and impact of nurses. Nursing roles are changing to encompass greater autonomy and skills (Maier & Aiken, 2016), and it is known that effective planning of the skill mix of nursing expertise is beneficial to patient outcomes (Blegen, Goode, Spetz, Vaughn, & Park, 2011; Griffiths, Murrells, Maben, Jones, & Ashworth, 2010) and that access to primary care is a factor in improving children's health outcomes (see Chapter 3).

In order to identify an optimal service, there is a need for accurate and comparable data about the proportion and distribution of nurses across the MOCHA countries within the healthcare workforce and more specifically those with a remit for child health. Furthermore, there is a need to anticipate emerging healthcare issues to ensure primary care services are targeted appropriately and are responsive to the wider healthcare needs of children, as well as the needs of vulnerable groups such as marginalised populations, migrant children and children with complex care needs (CCNs).

However, research into nursing workforce and skill-mix in primary care is limited (Jackson, Wright, & Martin, 2016; Maier & Aiken, 2016). There is great variability in the type and quality of data collected about primary care structures, processes and outcomes across the participating countries, and children's data are frequently aggregated with whole population data (see Chapter 7). The proportion of nurses across MOCHA countries varies considerably, ranging from 355 per 100,000 population in Greece to 1,631 per 100,000 population in Norway (World Health Organization, 2018). Nurses per 100,000 population are highest in combined systems of primary care (MacPepple & Gage, 2018). However, there are limitations to this data as some countries report the number of practising nurses providing direct care, while other countries report professionally active nurses which includes those who are not involved in direct care. Respondents to MOCHA surveys on SHS stated that only a minority of MOCHA countries ($n = 8$) specify a defined pupil-to-nurse ratio, which ranged from one nurse per 100 students (Latvia) to one nurse per 3,500 students (Malta) (see Chapter 11; Jansen et al., 2018). It is difficult to critique this variation in the nursing resource with respect to its relative impact on student health outcomes, due to the varying role of nurses in SHS across the MOCHA countries. However, international evidence does show that SHS can enhance access to health care, improve health and education outcomes and improve school attendance particularly among children with chronic health conditions (Baltag, Pachyna, & Hall, 2015; Bersamin, Garbers, Gaarde, & Santelli, 2016; Knopf et al., 2016; Leroy, Wallin, & Lee, 2017).

There is a need to develop systematic approaches to gathering data which reflect nursing in primary care and the outcomes they achieve. Developing a suite of nurse-sensitive indicators that are sufficiently broad to have utility across the various types of primary care workforce configurations would contribute to illuminating the impact of the nursing contribution. Factors such as patient experience, satisfaction, quality of life and engagement with treatment plans should also be evaluated to determine whether developments in nursing practice and service delivery add value to patients' care.

Nurses' Training and Skills

It is important that nurses working with children have the necessary skills and knowledge to deliver high-quality nursing care to all children and their families and are able to meet children's changing needs across their life course from infancy to adolescence. However, it is known that there is a great variation in the type, duration and availability of paediatric nursing programmes (Paediatric Nursing Association of Europe, 2011). In the MOCHA project, we explored nurses' preparedness for caring for children in primary care and found that a general nurse qualification is the minimum requirement for working with children in the community in the majority of responding MOCHA countries (Clancy, Montañana Montañana-Olaso, & Larkin, 2017). However, the educational preparation of general nurses across the MOCHA countries can vary from three years (e.g. France, Norway and Poland) to four years (e.g. Iceland, Ireland, Lithuania and Spain), which has an influence on both the theoretical and clinical content of these programmes. Specialised qualifications prior to working with children are required only in a minority of countries. These include paediatric nursing, public health or community nursing. However, five of the respondent countries (Estonia, Finland, Lithuania, Malta and Romania) had no paediatric options available for specialised training. In primary care, there are also differences. Nurses working in SHS, for example, are required to undergo specialised training in only half the responding countries ($n = 14/28$); yet, these nurses are increasingly encountering children and adolescents with chronic conditions, CCNs or psychosocial needs. Furthermore, despite the specific healthcare needs of children with CCNs, 73.9% ($n = 17$) of MOCHA countries reported that specialised training was not required by nurses caring for these children in primary care; this is shown in Figure 13.2 (Clancy et al., 2017).

Children with CCN offer a good example of how the disparity in nurses' educational preparation manifests itself across the MOCHA countries. These children are cared for by nurses whose minimum education ranges from a three-year undergraduate programme in countries where additional qualifications or specialisation are not required (Croatia, France, Italy, Malta, Norway, Poland and Romania) to five years in Sweden, for example, where nurses must have one year of nursing experience following a three-year undergraduate degree, after which they undertake a one-year postgraduate training in paediatric or community nursing. It is within this context that Brenner and colleagues in WP2 defined the need for all primary care providers caring for children with CCN to have specialist training as a standard of care for these children (Brenner et al., 2017) (see Chapter 10).

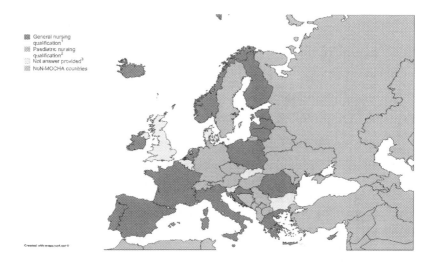

Figure 13.2.   Nursing training requirements to look after children with CCN. *Source:* Clancy et al. (2017). *Notes:* [1]Cyprus stated that paediatric nursing was not offered in the community. [2]Sweden stated that either community or paediatric nursing training was required to look after children with CCN in the community. [3]Danish data not available for this analysis.

The Need for Specialised Knowledge

MOCHA highlights concerns related to the divide between nurse education and current and future needs in clinical practice. As outlined in Chapter 1, children have distinct and evolving health, developmental, educational, emotional and social needs as they journey through childhood into adolescence and transition to adulthood. Nurses in primary care meet children at various stages in their life course and across a variety of settings, and must have the knowledge and expertise to identify and be responsive to children's needs within the context of their role. This is of critical importance when they are the first point of contact, particularly in the light of the emerging epidemiological trends in health and illness in children.

Paediatric expertise and access to specialised education are important factors in the appropriateness of referrals from primary to secondary care and in the integration of care for children with CCN (see Chapters 10 and 15). Relational ethics and healthcare providers' communication skills are repeatedly identified in the literature as contributing to positive patient experiences and therapeutic relationships in paediatric health care (Daley, Polifroni, & Sadler, 2017; Schaeuble, Haglund, & Vukovich, 2010) underlined by MOCHA's interviews with young people (see Chapter 3; Alma et al., 2017) This is of critical importance in the context of MOCHA's finding that young people (16–24 years), although satisfied with health care, consistently report poorer experience of care than older adults and are less likely than adults to feel respected or have necessary confidence and trust in their doctors (Alma et al., 2017).

However, Clancy and colleagues' analysis of the curricular content of under-graduate general nursing programmes across the MOCHA countries revealed wide variation in the focus on child health, paediatrics and children with CCN. Almost three-quarters of the curricula analysed (70.6%, $n = 12$) contained one or more compulsory core modules that focused on the care of children as can be seen in Figure 13.3 (Clancy et al., 2017). The workload assigned to each module was variable, and elements of child health primarily appeared in other modules, for example pharmacology, rather than as stand-alone modules, and largely represented a biomedical focus with little visibility of the psychosocial and holistic care needs of children. As described in the context of medical education, earlier in this chapter, content related to the healthcare needs of adolescents was similarly varied and did not emerge as a distinct stand-alone topic within the curricula of general nursing programmes and was either absent or taught within the wider context of children's health care.

The EU Directive on recognition of professional qualifications provides a broad framework for general nursing curricula across Europe, but does not offer guidance on the specific content and skills that are necessary for the nursing care of children (European Parliament and European Council, 2005; European Parliament and European Council, 2013). The implications of this broad directive are visible in the results of MOCHA which illustrate the great variations in both the emphasis placed on children in general nursing programmes across Europe and the extent to which nurses are educationally prepared to care for children in primary care.

Preparing Nurses for the Emerging Models of Care

Despite previous calls for change (Benner, Sutphen, Leonard, & Day, 2010), MOCHA could not identify a current European competence framework for how the nursing care of children should be taught or what content on child health

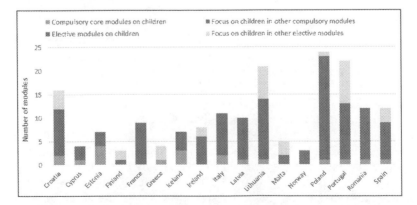

Figure 13.3.   Distribution of child-related content across the different modules in the curriculum. *Source*: Clancy et al. (2017).

should be included in general nursing programmes. There remains no consensus on the minimum standard and content of postgraduate nurse education in relation to children's specific healthcare needs. This, combined with differences in legislation and regulation on advanced roles, makes it difficult for nations to change nursing roles to adapt to new models of care (Maier & Aiken, 2016). Consequently, our capacity in MOCHA to determine which primary care nursing model confers the best outcomes for children is impeded by the current variation in educational preparation and minimum requirements for nurses caring for children. While a competence framework for the wider contexts of nursing children was not identified, the WHO has defined core competencies for all primary healthcare providers caring for adolescents under three domains: (1) adolescent health and development and effective communication, (2) laws, policies and quality standards, and (3) clinical care of adolescents with specific conditions (World Health Organization, 2015). The incorporation of these competencies within both undergraduate and specialist programmes would contribute to developing a nursing workforce that is responsive to the needs of this particular group.

The extent to which healthcare professionals listened, were caring, sympathetic, non-judgemental and respectful, and '*knew how to communicate with* [...] *children*' (p. 77) (Alma et al., 2017), influenced the establishment of a trusting relationship between professionals, children and parents. This corroborates the evidence of other researchers who found that children and adolescents viewed the building of trust as critical to the quality of their relationship with their healthcare providers, (Robinson, 2010). Professional competence and a willingness to seek additional training are further attributes of all healthcare professionals that are valued by children and families (Alma et al., 2017), as can be seen in MOCHA's analysis of medical training for children and adolescents described earlier in this chapter. Children also called for a more holistic approach to their health, to include their feelings and experiences of their illness, rather than solely focusing on the physical manifestations of their condition (Alma et al., 2017). This is of particular importance for the increasing number of children who are living with chronic and/or CCNs. The experiences of the children described in the DIPEx report highlight the need for generalist and specialist nursing curricula to include an emphasis on the psychosocial elements of children's healthcare experiences and the interpersonal competencies necessary to meet these.

A requirement now exists to consider the outcome measures which would lend themselves to evaluating the effect of nursing education on a holistic approach to children's health care in the primary care setting and the added value which specific education in children's nursing may contribute.

Summary

Our appraisal of the models of medical and nursing workforce – the operational backbone – for primary care for Europe's children shows unacceptable variation in terms of both numbers and adequacy of training required to meet the needs of Europe's children. The rapid reduction in numbers of primary care paediatricians in Europe with an increase in the number of family doctors and mixed systems necessitates a radical review of workforce planning in the EU and EEA for this large population group (van Esso et al., 2010). It is likely that a common set of uni- and multidisciplinary competencies needs to be developed for nursing in particular but also a much greater focus given to child health issues of most relevance in the twenty-first century highlighted in this report in both basic and postgraduate medical and nursing education. The preparation of medical students to work with children in primary care is varied and from our sample is, in many cases, lacking against defined essential knowledge for practice which may result in such career paths being less attractive and compound the workforce issues. The situation for nursing — the larger workforce having more interpersonal interaction with both well and ill children — is even more varied. But worse, there seems to be no basis of comparison or harmonisation, and little study of what is optimally required.

Within Europe, there is a common commitment and public expectation of quality of health care for children, but this does not manifest in professional education in key health professions. Europe has mutual recognition of qualifications, yet this is in effect mutual recognition of unequal knowledge and competencies. There is harmonisation of third-level educational structures through the Bologna framework, but no harmonisation of the content when applied to life-critical professions. There is work by the European Skills Council (ESCO) to harmonise skills and competencies across many employment sectors in Europe, but the application to medicine and nursing is low. Other than the paediatric associations' initiatives reported in this chapter, the health professions do not seem united or vocal in addressing standards of training for the health care of children. WHO has advocated standards for those working with adolescents (World Health Organisation 2015b), but not significantly for other groups. Thus, our appraisal of models of primary care for children has, unfortunately but importantly, discovered an indefensible lack of study or standards for educating Europe's doctors and nurses to care effectively for Europe's children in all 30 countries, and thus, there is no model of medical or nursing education over which we can stand — but several initiatives we can commend and a research need which we can articulate vigorously.

Adolescents are an important cohort of children (see Chapter 11). However, it is a concern that only seven countries in the MOCHA group provide some mandatory training in adolescent healthcare, which coupled with optional or ad hoc training available in other countries, could lead to sub-optimal care for this group of young people. Encouraging medical and nursing schools to progressively endorse and implement a minimal set of training objectives about adolescent health within stand-alone, mandatory sessions is an important aim. These sessions should include specific issues such as sexual and reproductive health, mental health or substance use and also address essential skills such as effective communication and ethical issues.

References

Alma, M., Mahtani, V., Palant, A., Klůzová Kráčmarová, L., & Prinjha, S. (2017). *Report on patient experiences of primary care in 5 DIPEx countries.* Retrieved from http://www.childhealthservicemodels.eu/publications/technical-reports/

Ambresin, A. E., Bennett, K., Patton, G. C., Sanci, L. A., & Sawyer, S. M. (2013). Assessment of youth-friendly health care: A systematic review of indicators drawn from young people's perspectives. *Journal of Adolescent Health, 52*, 670−681. doi:10.1016/j.jadohealth.2012.12.014

Baltag, V., & Mathison, A. (2010). *Youth-friendly health policies and services in the European region: Sharing experiences* (p. 267). Copenhagen: World Health Organization. Retrieved from http://www.euro.who.int/__data/assets/pdf_file/0017/123128/E94322.pdf

Baltag, V., Pachyna, A., & Hall, J. (2015). Global overview of school health services: Data from 102 countries. *Health Behavior and Policy Review, 2*(4), 268−283.

Benner, P., Sutphen, M., Leonard, V., & Day, L. (2010). *Educating nurses: A call for radical transformation.* Stanford, CA: The Carnegie Foundation for the Advancement of Teaching.

Bersamin, M., Garbers, S., Gaarde, J., & Santelli, J. (2016). Assessing the impact of school-based health centers on academic achievement and college preparation efforts: Using propensity score matching to assess school-level data in California. *The Journal of School Nursing, 32*(4), 241−245.

Blair, M., Rigby, M., & Alexander, D. (2017). *Final report on current models of primary care for children.* Retrieved from www.childhealthservicemodels.eu/wp-content/uploads/2017/07/MOCHA-WP1-Deliverable-WP1-D6-Feb-2017-1.pdf

Blegen, M. A., Goode, C. J., Spetz, J., Vaughn, T., & Park, S. H. (2011). Nurse staffing effects on patient outcomes: Safety-net and non-safety-net hospitals. *Medical Care, 49*(4), 406−414.

Brenner, M., Alma, M., Clancy, A., Larkin, A., Lignou, S., Luzi, D., ... Blair, M. (2017). *Report on needs and future visions for care of children with complex conditions.* Retrieved from http://www.childhealthservicemodels.eu/wp-content/uploads/20171130_Deliverable-D11-2.4-Report-on-needs-and-future-visions-for-care-of-children-with-complex-conditions.pdf

Clancy, A., Montañana Montañana-Olaso, E., & Larkin, P. (2017). *Work package 2: Nurses' preparedness for practice.* Internal Deliverable 2.10. MOCHA: Models of Child Health Appraised. Retrieved from http://www.childhealthservicemodels.eu/publications/technical-reports/

Daley, A. M., Polifroni, E. C., & Sadler, L. S. (2017). "Treat me like a normal person!" A meta-ethnography of adolescents' expectations of their health care providers. *Journal of Pediatric Nursing, 36*, 70−83. doi:10.1016/j.pedn.2017.04.009

European Academy of Paediatrics E.A.P. (2018). Retrieved from http://eapaediatrics.eu/

European Confederation of Primary Care Paediatricians (ECPCP). (2018). Retrieved from https://www.ecpcp.eu/

European Parliament and European Council. (2005). Directive 2005/36/EC of the European Parliament and of the Council of 7 September 2005 on the recognition of professional qualifications. *Official Journal of the European Union.* L255/22,

Article 31. Retrieved from https://eur-lex.europa.eu/LEXUriServ/LexUriServ.do? uri=OJ:L:2005:255:0022:0142:EN:PDF

European Parliament and European Council. (2013). Directive 2013/55/EU of the European Parliament and of the Council amending Directive 2005/36/EC on the recognition of professional qualifications and Regulation (EU) No 1024/2012 on administrative cooperation through the International Market Information System ('the IMI Regulation'). *Official Journal of the European Union*. L 354/132. Available at: http://eur-lex.europa.eu/legal-content/EN/TXT/PDF/?uri=CELEX:3 2013L0055&from=EN

European Union Medical Specialties (UEMS). (2013). Retrieved from https://www.uems.eu/

Griffiths, P., Murrells, T., Maben, J., Jones, S., & Ashworth, M. (2010). Nurse staffing and quality of care in UK general practice: Cross-sectional study using routinely collected data. *British Journal of General Practice*, *60*(570), e36–e48. doi:10.3399/bjgp10X482086

Hardoff, D., S. Benita, S., & Ziv, A. (2008). Simulated-patient-based programs for teaching communication with adolescents: The link between guidelines and practice. *Georgian Medical News*, 156, 80–83.

Hilliard, C., Clancy, A., Hollywood, E., & Brenner, M. (2018). *Children's nursing workforce and educational preparation in primary care in 30 European countries*. Retrieved from http://www.childhealthservicemodels.eu/publications/technical-reports/

International Federation of Medical Student Associations (IFMSA). (2017). Retrieved from https://ifmsa.org/

Jackson, C., Wright, T., & Martin, A. (2016). *Safe caseloads for adult community nursing services—An updated review of the evidence*. Canterbury Christ Church University, Canterbury. Retrieved from http://create.canterbury.ac.uk/15373/1/ Final%20Version%20Managing%20Safe%20Caseloads%20in%20Adult%20Community %20Nursing%20Settings%20with%20ISBN.pdf

Jansen, D. E. M. C., Visser, A., Vervoort, J. P. M., van der Pol, S., Kocken, P., Reijneveld, S. A., & Michaud, P. (2018). *School and adolescent health services in 30 European countries: A description of structure and functioning, and of health outcomes and cost*s. Retrieved from http://www.childhealthservicemodels.eu/wp-content/uploads/Deliverable-173.1_Final-report-on-the-description-of-the-various-models-of-school-health-services-and-adolescent-health-services.pdf

Klaber, B., & Watson, M. (2015). *Child health general practice hubs*. Retrieved from https://www.slideshare.net/NuffieldTrust/bob-klaber-and-mando-watson-child-health-general-practice-hubs

Knopf, J. A. 1., Finnie, R. K. 1., Peng, Y. 1., Hahn, R. A. 2., Truman, B. I. 3., Vernon-Smiley, M. 4., … Community Preventive Services Task Force. (2016). School-based health centers to advance health equity: A Community Guide systematic review. *American Journal of Preventive Medicine*, *51*(1), 114–126. doi:10.1016/j.amepre.2016.01.009

Kokotailo, P. K., Baltag, V., & Sawyer, S. M. (2018). Educating and training the future adolescent health workforce. *The Journal of Adolescent Health*, *62*(5), 511–524. doi:10.1016/j.jadohealth.2017.11.299

Leroy, Z. C., Wallin, R., & Lee, S. (2017). The role of school health services in addressing the needs of students with chronic health conditions: A systematic review. *The Journal of School Nursing*, *33*(1), 64–72. doi:10.1177/1059840516678909

MacPepple, E., & Gage, H. (2018). *Short report on financing mechanisms and health outcomes.* Retrieved from http://www.childhealthservicemodels.eu/wp-content/uploads/Deliverable-D16-6.1-Short-report-on-financial-systems-and-their-impact-on-outcomes.pdf

Maier, C. B., & Aiken, L. H. (2016). Task shifting from physicians to nurses in primary care in 39 countries: A cross-country comparative study. *European Journal of Public Health, 26*(6), 927–934. doi:10.1093/eurpub/ckw098

Michaud, P. A., Berg-Kelly, K., Macfarlane, A., & Lazar, B. (2010). Ethics and adolescent care: An international perspective. *Current Opinion in Paediatrics, 22*(4), 418–422. doi:10.1097/MOP.0b013e32833b53ec

Michaud, P. A., Blum, R. W., Benaroyo, L., Zermatten, J., & Baltag, V. (2015). Assessing an adolescent's capacity for autonomous decision-making in clinical care. *The Journal of Adolescent Health, 57*(4). doi:10.1016/j.jadohealth.2015.06.012

Michaud, P. A., Schrier, L., Ross-Russel, R., van der Heijden, L., Dossche, L., Copley, S., Alterio, T., Mazur, A., Dembinski, L., Hadjipanayis, A., Del Torso, S., Fonseca, H., Ambresin, A. E. (2018). Paediatric departments need to improve residents' training in adolescent medicine and health: A position paper of the European Academy of Paediatrics. *European Journal of Paediatrics, 177*(4), 479–487. doi:10.1007/s00431-017-3061-2

Michaud, P., & Baltag, V. (2015). *Core competencies in adolescent health and development for primary care providers.* Retrieved from http://www.who.int/maternal_child_adolescent/documents/core_competencies/en/

Michaud, P., Weber, M., Namazova-Baranova, L., & Ambresin, A. (2018). Improving the quality of care delivered to adolescents in Europe: A time to invest. *Archives of Disease in Childhood, 104*, 214–216. doi:10.1136/archdischild-2017-314429

Nair, M., Baltag, V., Bose, K., Boschi-Pinto, C., Lambrechts, T., & Mathai, M. (2015). Improving the quality of health care services for adolescents, globally: A standards-driven approach. *The Journal of Adolescent Health, 57*(3), 288–298. doi:10.1016/j.jadohealth.2015.05.011

Paediatric Nursing Association of Europe. (2011). *Paediatric nurse education across Europe 2010: Summary of key findings. PNAE.* Retrieved from https://www.nsf.no/Content/801048/Findings%20Paediatric%20Nurse%20Education%20across%20Europe%202010.pdf

Robinson, S. (2010). Children and young people's views of health professionals in England. *Journal of Child Health Care, 14*(4), 310–326. doi:10.1177/1367493510381772

Sawyer, S. M., Ambresin, A. E., Bennett, K. E., & Patton, G. C. (2014). A measurement framework for quality health care for adolescents in hospital. *The Journal of adolescent health, 55*(4), 484–490. doi:10.1016/j.jadohealth.2014.01.023

Schaeuble, K., Haglund, K., & Vukovich, M. (2010). Adolescents' preferences for primary care provider interactions. *Pediatric Nursing, 15*(3), 202–210. doi:10.1111/j.1744-6155.2010.00232.x

Tylee, A., Haller, D. M., Graham, T., Churchill, R., & Sanci, L. A. (2007). Youth-friendly primary-care services: How are we doing and what more needs to be done? *Lancet, 369*(9572), 1565–1573. doi:10.1016/S0140-6736(07)60371-7

UEMS. (2015). *Training requirements for the specialty of paediatrics.* Retrieved from https://www.uems.eu/__data/assets/pdf_file/0016/44440/UEMS-2015.30-European-Training-Requirements-in-Paediatrics.pdf

United Nations. (1989). *Convention on the rights of the child, New York.* Retrieved from https://downloads.unicef.org.uk/wp-content/uploads/2010/05/UNCRC_united_nations_convention_on_the_rights_of_the_child.pdf?_ga=2.209651665.274437633. 1540996300-199092997.1540996300

van Esso, D., del Torso, S., Hadjipanayis, A., Biver, A., Jaeger-Roman, E., Wettergren, B., ... Primary-Secondary Working Group (PSWG) of European Academy of Paediatrics (EAP). (2010). Paediatric primary care in Europe: Variation between countries. *Archives of Disease in Childhood,* 95. doi:10.1136/adc.2009.178459

World health Organization. (2013). *Health 2020: A European policy framework and strategy for the 21st century.* WHO Regional Office for Europe, Copenhagen.

World Health Organization. (2014). *European framework for quality standards in school health services and competences for school health professionals.* Retrieved from http://www.euro.who.int/__data/assets/pdf_file/0003/246981/European-framework-for-quality-standards-in-school-health-services-and-competences-for-school-health-professionals.pdf?ua=1

World Health Organization. (2015a). *Core competencies in adolescent health and development for primary care providers: Including a tool to assess the adolescent health and development component in pre-service education of health-care providers.* Geneva: World Health Organization. Retrieved from https://www.who.int/maternal_child_adolescent/documents/core_competencies/en/

World Health Organization. (2015b). *Global standards for quality health-care services for adolescents: a guide to implement a standards-driven approach to improve the quality of health care services for adolescents.* Volume 1: Standards and criteria. Retrieved from http://apps.who.int/iris/bitstream/10665/183935/1/9789241549332_vol1_eng.pdf

World Health Organization. (2016). *Improving the quality of care for reproductive, maternal, neonatal, child and adolescent health in the WHO European region.* Retrieved from http://www.euro.who.int/__data/assets/pdf_file/0009/330957/RMNCAH-QI-Framework.pdf?ua=1

World Health Organization. (2018). *Practising nurses, per 100,000 population.* European Health Information Gateway, World Health Organization Regional Office for Europe. Retrieved from https://gateway.euro.who.int/en/indicators/cah_17-practicing-nurses-per-100-000-population/visualizations/#id=27487&tab=table

Završnik, J., Stiris, T., Schrier, L., Russell, R.R., Del Torso, S., Valiulis, A., Mercier, J.C., Illy, K., & Hadjipanayis, A. (2018). Basic training requirements for health care professionals who care for children. *European Journal of Paediatrics, 177,* 1413. doi:10.1007/s00431-018-3150-x

Chapter 14

e-Health as the Enabler of Primary Care for Children

Michael Rigby, Grit Kühne and Shalmali Deshpande

Abstract

Information and communication technologies can transform how services can be and are delivered as has already happened in other arenas, such as civil aviation, financial services and retailing. Most modern health care is heavily dependent on e-health, including record keeping, targeted information sharing and digital diagnostic and imaging techniques. However, there remains little scientific knowledge base for optimal system content and function in primary health care, particularly for children. Models of Child Health Appraised (MOCHA) aimed to establish the current e-health situation in children's primary care services. Electronic health records (EHRs) are in regular use in much of northern and western Europe and in some newer European Union Member States, but other countries lag behind. MOCHA investigated the use of unique identifiers, the use of case-based public health EHRs and the capability of record linkage, linkage of information with school health data and monitoring of social media influences, such as health websites and health apps. A widespread lack of standards underlined a lack of research enquiry into this issue in terms of children's health data and health knowledge. Health websites and apps are a growing area of healthcare delivery, but there is a worrying lack of safeguards in place. The challenge for policy-makers and practitioners is to be aware and to lead on the innovative harnessing of new technologies, while protecting child users against new harms.

Keywords: Health information and communication technologies; child health; electronic health record; apps; websites; e-health

Introduction

Most modern health care is heavily dependent on e-health, including record keeping, targeted information sharing and digital diagnostic and imaging techniques. The Models of Child Health Appraised (MOCHA) project therefore contained a special work package looking at this issue.

The foundations are strong. The first electronic health record (EHR) application in child health in Europe was for immunisation scheduling and recording more than 55 years ago in the United Kingdom (Galloway, 1963). Moreover, it was fully operational as opposed to a trial, and was evaluated and found to have a sound economic case as it reduced health service costs as well as reducing morbidity (Saunders, 1970). This success attracted attention and was soon replicated in other localities across the UK, and for other preventive child health services where it showed major equity achievements (Chesham, Rigby, & Shelmerdine, 1975). It was then rationalised as a national system for the UK covering immunisation, preschool screening and school health (Rigby, 1987). The value of electronic records in ensuring that children (and other vulnerable patients) were not overlooked in service was highlighted (Rigby, 2004), and principles specifically related to child health informatics were promoted (Blair & Rigby, 2004).

However, the good news story did not last. Within the UK, political fashions came to prevail, and the national system was abandoned in favour of devolving computing policy to regions and also reducing central programmes in favour of embedding children's preventive care into generic primary care services and their generic computer support. Meanwhile in many locations across parts of the rest of Europe, similar systems were apparently steadily developed. However, as this was not seen at the time as significant health service innovation or scientific application, and evaluation was not considered necessary (Rigby, 2001), nothing entered the scientific health literature, and the national scenarios cannot readily be reconstructed.

The Current Limited Evidence and Knowledge Base

The current situation is that the impetus and scientific lead have been lost, and primary care child health computing is gaining modest ground as a new subject. So much so, in fact, that new pilots are being conducted and published which unknowingly rediscover facts of earlier decades, such as Atchison, Zvoc, and Balakrishnan (2013). However, there is still no scientific knowledge base for optimal system content and function in child primary care.

The MOCHA team has undertaken a literature review. Within Europe, there is no comprehensive knowledge base and very little literature on validated benefits of use or guidance on design. From the United States, the literature is mainly from professional sources seeking agreement and proof-in-use of a children's EHR data and design set, for example Dufendach et al. (2015), Spooner (2012), and Wald, Haque, and Rizk (2018), though primarily from a hospital viewpoint, but again underpinning the lack of assessed evidence-based approaches. The MOCHA project has therefore sought to find out the current situation.

Use of EHRs for Children in Primary Care

An initial action for MOCHA was to assess current use of EHRs in children's primary care. An early enquiry though the project's Country Agents was therefore of the extent of usage of EHRs in primary care practice for children. The answers were collated and published (Rigby, Kühne, Greenfield, Majeed, & Blair, 2018), and the key finding is shown in Figure 14.1. They correlate well with the findings of a slight earlier study by Grossman et al. (2016) for a smaller number of countries and using a different data gathering network.

This shows that for much of Northern and Western European countries EHRs are in regular use, as applies also in some new member states, but Greece and the Baltic countries were lagging behind. However, the methodology was not able to assess the nature and intensity of use, nor the functionality. But it was able to ask about the design or specification process, and whether commercial acquisition or in-house design; only one country was able to say that children's services and data needs had been a prime consideration.

But the project also looked at the use of case-based child public health EHRs, namely, systems that kept key immunisation and public health data but not a full medical record of illness and treatment.

Figure 14.2 shows the pattern of provision of these, and it is more varied but not complimentary in that countries without one system are not stronger with the other. Indeed, two of the countries with no primary care EHR use shown in Figure 14.1, Greece and Latvia, do not have a public health EHR system either.

For these systems, the study was able to ask for a summary of functionality, and the map shows that most covered health screening examinations and immunisation.

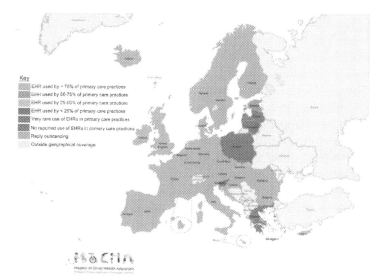

Key
- EHR used by > 75% of primary care practices
- EHR used by 50-75% of primary care practices
- EHR used by 25-50% of primary care practices
- EHR used by < 25% of primary care practices
- Very rare use of EHRs in primary care practices
- No reported use of EHRs in primary care practices
- Reply outstanding
- Outside geographical coverage

Figure 14.1.   Use of EHRs in delivery of primary care for children. *Source:* MOCHA survey data; Base map from FreeVectorMaps.com

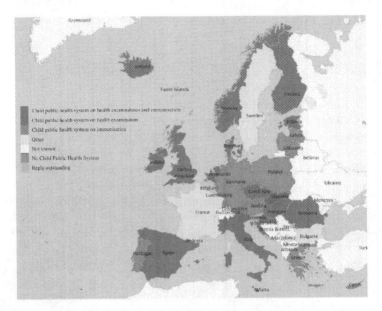

Figure 14.2.   Use of child public health EHRs in Europe. *Source:* MOCHA
survey data; Base map from FreeVectorMaps.com

Table 14.1. Functionality and data exchange of child public health systems.

System Directly Schedules Appointments	System Advises Provider of Children Overdue	Passive Record
Czech Republic	Czech Republic	Croatia (SA)
Denmark	Denmark	Finland
Estonia	Estonia	Malta (SA)
Iceland	Hungary (SA)	UK (Wales)
Spain	Iceland	
UK (Northern Ireland and Scotland) (SA)	Ireland (SA)	
	Italy	
	Norway	
	Romania	
	Spain	
	UK (England) (SA)	

Note: All use a form of automated data exchange unless marked Stand Alone (SA).

Table 14.1 then shows whether the systems were active in supporting attendance
monitoring or were merely passive repositories. In the light of the early UK case
study earlier in the chapter, it is noteworthy that England and Wales have a lower
level of e-health support in this field than half a century earlier.

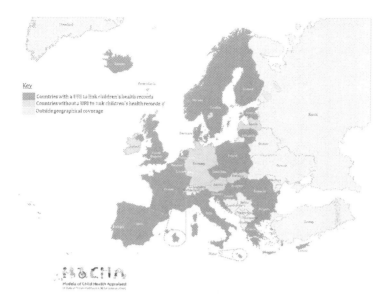

Figure 14.3.   Overview of countries with URIs to link children's health records in the EU/EEA. *Source:* MOCHA survey data; Base map from FreeVectorMaps.com

Unique Identifiers and Record Linkage

To be safe and effective, electronic record systems need to be able to link data and to be accessible to a concerned clinician, and for this, a national policy and provision of unique record identifier (URI) are important. Furthermore, if these are not issued at birth, there is a serious risk that key data will not be captured and passed on to the primary care provider. The MOCHA team has reported on the current picture and the implications (Kühne & Rigby, 2016; Kühne, Rigby, Majced, & Blair, 2017). The map shown as Figure 14.3 shows the wide coverage of the use of URIs, with only five countries not having these currently; of these five in Austria, Germany and Ireland there are concrete plans and a set timescale for implementation of a URI including for children.

However, not just having a URI in use, but its time of issue is important as mentioned. Figure 14.4 shows the time of issue, with only nine European countries commencing URI-based record linkage form birth. This implies significantly compromised record linkage in the remaining 21 countries.

The final aspect of record linkage is the files or records that can be linked using the one number. In some countries, there is a tradition, and public acceptance, of a comprehensive public services number; in other countries, this is viewed with anxiety, with health and related care being seen as separate and even more confidential. Figure 14.5 shows that just Cyprus and the UK keep health ring fenced, while Croatia, Czech Republic, Greece, Luxembourg and Spain have health and social care or welfare services within the group.

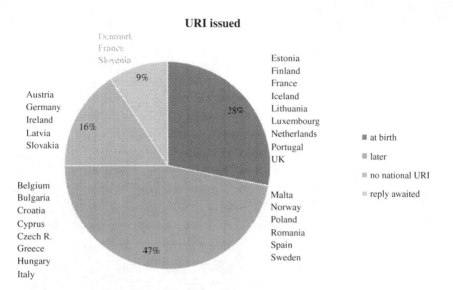

Figure 14.4. Overview on when the URI is issued.

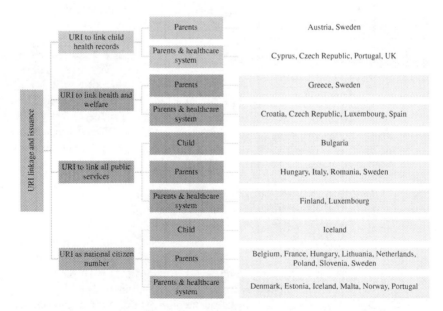

Figure 14.5. Overview on national issuing process and URI function.

The remaining 18 countries have either a public services number or a citizen identifier used for all purposes.

The final item that can be drawn from Figure 14.5 is that some countries issue the number in parallel to the health system, but none informs only the health system. Bulgaria and Iceland issue it to the newborn child, which may seem perplexing initially, but it is in fact an underscoring of the parents' role as custodians with a duty of care for the child as opposed to 'owning' the child. All of the other countries issue the Identifier to the parents or the parents and the healthcare system.

Practical and Operational Record Linkage

Electronic Health Data Exchange is the automated transfer (within strict protocols) of electronic data from one system to another (e.g. from maternity hospital to primary care practitioner, from practitioner immunising a child to a public health monitoring system, or between professionals sharing care for a child). It may be by electronic messaging, regular downloads and uploads or by ongoing real-time linkage. The purpose is to ensure that complementary systems are rapidly, reliably and accurately updated, without the need for data re-entry. To this end, the MOCHA team enquired whether there were any nationally specified electronic data messaging or structured data transfer regarding children's health records based on standards and whether there were any established means of sharing electronic records data among care providers. Table 14.2 reports the organisational linkages for data exchange reported for each country, and Table 14.3 reports the types of child health data exchanged; these have also been published (Rigby, Greenfield et al., 2018).

However, a different view on the same topic comes from the operational viewpoint. School health services (SHSs) provide a useful study area. Chapter 11 has quoted liaison with health services, and data management and records, as SHS quality standards, yet Table 14.2 shows that only four countries have structured data exchange with SHSs. So we also enquired about school health record keeping (not solely electronic records). Table 14.4 shows the data received:

Of the countries reporting, all but one keep records within school health, and three have a form of sharing with primary care. However Figures 14.6 and 14.7 show that there is practical liaison in some countries.

These results show the pattern for general health issue liaison, with variation between those countries which have a high degree of separation and those with some intended linkage to seek a holistic approach. Enquiries were also made as to the existence and use in countries of data standards. Many countries reported agreed national standards or protocols of the design of EHRs and data exchange, but very little use of international standards (Rigby, Kühne, Greenfield, & Deshpande, 2018). The lack of use of standards underscores how little has been completed regarding children's health data and, as covered in the literature review and the issues, raised in the American policy literature cited there.

The real test, though, can be in practical situations. The case of access to immunisation history for a child injured at school was taken by the MOCHA project as a suitable policy-framing vignette. The picture which resulted is shown in Figure 14.8.

Table 14.2. Overview on organisational linkages electronic record data sharing.

Country	Hospitals	Home/ Community Care Providers	Social Care	Schools	Any Other Agency (Mainly Registries Local Systems Funding)
Austria					
Bulgaria					✓
Croatia					
Cyprus					
Czech Republic	✓				✓
Denmark					
Estonia	✓			✓	✓
Finland	✓	✓	✓	✓	✓
France			✓		
Germany					
Greece					
Hungary					✓
Iceland	✓			✓	✓
Ireland	✓				✓
Italy	✓	✓			✓
Latvia					
Lithuania					
Malta					
Netherlands	✓				
Norway	✓				✓
Poland					
Portugal	✓				
Romania	✓			✓	✓
Slovakia					
Spain	✓				
Sweden	✓				✓
United Kingdom					
Total	12	2	2	4	11

Table 14.3. Overview on types of electronic health data exchanged.

Country	No Reported Data Exchange	Data Set Exchange or Messaging					
		Data on Newborn	Data on Hospital Discharge	Home Visiting Nurses	Immun.	Preventive or Routine Exams	Possible Maltreatment
Austria	✓						
Bulgaria	✓						
Croatia					✓		
Cyprus	✓						
Czech Republic	✓						
Denmark		✓	✓	✓	✓	✓	
Estonia		✓	✓	✓	✓	✓	
Finland	✓						
France	✓						
Germany	✓						
Greece	✓						
Hungary		✓					
Iceland		✓	✓		✓		
Ireland				✓	✓		
Italy	✓						
Latvia	✓						
Lithuania	✓						

Table 14.3. (*Continued*)

Country	No Reported Data Exchange	Data Set Exchange or Messaging					
		Data on Newborn	Data on Hospital Discharge	Home Visiting Nurses	Immun.	Preventive or Routine Exams	Possible Maltreatment
Malta	✓						
Netherlands		✓	✓	✓	✓	✓	✓
Norway					✓		
Poland	✓						
Portugal		✓	✓	✓	✓	✓	✓
Romania	✓						
Slovakia	✓						
Spain		✓	✓				
Sweden							
UK	✓						
Total	16	8	6	5	8	4	2

Table 14.4. What is the policy in your country for health professionals of the school health service (SHS) in keeping their own health records?

Country	They Keep Separate SHS Records to Those of the Main Primary Healthcare Service	They Contribute to a Shared Primary Care Record – in Which School Health and Primary Care Professionals Can See All Parts	They Contribute to a Shared Primary Care Record – in Which Each Service Can See Only Parts of the Partner Service's Record	No Records Are Kept Within the School Health Service	There Is No School Health Service
Austria	✓				
Bulgaria	✓	✓			
Croatia	✓				
Cyprus	✓				
Czech Republic					✓
Denmark	✓				
Estonia	✓				
Finland		✓			
France	✓				
Germany	✓				
Hungary	✓				✓
Iceland	✓				
Ireland	✓				
Italy				✓	

Table 14.4. (*Continued*)

Country	They Keep Separate SHS Records to Those of the Main Primary Healthcare Service	They Contribute to a Shared Primary Care Record – in Which School Health and Primary Care Professionals Can See All Parts	They Contribute to a Shared Primary Care Record – in Which Each Service Can See Only Parts of the Partner Service's Record	No Records Are Kept Within the School Health Service	There Is No School Health Service
Latvia	✓				
Lithuania	✓				
Malta	✓				
Netherlands	✓				
Norway	✓				
Poland	✓				
Portugal	✓				
Romania			✓		
Slovakia					✓
Slovenia	✓				
Spain					✓
Sweden	✓				
United Kingdom	✓				
Total numbers	21	2	1	1	4

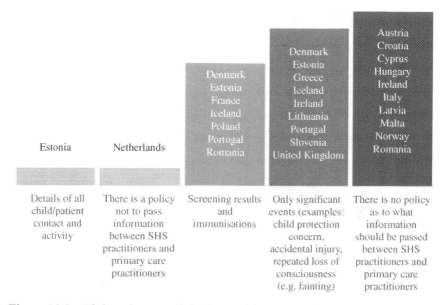

Estonia	Netherlands	Denmark Estonia France Iceland Poland Portugal Romania	Denmark Estonia Greece Iceland Ireland Lithuania Portugal Slovenia United Kingdom	Austria Croatia Cyprus Hungary Ireland Italy Latvia Malta Norway Romania
Details of all child/patient contact and activity	There is a policy not to pass information between SHS practitioners and primary care practitioners	Screening results and immunisations	Only significant events (examples: child protection concern, accidental injury, repeated loss of consciousness (e.g. fainting)	There is no policy as to what information should be passed between SHS practitioners and primary care practitioners

Figure 14.6.   If there is not a linked record between primary care services and school health services, what type of information is it policy to pass *from* the SHS practitioner *to* the primary care practitioner?

There are quite important societal, ethical and child well-being issues contained in these varied national responses.

Finally, on the topic of Electronic Records, the study within MOCHA considered the ability of a child to see his/her own records. The answers are shown in Figure 14.9.

However, a different situation arises when a child (up to age 18) feels that there are sensitive items in his/her health record which he/she would not want his/her parents to see. Indeed, this might be a barrier to seeking medical help. The reverse situation therefore addresses whether a child could block parental access. The answers to this are shown in Figure 14.10.

New e-Health Media

Recognising that new media and social media have an increasingly important role in enabling children and young people to access advice, and on occasions, virtual services, this field has been one of the objects of study for the MOCHA project.

Websites

There are numerous websites that children can access regarding health matters, whether or not designed for children. It is also known that many websites can be

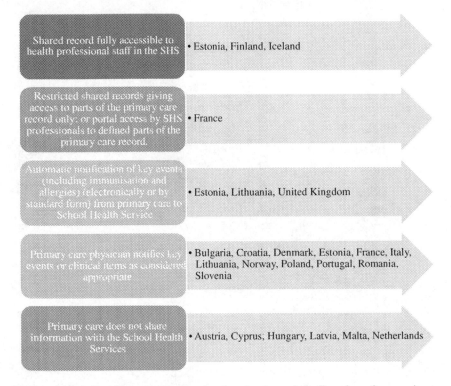

Figure 14.7.   Looking at communication in the other direction, from primary care to school health service professionals, what is the policy of information sharing *from* primary care *to* the school health service?

malicious, and others can be ineffectual or containing poor advice (Forsström & Rigby, 2000). Significant years later, few countries have developed means of validating and protecting children against poor or dangerous websites. Enquiries of the MOCHA countries identified seven with processes in place, as shown in Table 14.5.

The HON Code refers to a generic initiative run by the Health on the Net Foundation (https://www.hon.ch/en/).

Apps

An even more modern form of health advice and interaction is via smartphone apps. While these can be innovative and helpful, they can also be unscientific or even malicious, and they can surreptitiously gather use data. There has been some discussion with the European Commission as to whether to seek to create standards. MOCHA studied how many countries already had safeguards in place and found that was only in five countries and some of these were not particularly robust (Table 14.6):

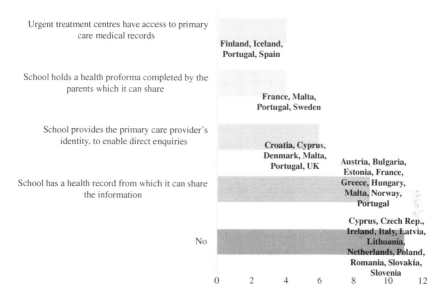

Figure 14.8.   If a pupil sustains an injury in school that needs urgent medical treatment, is the school able to supply to the urgent treatment centre: the child's tetanus immunisation status?

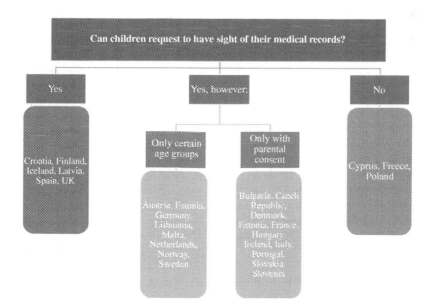

Figure 14.9.   According to the policy for record keeping in your country, can a child request to have sight of their medical records?

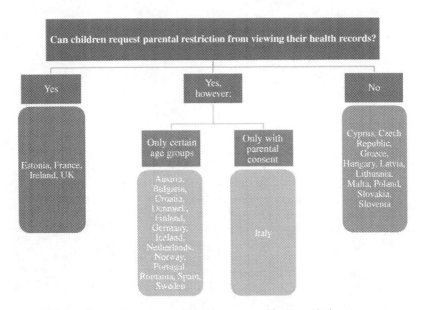

Figure 14.10.   Countries where a child can specify that their parents *may not* see part of their medical records.

External Collaboration

Finally, this work can be contextualised in two respects. The European Centre for Disease Control (ECDC) has a major interest in Immunisation Information System (IIS) provision. IISs keep records of individuals' immunisation history across all ages and including travel and occupational vaccine protections. But childhood immunisation forms a core part of this. In 2017, ECDC undertook a Europe-wide survey, which not only included the use of IISs in each country, but also included study of URIs (ECDC, 2017). The findings of ECDC have been matched against the MOCHA findings, and the results are mutually supportive. This not only strengthens the perception of the importance of these practical e-health principles, but also enables joint consideration.

HL7 Foundation and Trillium II Project

The HL7 Foundation is a key international body in the setting of health data standards. It is also currently running the Trillium II project, (https://trillium2.eu/) to develop data and content standards for an International Patient Summary. This project has seen the omission from its work hitherto of child-specific summaries and has agreed a formal collaboration with the MOCHA project to pursue joint work on standards for child health records, data items and processes. This is important in its own right and starts to address what has already been identified as an unmet need. As the MOCHA project comes to an

Table 14.5. MOCHA countries with website accreditation process in place.

Country	Accreditation Process Reported
Austria	HON code
Croatia	No specific details given
Estonia	No specific details given
France	HON code
Germany	HON code
Portugal	Institutional websites, accredited by providers
Spain	HON code, MedCIRCLE [...]
United Kingdom	The Information Standard

Table 14.6. MOCHA countries with apps accreditation process reported.

Country	Accreditation Process Reported
Estonia	Child helpline service app
Germany	Unofficial, internal regulation
Portugal	No specific details given
Slovenia	Slovenian Institute of Quality and Metrology (SIQ) certifies apps as any other medical equipment
Spain	Processes vary across autonomous regions
United Kingdom	MHRA, National Information Board

end, joint workshops with the Trillium II project, and with ECDC, are seeking to take forward this work, and for some of the objectives of MOCHA to be continued in that forum.

Conclusion

e-Health is a large subject. It also sits in a peculiar position in policy development. IT services should always be in the background, as supporters of modern care delivery. However, new information technologies have the power to transform radically how services can be and are delivered – as has already happened in particular with civil aviation, financial services and retailing. New opportunities and mobilities arise, and information silos can be broken down – though new inequalities and other perverse effects have to be anticipated and avoided.

More recently, online services of the Internet and smartphone apps have enabled the citizen (including children) to access information, and initiate actions, in ways which can be enlightening and empowering, or which can be dangerous and disruptive. The challenge for policy-makers and practitioners is to be aware and to lead on innovative harnessing of new technologies and to protect the citizen and patient against new harms.

The work of MOCHA on e-health to support modern models of primary care for children has shown a largely worrying picture. Though basic electronic records are widespread in much of Europe, opportunities to initiate positive innovation seems restricted to just a few countries. Protection against harm is even more unusual. Yet out of this, and the compilation and publication of situation analyses, some synergy is emerging of a wish to be more positive in developing e-health to support primary care for children.

References

Atchison, C., Zvoc, M., & Balakrishnan, R. (2013). The evaluation of a standardized call/recall system for childhood immunizations in Wandsworth, England. *Journal of Community Health, 38*(3), 581−587. doi:10.1007/s10900-013-9654-4.

Blair, M., & Rigby, M. (2004). Principles and purpose for child health informatics. In M. Rigby (Ed.), *Vision and value in health information* (pp. 108−120). Oxford: Radcliffe Medical Press (ISBN 1 85775 863 3).

Chesham, I., Rigby, M. J., & Shelmerdine, H. R. (1975). Paediatric screening. *Health and Social Service Journal, 85*, 293−294.

Dufendach, K. R., Eichenberger, J. A., McPheeters, M. L., Temple, M. W., Bhatia, H. L., Alrifai, W., et al. (2015). *AHRQ comparative effectiveness technical briefs. Core functionality in pediatric electronic health records.* Rockville, MD: Agency for Healthcare Research and Quality. Retrieved from https://www.ncbi.nlm.nih.gov/books/NBK293626/

European Centre for Disease Control. (2017). *Technical report − Immunisation information systems in the EU and EEA results of a survey on implementation and system characteristics ECDC Stockholm.* Retrieved from https://ecdc.europa.eu/sites/portal/files/documents/immunisation-systems.pdf

Forsström, J., & Rigby, M. (2000). TEAC-health − Research-based recommendations for European certification of health telematics services. In A. Hasman, B. Blobel, D. Dudeck, R. Engelbrecht, G. Gell, H. U. Prokosch (Eds.), *Medical infobahn for Europe: Proceedings of MIE2000 and GMDS2000* (pp. 288−292). Amsterdam: IOS Press.

Galloway, T. McL. (1963). Management of vaccination and immunization procedures by electronic computer. *Medical Officer, 109*, 232.

Grossman, Z., del Torso, S., van Esso, D., Ehrich, J. H. H., Altorjai, P., Mazur, A., … Hadjipanayis, A. (2016). Use of electronic health records by child primary healthcare providers in Europe; Child: Care, health and development. *Child Care Health and Development, 42*(6), 928−933. doi:10.1111/cch.12374. Epub 2016 Jul 10.

Kühne, G., & Rigby, M. (2016). *Description and analysis of current child health electronic record keeping across Europe.* Retrieved from http://www.childhealthservicemodels.eu/publications/technical-reports/

Kühne, G., Rigby, M. J., Majeed, A., & Blair, M. E. (2017). Towards safe and efficient child primary care − Gaps in the use of unique identifiers in Europe.

In A. Ugon et al. (Eds.), *Informatics for health: Connected citizen-led wellness and population health* (pp. 930–934). Amsterdam: IOS Press.

Rigby, M. (2001). Evaluation: 16 powerful reasons why not to do it – And 6 overriding imperatives. In V. Patel, R. Rogers, R. Haux (Eds.), *Medinfo 2001: Proceedings of the 10th. world congress on medical informatics* (pp. 1198–1202). Amsterdam: IOS Press.

Rigby, M. (2004). Information as the patient's advocate. In M. Rigby (Ed.), *Vision and value in health information* (pp. 57–67). Oxford: Radcliffe Medical Press (ISBN 1 85775 863 3).

Rigby, M. J. (1987). The national child health computer system. In A. Macfarlane (Ed.), *Progress in child health* (Vol. 3). Abingdon: Churchill Livingstone.

Rigby, M., Greenfield, R., Majeed, A., & Blair, M. (2018). *Variation of national policies on controlled sharing with partner services of children's primary care data.* Retrieved from http://www.childhealthservicemodels.eu/publications/technical-reports/

Rigby, M., Kühne, G., Greenfield, R., & Deshpande, S. (2018). *Future achievable potential models of child health electronic record systems to support care delivery.* Retrieved from http://www.childhealthservicemodels.eu/publications/deliverables/

Rigby, M., Kühne, G., Greenfield, R., Majeed, A., & Blair, M. (2018). Extent of use of electronic records in children's primary care and public health in Europe. *Studies Health Technology and Informatics, 247*, 930–934 (PMID: 29678097).

Saunders, J. (1970). Results and costs of a computer-assisted immunization scheme. *British Journal of Social and Preventive Medicine, 24*, 187–191.

Spooner, S. A. (2012). We are still waiting for fully supportive electronic health records in pediatrics. *Pediatrics, 130*(6).

Wald, J., Haque, S., & Rizk, S. (2018). Enhancing health IT functionality for children the 2015 children's EHR format. *Pediatrics, 141*, 1–7.

Chapter 15

Affiliate Contributors to Primary Care for Children

Denise Alexander, Uttara Kurup, Arjun Menon,
Michael Mahgerefteh, Austin Warters, Michael Rigby and
Mitch Blair

Abstract

There is more to primary care than solely medical and nursing services. Models of Child Health Appraised (MOCHA) explored the role of the professions of pharmacy, dental health and social care as examples of affiliate contributors to primary care in providing health advice and treatment to children and young people. Pharmacies are much used, but their value as a resource for children seems to be insufficiently recognised in most European Union (EU) and European Economic Area (EEA) countries. Advice from a pharmacist is invaluable, particularly because many medicines for children are only available off-label, or not available in the correct dose, access to a pharmacist for simple queries around certain health issues is often easier and quicker than access to a primary care physician or nursing service. Preventive dentistry is available throughout the EU and EEA, but there are few targeted incentives to ensure all children receive the service, and accessibility to dental treatment is variable, particularly for disabled children or those with specific health needs. Social care services are an essential part of health care for many extremely vulnerable children, for example those with complex care needs. Mapping social care services and the interaction with health services is challenging due to their fragmented provision and the variability of access across the EU and EEA. A lack of coherent structure of the health and social care interface requires parents or other family members to navigate complex systems with little assistance. The needs of pharmacy, dentistry and social care are varied and interwoven with needs from each other and from the healthcare system. Yet, because this inter-connectivity is not sufficiently recognised in the EU and EEA countries, there is a need for improvement of coordination and with the need for these services to focus more fully on children and young people.

Keywords: Child; adolescent; community pharmacy; dentistry; social care; coordination

Introduction

This chapter looks at some of the many other professions that provide primary care for children, keeping them well and helping them achieve optimum health. As discussed in Chapters 9 and 16, there is evidence to suggest that the health problems triggering many primary care visits by children and young people could have been treated successfully by other professionals (Gill et al., 2013). Specifically, in Models of Child Health Appraised (MOCHA), we looked at the contribution of, and interface with, community pharmacy, dental health and social care services. Other professions in primary health care, including ophthalmologists, physiotherapists, gynaecologists and psychiatrists, fall outside MOCHA's scope either because of a lack of project capacity or because these services are not generally available in primary care in all of the 30 MOCHA countries; nevertheless, they play an important role. The interface of primary care health services and other professional contributors is not a fixed boundary – but rather, the child's progress between them is fluid. Essential, therefore, in successfully providing these services to the benefit of the child is the need for the primary care health system, and the other systems, to facilitate multidisciplinary communication and working.

The Contribution of Community Pharmacy to Primary Care

Community pharmacy provides an important primary care service for infants, children and young people and their parents (Alexander & Blair, 2018; Blair & Menon, 2018). We know that in many countries, pharmacy is considered an important source of health advice and is used widely before visiting traditional primary care services, and pharmacies have the potential for easier access because of longer opening hours. What has been unknown until now is the extent to which community pharmacy recognises the needs of children and young people, including communication needs, and how it contributes to primary care services as an overarching concept in the different countries of the European Union (EU) and European Economic Area (EEA). MOCHA, therefore, explored how children, young people and their families seek advice about medication, consult over an illness and obtain health advice, including advice about diet, sexual health and so on (Alexander & Blair, 2018). MOCHA's task was not to appraise pharmacy services themselves, but to investigate their contribution to wider primary care services that can be and are accessed by the children and families of Europe.

The MOCHA Survey into Pharmacy Use

Twenty-nine out of the 30 MOCHA country agents (see Chapter 1) returned completed surveys about the accessibility and use of pharmacy by children, young people and their families in their countries and also the quality of service from the pharmacy.

Increasing Access for Children and Young People

We asked specifically about out-of-hours' accessibility, the presence of private consulting rooms that would allow children to talk to a pharmacist in private, and whether it was seen as usual in the country to visit the pharmacist before seeing a doctor or other health professional.

In most countries, pharmacies provide both dispensing and advice outside of normal business hours. Only a small proportion of countries provide dispensing of medicines ($N = 3$) or over the counter advice only ($N = 3$) out of hours. One country was unable to provide a clear answer to this question, due to the variability of services.

The use of a consulting room in a pharmacy is increasingly viewed as good practice and good for business. Certainly, privacy and confidentiality are very important to children and young people (see also Chapter 3; Alma, Mahtani, Palant, Klůzová Kráčmarová, & Prinjha, 2017; Blair & Menon, 2018). If the pharmacy is to be increasingly used as a source of initial primary care advice, prioritising the privacy of the customers raises the standard of care in pharmacies. Sixteen out of the 29 MOCHA countries that responded to this survey question stated that most pharmacies had a consulting room. This is shown in Table 15.1.

Belgium, Germany, Ireland, Norway, Portugal and Romania all stated that pharmacists are legally required to provide separate rooms for confidential consultation. In Portugal, a minimum size of room is also specified in law. In Romania, anecdotally, it was reported that not all pharmacies have the physical space for such a room, despite it being a legal requirement. Austria, Czech Republic, Estonia, France, Iceland, Malta, Netherlands, Spain and the UK have voluntary provision of consulting rooms. In France and Iceland, the provision of a separate space is recommended, and in the UK, it is possible to discuss issues with the pharmacist on the telephone. In many smaller pharmacies,

Table 15.1. Policy for provision of consulting rooms in pharmacies.

Countries with Consulting Rooms Present	No Consulting Rooms
Austria, Belgium, Czech Republic, Estonia, France, Germany, Greece, Iceland, Ireland, Malta, Netherlands, Norway, Portugal, Romania, Spain and the UK	Bulgaria, Croatia, Cyprus, Denmark, Finland, Hungary, Italy, Latvia, Lithuania, Luxembourg, Poland, Slovenia and Sweden

however, it is not possible to include a separate room for private consultations with the pharmacist. In the Czech Republic and Estonia, consulting rooms exist in very few pharmacies, but work is underway to increase that number, and actively encourage the provision of private rooms. Cyprus. Denmark and Finland have no formal requirement for consulting rooms, but they nevertheless exist in some pharmacies. A major barrier to their presence is physical space. In Bulgaria, Greece, Hungary, Italy, Latvia, Lithuania, Poland and Slovenia, there is generally no separate room, but privacy is encouraged by means of a distance between the counter and a queue, or separate counters to consult with a pharmacist.

The majority of countries reported that it was quite usual for the pharmacy to be consulted as a first port of call for health care and advice instead of, or before going to see a physician in primary care. In Spain and Iceland, it was unusual to go to a community pharmacy before visiting a doctor, while conversely in Denmark, Belgium, Bulgaria, Cyprus, Slovenia and the UK, it was becoming increasingly common or it was more common in some areas than others. No country stated that it wasn't possible to visit a pharmacy for initial advice or treatment of general illness.

Some countries had conducted specific surveys about this issue. In Germany, for example, a sample survey of population aged over 15 found that 70% would consult a pharmacist for advice on medication and that 70% would judge the pharmacist's advice on medication to be the most important (B.A.H., 2016).

The majority of countries reported that it was normal for a family or a young person to visit the pharmacist as a first port of call particularly for minor ailments such as fever, cough, flu or minor stomach issues before visiting more traditional primary care services. Most country agents said that in their country, people visited the pharmacist in the first instance because it was easier, quicker and, in some countries, cheaper than contacting a physician. One country, Bulgaria, felt it was impossible to answer this question, because of the variation in pharmacy provision in the country, and also the professional competencies of the pharmacist, which might influence the use of the pharmacy.

Quality of Pharmacy Services

MOCHA's remit was not to appraise pharmacy services, but to look at their role in primary care provision; nevertheless, we aimed to assess how well pharmacy responds to children and young people's needs in particular. We asked about the training of pharmacists specifically in childhood illness and whether any previous national research had been undertaken that described the use of pharmacy by children and young people (Alexander & Blair, 2018).

We found that the majority of country agents reported that pharmacists in their countries are trained specifically in common childhood illnesses, but the length and type of training vary from country to country. Some reported that it was a compulsory part of pharmaceutical training; in other countries, it is a mandatory post-graduate or continuing professional development requirement. In six countries, no specific training in childhood is needed. This disparity in

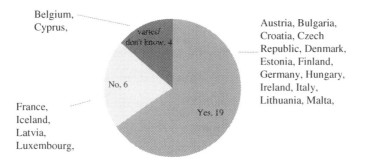

Figure 15.1. Training in the management and treatment of common illnesses in childhood.

child centricity is also reflected in the training of nurses and physicians in child-specific care (see Chapter 13). The breakdown is shown in Figure 15.1.

In most of the countries surveyed, no research had been carried out specifically about young people's use of pharmacy. Children were the focus of research or of community pharmacy initiatives in 11 countries (Czech Republic, Estonia, Finland, Germany, Greece, Hungary, Ireland, Latvia, Romania, Spain and England (as part of the UK)); this included pharmacists being sources of specific health campaigns or health education. For example, the Czech Republic country agent described a campaign initiated in pharmacies to improve the amount of liquid a child drinks as a contribution to fostering good health habits in childhood. In Spain, research focused on the provision of emergency contraception by pharmacists for young women aged older than 15 years. In Estonia, attention was directed towards medicine awareness among children, including its safe use and possible side effects. This initiative was apparently conducted after it was found that only 28% of the population (all ages) took medicines correctly. In Finland, pharmacy use was the subject of doctoral studies: such as the use of children's medicines (Ylinen, Hämeen-Anttila, Sepponen, Lindblad, & Ahonen, 2010) and self-medication among children (Siponen, 2014). In Latvia, research took the form of an international survey; the Health Behaviour in School-aged children study reported on teenage use of medication in Latvia in 2013/2014 (Gobina et al., 2014). The Irish Pharmacy Union (2015) and the Pharmaceutical Society of Ireland (2016) identified that children make up around 30% of pharmacy users (either alone or as part of a family) and young people aged 12–30 made up another 16% of users – underlining the extent to which pharmacy is used by young people.

A number of countries responded that surveys and research existed into pharmacy use in general, which potentially was of relevance to young people. In Greece, for example, the country reported a survey about people's satisfaction levels with pharmacy, showing that most people were satisfied despite the current economic challenges, and in Portugal, the results of a general survey about pharmacy services by the National Association of Pharmacies were published, but it did not contain specific to parents of young children or adolescents.

In Poland, the country agent reported that a 2009 survey identified public perception of a pharmacist has having a lack of status as a healthcare professional, even though they are often used as a source of initial advice in the sense of unofficial triage before visiting a doctor. This initial research led to an expert group being set up in Poland to increase the quality of the pharmacists' work and to improve communication with patients (Waszyk-Nowaczyk & Simon, 2009).

Themes of Pharmacy Use by Children and Young People

Resulting from this exercise we were able to identify three themes about pharmacy use by children, young people and their families: accessibility, appropriateness and approachability. As described in Chapters 3 and 4, these are of particular importance to children and young people and what we know about optimal primary care services.

Accessibility

Our questions about access to pharmacy out of hours were important for a number of reasons. The rapid progression of childhood illnesses mean urgent advice is often sought when standard primary care services are unavailable; because young people may want to consult about a health issue without their parents knowing (see also Chapter 11), and because it is quicker, cheaper and easier to talk to a pharmacist about an issue and potentially avoiding the cost or time to see a doctor. In all responding countries, pharmacy has a significant role to play in increasing accessibility in primary care on these terms.

We found differences in the definition of 'out of hours' and our results suggested that it is, in general, much easier to find pharmacies with extended or 24-hour service in larger cities than in rural areas. Most countries have systems in place to ensure that pharmacies are accessible to some extent in all parts of a country, but in very rural areas, the distance and fewer opening hours may prove prohibitive to an adolescent seeking advice or treatment.

Another aspect of accessibility is the need to pay out-of-pocket costs. This can be a particularly worrying issue for a child or young person seeking advice, particularly if they are acting independently. Conversely, if a pharmacist provides immediate and free advice, while the medical primary care makes an out-of-pocket charge, the community pharmacy is a source of greater accessibility to a child in need.

Appropriateness

Three separate issues contribute to our knowledge of appropriateness: the extent to which pharmacists are trained in children's illnesses, whether national surveys had been carried out into the use of pharmacy by children and young people and how people, including families and young people, use community pharmacy services in general.

Most pharmacists are trained to recognise and medicate for normal childhood illnesses, although the extent of the training varies between countries.

In some countries, learning is more ad hoc and undertaken through experience of working in a pharmacy over a period of time. However, the conclusion can be drawn that in those countries where training is compulsory; either as part of general pharmaceutical training or as continuing professional development; the unique needs of children are recognised. Their importance in terms of the population using pharmacies for advice and treatment is also appreciated. Similarly, the absence of surveys about pharmacy use by children and young people in many countries gives a worrying indication of the lack of priority that is given to children. This is particularly acute in the current context of constraints on primary care and economic hardship that is faced by many families across Europe. Such a situation may also reflect a lack of national focus on the role of pharmacy in primary health care for children and young people, despite their unique needs and high use of primary care systems (see also Chapter 6).

The perception of community pharmacy by the general public can be seen as a combination of the results of accessibility and appropriateness of the service. This, to some extent can be seen in those countries that reported it was normal for a young person to visit the pharmacist as a port of call. This could be because there is a general expectation of useful advice and good service from a family, or the fact that primary medical care is not so easily accessible to young people. The majority of countries answered that it was easier to see a pharmacist than it was to book an appointment with a doctor. Within the constraints of this exercise, it is impossible to know, but there is certainly a role for both services, and also warrants serious consideration of greater collaboration or communication between pharmacies and traditional primary care to achieve better coordination of care.

Approachability
In our survey, the second most popular reason for visiting a pharmacy before medical primary care services was that the pharmacist was more approachable. In addition to this direct question, our question about the presence of separate consulting rooms in a pharmacy addressed an aspect of approachability important to children and young people. This hypothesis was based on the fact that young people value privacy and confidentiality, particularly when seeking advice independently (Alma et al., 2017). Young people stressed that confidentiality and a lack of clarity that their information would remain private was a barrier to primary care for them (see Chapter 4); if young people are not confident that they can discuss issues in private, they are very reluctant to seek help from any professional (Alma et al., 2017). Our survey has highlighted a great deal of variability based on either legal requirements or practical space issues. In many countries, the trend to increasing consulting room facilities has been welcome particularly for adolescents who are seeking a confidential service outside their traditional primary care provider. Despite this, however, it was interesting to note that in five out of the nine countries where it is common to have a separate consulting area in pharmacies, the country agents also said that the pharmacist was approachable and gave health advice.

The Contribution of Dental Services to Primary Care

The role of the dentist is also one of great importance as a 'first point of contact' in primary care. Good dental health not only contributes to overall good health, but a dentist may well identify underlying disease as a result of a consultation. In addition to this, dentistry has a strong preventive role, on an individual level in terms of health education and preventive actions, and on a population level, as poor dental health has been used as an indicator for deprivation, low socio-economic status and even child abuse (Platform for Better Oral Health, 2012) (see also Chapter 5).

We explored how the dental health services address children's primary dental needs and whether there is a close connection between other primary care services. The MOCHA country agents were asked a number of questions about dental services in their countries, particularly focusing on accessibility and availability of dental services, including for children with additional or complex needs.

Accessibility

In order for dental health services to play a useful role in primary care, they need to be accessible to all. We asked if there is a policy for children to be able to access basic dental care free of charge and if these services were for inspection, and for basic treatment, such as a filling. All countries had free access for inspection purposes; France and Slovakia do not provide free basic treatment to children. There was no data received from Belgium (Table 15.2).

Table 15.2. Is there a policy that all children have access to a dentist free of charge?

Free Service to Children for Inspection	Free Service to Children for Basic Treatment (e.g. Fillings)	No Free Dental Service	Free Inspection but not Treatment
Austria, Bulgaria, Croatia, Cyprus, Czech Republic, Denmark, Estonia, Finland, France, Germany, Greece, Hungary, Iceland, Ireland, Italy (up to age 14), Latvia, Lithuania, Luxembourg, Malta, Netherlands, Norway, Poland, Portugal, Romania, Slovakia, Slovenia, Spain, Sweden and UK	Austria, Bulgaria, Croatia, Cyprus, Czech Republic, Denmark, Estonia, Finland, Germany, Greece, Hungary, Iceland, Ireland, Latvia, Lithuania, Luxembourg, Malta, Netherlands, Norway, Poland, Portugal, Romania, Slovenia, Spain, Sweden and UK		France, Slovakia

The majority of countries had a system that ensured every child has a dental examination at set ages. However, in Austria, Bulgaria, Malta, Netherlands, Romania, Poland and the United Kingdom, no specific ages were specified, but in the United Kingdom, for example, guidelines recommend the first dental check-up around the time of the first tooth eruption. Despite no recommendations set at ages, the service is free and children can attend regularly until they reach the age of 18 years. Current evidence has shown this to be a weak incentive, because even in countries where there is a free system, it is known that children of lower socio-economic status do not attend the dentist regularly (Platform for Better Oral Health, 2012). The Estonian country agent reported that many parents in rural areas do not attend the dental service, which seems to reflect this research knowledge. Austria, Cyprus and Luxembourg provide regular dental service through the school system. In Greece and Lithuania, it is compulsory to have a dental check-up before eligibility to preschool. Only Germany, Iceland, Netherlands, Poland and the United Kingdom have no set programme to ensure children have dental examinations at certain ages.

In the countries that do not provide a programme to ensure access to primary dental care, we asked if children with disability or children with a specific clinical risk have facilities available to them to make visiting a dentist easier. In addition to this, country agents that do have set programmes gave further information about access to primary dental care for disabled children or those with a specific clinical risk. These are summarised in Table 15.3. There were no data from Belgium.

We also asked if it was routine for primary care dental practitioners including those working in schools routinely have the facilities to see disabled children in their practices, without referring to specialist hospital services.

In 13 countries (Croatia, Cyprus, Czech Republic, France, Greece, Italy, Lithuania, Luxembourg, Netherlands, Romania, Slovakia and Spain), it was not routine for the facilities to exist in primary care dental practices. Norway answered both 'yes' and 'no' to the question as it was difficult to answer on a nationwide scale. The Czech Republic country agent pointed out that primary care dentistry does not exist in that country in the same way as in other countries, but is carried out in schools via the PLDD doctor (see Chapter 13) who refers to a dentist if necessary; thus, for the Czech Republic, this was an unanswerable question. In Poland, there is no distinction in law between dental services for disabled and non-disabled children. Many of the country agents that stated they did not routinely have such facilities in their countries mentioned that this was the case when a disability warranted any dental examinations or treatment to be carried out under general anaesthetic, and this would need a specialist team in a hospital. Most countries, however, stated that they could provide services to almost all disabled children in primary care, with some exceptions (as would be the case with any condition).

Preventive Care

An important element in dental primary care is the focus on prevention. Research by the Platform for Better Oral Health (2012) found that children who

Table 15.3. Access for children with a disability or with a specific clinical risk.

	Provision for Children with a Disability or Specific Clinical Risks
Cyprus	Children with disabilities or with a specific clinical risk who are unable to receive oral health care on a dental chair are treated under general anaesthesia
Czech Republic	Children with a disability which makes access to normal dental services difficult and children with a specific clinical risk are advised about a dentist able to provide such care by their registering PLDD (General Practitioner for children and Adolescents)
Estonia	All children (including disabled children) are free to visit any dentist that has signed a contract for financing medical treatment
France	These children have the same theoretical access to screening and care as other children. There is a module devoted to children in the course of university training for dentists, but there is nothing specifically dedicated to disability. In hospitals, there are slots (often restricted) for certain pathologies, including mental disabilities
Germany	Children with disabilities have the same access to dentistry as those without disability. Many practices are accessible, but sometimes dental care is challenging for the children involved
Italy	There is a decree from the Ministry of Health to provide appropriate care for all, but the extent to which this is adhered to in the different regions is unknown
Malta	Children with special needs are seen at the Dental Clinic, Mater Dei Hospital. There is a special clinic within Mater Dei Hospital which is dedicated to children with special needs
Netherlands	Specialised clinics provide care to these groups as far as these cannot be served in routine dental care. Conditions regarding costs are similar to those for general dental care and in addition covering the special arrangement
Poland	All children are treated equally, but disabled young people can have composite light-curing materials for fillings and general anaesthetics before dental procedures if necessary. There is access to highly trained dentists and nurses if necessary
Slovakia	Children with a disability and specific clinical risk diseases are treated in university hospitals. In many cases, the problem is in access to hospital due to a long distance. Treatment is done by specialists in cooperation – specialists for paediatric dentistry, anaesthesiologists, dento-alveolar surgeons, haematologists and other medical specialists depend on general diseases

Table 15.3. (*Continued*)

	Provision for Children with a Disability or Specific Clinical Risks
Sweden	Disabled children with special dental concerns because of behaviour problems as well as an underlying condition or medication which increases the risk of caries are often cared for in special programmes by specialist dentists, but this varies between counties. Secondary preventive programmes exist in several cities like Stockholm and Malmö
UK	• England: The Community Dental Service exists primarily to serve this purpose but provision is variable and access is not ensured. There are insufficient Specialists in Paediatric Dentistry in England.
	• Scotland: Variable across the 14 health board areas of Scotland, and it is up to each health board how it achieves this, but there are facilities available for all children to access dental care, albeit without sufficient specialists.
	• NI: Routine screening by the Community Dental Service (CDS) is now only applied to children with special care needs.
	• Wales: This is generally provided by the CDS.

brush their teeth twice a day by the age of 12 years are more likely to continue such habits throughout childhood and into adulthood. Regular brushing and other preventive regimes are known to be more common in families of higher socio-economic status (see Chapter 5), which means that having an established programme of preventive education and check-ups may mean that children from other socio-economic groups are actively encouraged to develop better dental habits.

We asked the country agents to tell us whether programmes exist in their country for oral health promotion and prevention of dental caries and gum disease. Only Hungary, Luxembourg and Romania responded that there was no such programme. In Hungary, several former programmes are no longer active. In Luxembourg, although national programmes do not exist, education in dental health and hygiene is carried out in kindergartens and primary schools by trained medical teams, educators and teachers. The programmes that do exist range from those that cover the entire country but are not nationally produced, rather they are devised and administered by regional health authorities (e.g. in Austria and Greece), a 'dental passport' is given to school-aged children in Croatia and programmes that are mainly administered through the school system, as in Slovenia or Italy.

Economics

As discussed in Chapter 9, the funding of dental care is important in ensuring its sustainability and accessibility. We asked how preventive dentistry is provided for children, giving three choices – a directly employed school dentist (who would in theory be not only very accessible to children in school, but also experienced in children's preventive dental care), a salaried community dentist or a general dental practitioner in their own premises (self-employed).

This is not a simple question to answer in some countries. For example, in Austria, it could be said that none and all of the options were available. Specialised dental physicians visit kindergartens and schools regularly to inspect the children's teeth, and such preventive services are provided by these specialist physicians in their own practices. This is also the case in Luxembourg, where a few dentists exclusively work for school health services, but many others are general dental practitioners who are contracted to work in schools on certain occasions.

In some countries, such as Germany and the United Kingdom, some dentists are working in their own premises, but also employ salaried dentists to work alongside them. In Spain, preventive services are sometimes provided by a salaried community dentist (Madrid Region) or by a general practitioner in their own premises, which is more common in other regions (e.g. Basque Country, or Andalusia Region).

Estonia does not have specialised school dentists, but dentists contract their services to schools as part of the Health Insurance Fund. In France, preventive dentistry is provided by a community dentist, as part of hospital services, or contracted as part of a targeted programme. This is also the case in Poland, where dentists are not employed by the schools, but are financed by the National Health Fund.

We also asked if any of these dental practitioners received additional remuneration for targeted preventive activity, such as fluoride paint, or dental hygiene work, which may show a prioritisation of preventive care, and a means of ensuring that preventive care is available to the child population. The majority of countries said that no such remuneration existed, and in two countries, there were strong regional differences which made it impossible to answer the question accurately (Sweden and the United Kingdom). In the countries that said there was additional remuneration, there were differences in the circumstances in which this could be provided. For example, in Croatia, dentists can contract with the National Insurance Fund to provide additional services such as preventive care and emergency services. In the Czech Republic, a dentist can be reimbursed for preventive care within the rules of the health insurance that covers the patient, and there is a limit as to the number of times a client can be seen in order to claim the costs incurred. Similarly in the Netherlands, dental care is paid for by healthcare packages, and if preventive activities are carried out, such as fluoride paint, they are reimbursed as and when they are provided. In Denmark, private dental practitioners receive extra remuneration for preventive work, as they are subsidised by municipality and by the patient themselves. Danish public dentists, who work in a clinic affiliated with schools, do not receive additional remuneration, as they receive a monthly salary. In Italy, preventive dental services are provided by private dentists. In some cases, they provide preventive services for the local health service, which are reimbursed partly by the national health service and partly by a co-payment from the client; those on a low income may be exempt from this co-payment. In Poland, additional remuneration for preventive work is only possible in exceptional circumstances, such as the presence of a particular scheme. In Lithuania, preventive dental care is financially incentivised, as each visit by a child for preventive care is remunerated in addition to normal payment. In Slovenia, payment is given for fluoride gel that is used at schools to routinely prevent caries.

The Interface of Social Care Services with Primary Care

Social support can be understood as providing assistance to address the everyday or ordinary needs of children so that they can lead full lives and as such are differentiated from health treatment or clinical support. Up until the MOCHA project, there has been very little research to examine the types of social care support in European countries for children with complex healthcare needs in particular (Kielthy, Warters, Brenner, & McHugh, 2017). The MOCHA project explored the extent to which countries navigate the dynamic and complex interface between social and primary healthcare services. This is discussed fully in (Kielthy et al., 2017).

Social care services are very closely aligned to healthcare services in a conceptual and a practical sense. Without good social care, children cannot live optimally healthy lives and as such, it is an essential part of primary care in its broadest sense. In the MOCHA project, the interface of social care services with primary care services was investigated by researching the experiences of a particularly vulnerable population group of children, those with complex care needs (see Chapter 10) as a tracer for all children who may need social care services for a variety of reasons. The United Nations Convention on the Rights of the Child (see also Chapters 4 and 17) states that all children have the right to additional support they need it, in order to allow them to live full lives. As such, they have the same right to a warm family environment, go to school, make friends and take part in leisure activities as do other children. Some children require the support of social care services to fulfil this right. In terms of the organisation and provision of services, some are universal, and some are targeted at children and young people who are in high-risk groups. These types of social services can vary, even within a country. In universal services, all families are eligible for support, whereas in targeted services, only those with the greatest need or most limited means are eligible. In some countries, such as the Nordic countries of Europe, a cascade model operates: universal services that encompass a preventive approach are available to all families, and more targeted, specialised and tailored support is also available to families and children with complex care needs (Lara Montero, van Duijn, Zonneveld, Minkman, & Nies, 2016). This is considered to be good practice, but it must be noted that there is an absence of evidence to prove that this improves the outcomes for children with complex care needs, as outcome data are difficult to define, and data are not available that can be compared across different systems (see also Chapters 7 and 8).

In the case of children with complex care needs, it can be difficult, or even impossible to disentangle the social care needs from healthcare needs, which is an extreme manifestation of the multifaceted relationship social care needs and healthcare needs may have in any child's life. Healthcare needs are so much a part of their everyday lives that dividing such needs into categories of 'health' and 'social care' is untenable (Marchant, Lefevre, Jones, & Luckock, 2007).

In addition to social care that provides for child welfare, social care also encompasses the safeguarding of children from abuse or neglect (see also Chapter 17). The Fundamental Rights Agency (European Union Agency for Fundamental Rights, 2015a) states that there are significant inadequacies in child protection systems in the EU member states, which often fail children with complex needs from abuse and violence (2015), which has also been reflected in the MOCHA findings (see Chapter 17). The vulnerability of children to being abused because of their dependency on adults is an important factor in ensuring a seamless interface with social care services to produce good health and well-being outcomes for the child. This has also been reflected in the MOCHA findings. We asked about procedures and policy for child safeguarding for a child with complex care needs and how these could be accessed. The MOCHA country agents responded to a questionnaire, which was designed to provide an understanding of the national context in which social care services are provided, and how they integrate with primary social care services. The questionnaire drew upon case studies and vignettes already developed in the MOCHA project (see Chapter 10, and Kielthy et al., 2017) and adapted them to enable an exploration of social care needs. The focus was on care for an individual with complex care needs, by emphasising the policy and legislative framework of social care in that country. The questionnaire responses allowed us to map social care services in the EU and EEA countries and how these link with primary healthcare services in the community. In addition, it provided us with the means to examine the interface between primary health care and child protection, recognising the specific roles that differentiate the need of social care to enable an 'ordinary life' for a child with additional needs, and the need to protect a child from an abusive environment. Specifically, we looked at social care in terms of whether it has a legal basis, the extent to which social care and primary healthcare services are integrated, the way in which social care services is implemented, and the level of participation in and costs of social services.

Legal Basis for Social Care

We found that all countries have a legal framework for social care, and a main law for the provision of social care services was present in most countries. In 13 countries, special entitlements were available for children with complex care needs, and these were included in social care legislation. Only 35% of responding countries had a central national authority to coordinate social care. Table 15.4 gives further information.

All countries reported they had a child protection framework, although the Fundamental Rights Agency (European Union Agency for Fundamental Rights, 2015b) reports that a main law for child protection is present in only

Table 15.4. Legal entitlement to social care for children with complex care needs in European countries.

	Social Care Legislation	Special Provision for Children with Complex Care Needs within Social Care Legislation	Measure to Promote the Welfare of Children with Complex Care Needs within Child Protection Legislation	Financial Entitlement in Social Care Legal Framework	Home Help OR Personal Care Entitlement in Social Care Legal Framework (HH) (PC)	Family Support Entitlement in Social Care Legal Framework	Educational Entitlement in Social Care Legal Framework	Psychosocial Entitlement in Social Care Legal Framework
Austria	Yes (Federal)[ab]	Yes[ab]	No[a]	No[a]	Yes (HH)[a]	Yes[a]	No[a]	Yes[a]
Croatia	Yes[ab]	Yes[ab]	No[a]	Yes[a]	Yes (HH)[a]	Yes[a]	Yes[a]	Yes[a]
Cyprus	Yes (across different laws)[ab]	Other[ab]	No[a]	Not applicable	Not applicable	Not applicable	Not applicable	Not applicable
Czech Republic	Yes[ab]	Yes[ab]	Other (recommendation applicable to children with physical disabilities)[ab]	Yes[ab]	Yes (HH)[ab]	Yes[ab]	Yes[ab]	Yes[ab]
Estonia	Yes[ab]	Yes[ab]	Yes[ab]	Yes[a]	No[a]	No[a]	No[a]	No[a]
Finland	Yes[ab]	No[ab]	No[ab]	Not applicable	Not applicable	Not applicable	Not applicable	Not applicable
Germany	Yes[ab]	Yes[ab]	No[a]	No[ab]	Yes (HH)[ab]	No[ab]	Yes[ab]	Yes[ab]
Greece	Yes[ab]	No[ab]	No[a]	Not applicable	Not applicable	Not applicable	Not applicable	Not applicable
Hungary	Yes (across different laws)[a]	No[a]	No[a]	Yes[ab]	No[ab]	Yes[ab]	Yes[ab]	Yes[ab]

Table 15.4. (*Continued*)

	Social Care Legislation	Special Provision for Children with Complex Care Needs within Social Care Legislation	Measure to Promote the Welfare of Children with Complex Care Needs within Child Protection Legislation	Financial Entitlement in Social Care Legal Framework	Home Help OR Personal Care Entitlement in Social Care Legal Framework (HH) (PC)	Family Support Entitlement in Social Care Legal Framework	Educational Entitlement in Social Care Legal Framework	Psychosocial Entitlement in Social Care Legal Framework
Iceland	Yes[ab]	Yes[ab]	*	Yes[ab]	No[ab]	Yes[ab]	Yes[ab]	Yes[ab]
Ireland	Yes (across different laws)[ab]	Other[ab]	Yes[ab]	Not applicable	Not applicable	Not applicable	Not applicable	Not applicable
Italy	Yes[ab]	No[ab]	No[ab]	Not applicable[ab]	Not applicable[ab]	Not applicable[ab]	Not applicable[ab]	Not applicable[ab]
Latvia	Yes[ab]	Yes[ab]	Yes[ab]	Yes[a]	Yes (HH)[a]	No[a]	No[a]	Yes[a]
Lithuania	Yes[ab]	Yes[ab]	Yes[ab]	Yes[ab]	No[ab]	Yes[ab]	No[ab]	Yes[ab]
Malta	*	*	*	*	*	*	*	*
Netherlands	Yes (across different laws)[ab]	No[ab]	No[ab]	Not applicable	Not applicable	Not applicable	Not applicable	Not applicable
Norway	Yes[ab]	Other[ab]	Other (the law allows the social welfare board to instigate a treatment order for children with disabilities or who need extra help if parents fail to ensure they receive necessary services)[ab]	Not applicable	Not applicable	Not applicable	Not applicable	Not applicable

Country								
Poland	Yes (across different laws)[a,b]	Other[a,b]	No[a,b]	Yes (Recent introduction of a law called Za życiem (For Life), which gives additional support to parents of children who have incurable, life-threatening conditions)[a]	No[a,b]	Yes[a,b]	Yes[a,b]	Yes[a,b]
Portugal	Yes[a,b]	No[a,b]	No[a,b]	Not applicable	Not applicable	Not applicable	Not applicable	Not applicable
Romania	Yes[a,b]	Yes[a,b]	Yes[a,b]	Yes[a,b]	Yes (HH)[a,b]	No[a,b]	No[a,b]	Yes[a,b]
Slovakia	Yes[a,b]	Yes[a,b]	*	Yes[a,b]	Yes (HH)[a,b]	Yes[a,b]	Yes[a,b]	Yes[a,b]
Spain	Yes (Regional)[a,b]	Yes[a,b]	No[a,b]	No[a,b]	No[a,b]	No[a,b]	No[a,b]	Yes[a,b]
Sweden	Yes[a,b]	Yes[a,b]	No[a,b]	Yes[a,b]	Yes (HH)[a,b]	No[a,b]	No[a,b]	Yes[a,b]
UK (England as a part of the United	Yes[a,b]	Yes[a,b]	Yes[a,b]	Not applicable	Not applicable	Not applicable	Not applicable	Not applicable

Notes: [a]Country agent response, [b]Policy documentation, [c]Research literature, [d]Other external information sources. *Insufficient information provided.

18 EU countries. Only six countries stated they had specific objectives regarding the safeguarding of children with complex care needs who have communication or cognitive difficulties.

Having a legal framework is important, but the fact that only half have special recognition for especially vulnerable children and young people, for example those with complex care needs, is potentially worrying. However, it is impossible to know if additional legal protection, which is the case in some countries, makes a difference to the outcomes of the child – because of the lack of comparable and applicable data that describe the physical and social well-being of the child (see Chapters 7 and 8).

Integration of Social Care with Primary Health Care

Denmark, France, Finland, Hungary, Ireland, Sweden and the UK (Léveillé & Chamberland, 2010) use the Assessment Framework (AF) (Department of Health, England et al., 2000) as a framework to establish a common language to understand children's needs, thus improving the possibility for effective integrated care This framework is essentially child-centric (see also Chapter 4) and recognises a child's health and social care needs as well as those of parents or carers. Figure 15.2 describes the framework in more detail.

In the MOCHA countries, the integration of care between the services takes the form of formal, legal integration and more informal integration and

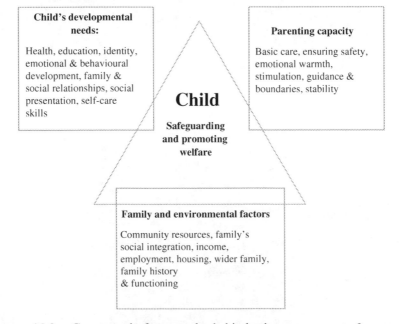

Figure 15.2. Conceptual framework behind the assessment framework.
Source; Department of Health, 2000.

networks between the two services. In 65% of countries, there were legal or policy frameworks that outline coordination between primary healthcare and social care services, and in 23% of countries (Croatia, Finland, Italy, Norway, Spain and England (as part of the UK)), they specify a legal and policy framework where both legal and policy documentations are in place to link primary health care and social care. In 19% of countries, legal frameworks only are described (Czech Republic, Greece, Latvia, Poland and Portugal) and in 19% of countries (Austria, Bulgaria, Denmark, Estonia and the Netherlands), policy frameworks only are described. In 31% of countries, neither a legal or policy framework was described to link primary health care and social care. Ireland has a single entity that is responsible for delivering primary and social care, the Health Service Executive – however, in practice, the links between the two remain informal and are not yet fully integrated. Similarly in Finland, it is planned that from 2018, newly identified counties will be in charge of implementing both primary health care and social care (Figure 15.3).

Aside from formal integration of primary care and social care services, there are a number of means by which informal integration takes place in the responding countries, such as co-location of services, coordination through formal networks and informal ad hoc coordination.

Co-location
Siting primary healthcare and social care professionals together in the primary care setting, on a whole population level is described by two respondents. In Spain, for example, a multidisciplinary primary care team consists of a social worker within a multidisciplinary primary care team, in the same location.

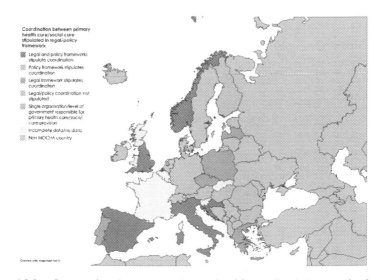

Figure 15.3.   Integration between primary health care/social care stipulated in legal/policy framework.

In some instances, this also occurs in Sweden, but this more often happens in the secondary care setting. In terms of integration of care for all children, co-location of primary healthcare and social care professionals in the primary care setting for children (and mothers) is planned in Bulgaria where maternal and child health centres are being implemented. However, we have interpreted our results on co-location with caution; not least because it is likely there are regional differences in each country, but also that the understanding of 'co-location' may be subtly different in separate countries. It is likely that this is more widespread than we have been able to ascertain in this exercise.

Formal Networks

In Cyprus and Estonia, the country agents described ongoing cooperation between primary healthcare and social care services in the care of children. There are also examples of virtual integration where coordination between primary health care and organisations responsible for providing social care is arranged through networks. This type of integration is reported in Denmark, Estonia, Italy, Norway, Portugal, Romania and England (as part of the UK). To target children with complex care needs, in Ireland, the newly created Children's Disability Network Teams consist of multidisciplinary teams of professionals working together to provide integrated care. In terms of targeted care for children with complex care needs, the Czech Republic primary care physician acts as a formal coordinator of care between the wider health service and social services for children with complex needs; the management of children with complex care needs in this way is part of their training. However, in Denmark, coordinating case workers are used for several target groups, including those with complex care needs, to navigate between social care as well as education, health care and employment.

Informal Networks or Communication

In some countries, links between primary health care and social care have been created as necessary or as a result of specific circumstances. In Greece, the primary care physician can refer service users to social services, and social services can provide information on health services; in Iceland, the country agent notes that when social counselling is offered, it must be in conjunction with healthcare services. In Germany, paediatricians and social services coordinate to deliver what is called an early-detection exam for all children. In terms of targeted care for children with complex needs, in the absence of formal networks of coordination, Hungary and Croatia described collaboration between services for these children (see Kielthy et al., 2017).

Implementation and Coordination of Social Care and Primary Care Services

Implementing good care can take the form of many different actions. We asked about the availability of different types of support in a broad sense; often the type and quality of supports provided varied hugely between countries. For example, when asked about the availability of supports for 'parenting skills', respondents pointed to provisions ranging from the availability of courses for parents on caring for a child with complex needs, where travel and other course expenses are paid, to online forums where parents can talk online to peers in similar situations.

Implementation of care also implies good coordination of care for the children needing health and social support. The degree to which primary health care and social care are coordinated varies considerably throughout the countries of the study. This coordinated support may be provided through a number of different means:

- coordination of primary health care and social care for the whole population;
- coordination of primary health care and social care for all children; and
- targeted coordinated support, which includes coordination of primary health care and social care, for children with complex needs.

Coordination of both services may be facilitated by the presence of coordinating laws and/or policies that specify how primary health care and social care should be linked, or again, it may be more informal. For children with complex care needs, it is not always primary health care which is a priority when it comes to coordination of care, although the need remains for integrated care. In some cases, the focus of care coordination can be to coordinate care between, for example, secondary hospital care and support in the community. In Denmark, for example, the country agent described how generalised established structures which support cooperation between different sectors and services have been implemented by several municipalities. A coordinating case worker is used for several target groups who receive support from several local government actors; the coordinating case worker navigates between the social area, the employment area and the areas of education and health care.

Flexible Support

The provision of a care coordinator or case manager for individual cases is recognised as good practice in providing support for children with complex care needs. Alongside the example of coordination of support by a professional, there are examples within MOCHA data of the provision of flexible support which facilitates equity of access. In Poland, for example, access to counselling is offered through the phone or online; the respondent also describes how rehabilitation can be made available at home for those who are unable to attend outpatient treatment centres. In the Czech Republic, the respondent describes how rehabilitation can be made available as a field service providing care in rural areas. On the whole, however, MOCHA data suggested that there is a degree of inequity of access of care coordination and of services in general. Location seemed to be an important factor that affected the availability of specialised rehabilitation care in the community. Reduced access to rehabilitative care was evident from 19% of responses, cited in Czech Republic, Greece, Hungary, Lithuania and Romania. Additionally, the role played by external organisations of various types, particularly not-for-profit organisations, in providing social care is considerable. Access to support in some countries was determined by the resources available to non-profit organisations, or from commercial services in lieu of statutory provided services, meaning that access for some families was dependent on financial resources (see Chapters 5, 6 and 9).

Using the tracer condition of acquired brain injury (ABI), the provision of social care support for a child with complex needs showed that a care coordinator or case manager, who can coordinate the required support for the child and family at home or in the community, was present in only 50% of the countries that responded. In one case, this refers to location-based coordination (Norway). In 38% of cases, the family was the main coordinator of support most of the time (see also Chapter 10). In Cyprus, no case coordination is available, meaning the family has the responsibility to contact the three government agencies and services that provide social support. In another country, coordination is available in day care centres, but only in certain localities, meaning some families are left unsupported depending on location. The lack of care coordination has the potential to be problematic and challenging for the families, as it relies upon a high level of capability of the parents or guardians. The Polish country agent acknowledged this by saying: '*A*ctivity, competence, awareness, and socio-economic status of parents are crucial in relation to further treatment and development of the child with health problems'. There is concern here because even in countries with a case coordinator role in place, it is possible that many parents are left to manage or coordinate the care for their child. This raises the risk that those parents without the capacity to do so, either because of stress or another reason, are unable to fulfil this role, leaving the child vulnerable – and possibly at risk of needing child protection support. Bulgaria, Finland and England (as a part of the United Kingdom) are notable as they are currently placing emphasis on achieving more comprehensive systems of integration. In Bulgaria, the respondent notes that a National Program for the Improvement of Maternal and Child Health was implemented in 2014, partly as a result of a lack of integrated medical and social approaches to serve children with chronic disease or disability. A number of measures to link social care services to primary health care have been identified and seem to reflect good practice. One measure is the creation of Centres for Maternal and Child Health; services will be provided by doctors specialising in obstetrics, gynaecology and paediatrics, as well as nurses, midwives, social workers and psychologists, both in the centre and in the family home. In Finland, greater integration will be achieved through the creation of autonomous counties which will be responsible for both primary healthcare and social care provision (at present, they are under control of the municipal level) from 2018. In England (as a part of the United Kingdom) meanwhile, the emphasis is on increasing the effectiveness of coordination of care through virtual integration with the creation of networks of clinical commissioning groups. A less extensive recent change in Romania has seen a law brought into effect to specify the manner in which the social and health sectors should coordinate care for children and adolescents with disabilities/and or special educational needs.

Child Protection

There is some evidence to suggest that the safeguarding needs of children with complex care needs are not being fulfilled (European Union Agency for Fundamental Rights, 2015a), even though we know that disabled children with complex care needs are three to four times more likely to be victims of violence, neglect and abuse than other children (Jones et al., 2012; Stalker & McArthur, 2012; Sullivan, 2009; Sullivan & Knutson, 2000) For more information, see Kielthy et al. (2017). All countries in the MOCHA study reported the presence of a child protection framework. However, the FRA reports that a main law for child protection is present in only 18 countries. No MOCHA respondent described a change in policy or legal framework prompted by failings in the child protection system by exposing a child with complex care needs or disability to risk, although, in Chapter 17, child abuse is identified as a cultural phenomenon that has been a stimulus for policy discussions in more than one country.

Access and Participation

Participation in a child's care from all parties, including from the child, is important for quality social care. An additional important element is good accessibility of services. In Denmark, for example, all children considered to be in need of special support are assessed for social care needs, in what is termed the Children's Specialist Examination. It is based on a holistic approach, as it includes parameters such as development and behaviour, family relationships, school, health, leisure time activities and friendships. The examination is used to assess whether there is a need for special support for the child and family and what kind of support is necessary.

Funding and Equity of Access

The delivery of social support is achieved via a complex array of organisational and funding structures across the MOCHA countries. We did not seek to establish the level of funding provided for these services (see also Chapters 7 and 9), but it seems reasonable to assume that there will be variations in the level of spending. It is thus challenging to establish how easy it is for a child and family to access support and whether funding or insurance coverage is sufficient to meet the need or if there exists some form of 'rationing' or prioritisation based on level of need, which limits a patient's access to care. What is evident from the Country Agent data is that most countries have an element of regional variation in the delivery of social care. For example, living in a rural area can disadvantage children with complex care needs and their families (something that is also reflected in a 2015 OECD report on integrated social services for vulnerable groups). It is important that existing policies must be facilitated in practice throughout each country in order to ensure equity of access.

Information Provision for Support to Parents

The provision of support services for parents/guardians may help to bridge the gap between those who find it easier to participate in the caregiving process and those who find it more difficult. An initiative in Norway which aims to meet the informational and support needs of parents of a child with a complex care needs is a weekend-long parenting course entitled *Hva med oss?* or *What about us?* The purpose is to strengthen relationships and family life, and provide families with the chance to swap experiences, to reflect and to celebrate. It is also noted that for parents of a child with complex care needs, meeting parents in a similar situation can be very beneficial. The Estonian Social Insurance Board is composed of 13 units and 17 customer service points around Estonia, and in addition, the Social Insurance Board has an informative website where important information and materials about activities, subunits and social insurance news are posted. The objective is to make sure that individuals anywhere in the country can find out exactly which customer service point or employee can address their concern and the legal basis for the granting of entitlement to state benefits.

Equity of Access to Supports
As reported previously, several country agencies reported that there were regional variations in some services; a disparity in availability of care is clearly apparent in rural areas compared to urban areas in many countries. A number of respondents reported that access to supports can vary depending on the funding priorities of the locality, municipality or region. This is effectively a determinant of access to services.

Compensation for Costs Associated with Care
In Denmark and Finland, the country agents outlined the availability of financial compensation for travel and accommodation for parents of a child with a complex care need. In Denmark, compensation may also be provided for additional costs, such as overnight stays at a hospital location, or for special diets that children may need, and travel expenses. Other examples of financial compensation include expenses paid to parents for taking parenting courses relevant to children with complex care needs. In Finland, compensation may be provided for travel and overnight accommodation costs to help with a child and an accompanying person's travel costs if the child needs to travel in order to undergo examination and receive treatment.

Summary

We have shown that primary care is more than the traditional medical and nursing health care services. Pharmacy, Dental services and Social care services perform or have the potential to provide essential roles for children and young people. Needs from pharmacy, dentistry and social care are varied and interwoven with needs from each other and from the healthcare system. Yet, because this inter-connectivity is not sufficiently recognised in the EU and EEA countries, there is a need for improvement of coordination and with the need for these services to focus more fully on children and young people.

Pharmacy

Pharmacies are very much used, but their value to children and young people seems not to be sufficiently recognised in EU and EEA countries. The relationship between community pharmacies and primary care services needs to be recognised and strengthened in order to substantially improve access and treatment for children's illnesses, especially for those children who are managing chronic conditions. Pharmacists are an extremely important part of primary care in the broadest sense, and the advice of a highly trained pharmacist is invaluable. Not least because medicines for children are often only available off-label, or not available in the correct dose. This skilled activity includes giving clear and accurate information about doses, how to take the medication and any interactions with other medications (Pharmaceutical Group of the European Union (PGEU), 2012). Pharmacies can potentially provide a much greater role in terms of improving self-management and well-being of generally healthy children. This could be further strengthened by the development of stronger links between pharmacists and other primary care professionals, such as physicians, nurses and allied health professionals to provide a truly comprehensive service to children and young people.

Dentistry

Preventive dentistry is available throughout the EU and EEA, but there are few targeted incentives to ensure that children receive the service. The presence of free service alone seems to be relied on as an incentive by many countries, even though this has not been shown to be effective in reducing inequalities. Services to children who are disabled or who have particular needs vary in their accessibility and availability across the EU and EEA.

Social Care Services

Mapping social care services to children with complex healthcare needs across all EU countries has presented significant challenges due to the different cultural contexts. In addition, the role played by multiple organisations of various types in the provision of social care throughout Europe is considerable. This represents fragmentation of social care provision and must present a challenge for coordination between primary health care and social care as state and non-state actors must cooperate. This also makes it more difficult to map the availability and accessibility of social care services within each country. It is also clear that, for many children, it is their parents or carers who will be responsible for making sure their social care needs are met. In many countries, parents may have to navigate various statutory and/or external organisations in order to access the additional supports that they and their child require.

Arrangements for coordination between primary health care and social care are common to a number of countries. As noted, some countries are investing significant policy and organisational development in further integrating health and social care systems. In Finland, real integration is prioritised with the creation of a model where systems will be more fully integrated by coming under the responsibility of one organisation. It should be kept in mind; however, Lewis, Rosen, Goodwin, and Dixon (2010) note that full organisational integration is not necessarily optimal and 'it may be that a care user's needs are better served through less organisational integration and more opportunity for choice and personalisation of care across a range of alternative providers that is well coordinated' (2010, p. 12). Leutz is of a similar opinion for a different reason; he asserts that coordination may be a better strategy when striving to meet the needs of the whole population (1999).

References

Alexander, D., & Blair, M. (2018). *Children and young people's use of pharmacy in primary care*. Retrieved from http://www.childhealthservicemodels.eu/wp-content/uploads/member-files/MOCHA-Pharmacy-in-primary-care-for-children-Confidential-Draft-May-2018.pdf

Alma, M., Mahtani, V., Palant, A., Klůzová Kráčmarová, L., & Prinjha, S. (2017). *Report on patient experiences of primary care in 5 DIPEx countries*. Retrieved from http://www.childhealthservicemodels.eu/wp-content/uploads/Patient-experiences-of-primary-care-in-five-countries.pdf

B.A.H. (2016). *Jeder Dritter möchte mehr Beratung bei der Medikamenteneinnahme*. Retrieved from www.bah-bonn.de/index.php?eID=dumpFile&t=f&f=9083&token=1a6b85418431b046266eac6327bfdd81b7ca79b0

Blair, M., & Menon, A. (2018). Community pharmacy use by children across Europe: A narrative literature review. *Pharmacy, 6*, 51. doi:10.3390/pharmacy6020051

Department of Health. (2000). *Framework for the assessment of the needs of children and their families*. London: The Stationery Office. Retrieved from http://webarchive.nationalarchives.gov.uk/20130123203811/ http://www.dh.gov.uk/en/Publicationsandstatistics/Publications/PublicationsPolicyAndGuidance/DH_4003256

European Union Agency for Fundamental Rights. (2015a). *Violence against children with disabilities: Legislation, policies and programmes in the EU*. Retrieved from http://fra.europa.eu/en/publication/2015/children-disabilities-violence

European Union Agency for Fundamental Rights. (2015b). *Mapping child protection systems in the EU*. Retrieved from http://fra.europa.eu/en/publications-and-resources/data-and-maps/comparative-data/child-protection

Gill, P., Goldacre, M. J., Mant, D., Heneghan, C., Thomson, A., Seagroatt, V., & Harnden, A. (2013). Increase in emergency admissions to hospital for children aged under 15 in England, 1999–2010: National database analysis. *Archieves of Disease in Childhood, 98*, 328–334. doi:10.1136/archdischild-2012-302383

Gobina, I., Villberg, J., Villerusa, A., Välimaa, R., Tynjälä, J., Ottova-Jordan, V., … Holstein, B. E. (2014). Self-reported recurrent pain and medicine use behaviours among 15-year olds: Results from the international study. *European Journal of Pain, 19*(1), doi:10.1002/ejp.524/pdf

Irish Pharmacy Union. (2015). *Review of the Irish community pharmacy sector 2013/14: Sustainability in a changing environment*. Retrieved from https://docplayer.net/

17926664-Review-of-the-irish-community-pharmacy-sector-2013-14-sustainability-in-a-changing-environment.html

Jones, L., Bellis, M. A., Wood, S., Hughes, K., McCoy, E., Eckley, L., ... Officer, A. (2012). Prevalence and risk of violence against children with disabilities: A systematic review and meta-analysis of observational studies. *Lancet*, *380*(9845), 899–907. doi:10.1016/S0140-6736(12)60692-8

Kielthy, P., Warters, A., Brenner, M., & McHugh, R. (2017). *Final report on models of children's social care support across the EU and the relationship with primary health care*. Retrieved from http://www.childhealthservicemodels.eu/publications/deliverables/

Lara Montero, A., van Duijn, S., Zonneveld, N., Minkman, M., & Nies, H. (2016). *Integrated social services in Europe. European Social Network*. Retrieved from www.esn-eu.org/raw.php?page=files&id=1910

Leutz, W. N. (1999). Five laws for integrating medical and social services: Lessons from the United States and the United Kingdom. *Milbank Quarterly*, *77*(1), 77–110.

Léveillé, S., & Chamberland, C. (2010). Toward a general model for child welfare and protection services: A meta-evaluation of international experiences regarding the adoption of the framework for the assessment of children in need and their families (FACNF). *Children and Youth Services Review*, *32*(7), 929–944. doi:10.1016/j.childyouth.2010.03.009

Lewis, R., Rosen, R., Goodwin, N., & Dixon, J. (2010). *Where next for integrated care organisations in the English NHS?* London: The Nuffield Trust. Retrieved from https://www.nuffieldtrust.org.uk/research/where-next-for-integrated-care-organisations-in-the-english-nhs

Marchant, R., Lefevre, M., Jones, M., Luckock, B. (2007). *Knowledge review: Necessary stuff – The social care needs of children with complex health care needs and their families*. Project Report, 18. Social Care Institute for Excellence (Scie), London. Retrieved from https://www.scie.org.uk/publications/knowledgereviews/kr18.asp

Pharmaceutical Group of the European Union. (2012). *European community pharmacy blueprint*. Retrieved from https://pgeu.eu/en/policy/19-the-european-community-pharmacy-blueprint.html

Pharmaceutical Society of Ireland (PSI). (2016). *Future pharmacy practice in Ireland PSI Irish pharmacy regulator*. Retrieved from https://www.thepsi.ie/Libraries/Pharmacy_Practice/PSI_Future_Pharmacy_Practice_in_Ireland.sflb.ashx

Platform for Better Oral Health. (2012). *The state of oral health in Europe*. Retrieved from http://www.oralhealthplatform.eu/our-work/the-state-of-oral-health-in-europe/

Siponen, S. (2014). *Children's health, self-care and the use of self-medication – A population-based study in Finland*. University of Eastern Finland. Retrieved from http://epublications.uef.fi/pub/urn_isbn_978-952-61-1418-7/urn_isbn_978-952-61-1418-7.pdf

Stalker, K., & McArthur, K. (2012). Child abuse, child protection and disabled children: A review of recent research. *Child Abuse Review*, *21*(1), 24–40. doi:10.1002/car.1154

Sullivan, P. M. (2009). Violence exposure among children with disabilities. *Clinical Child and Family Psychology Review*, *12*(2), 196–216.

Sullivan, P. M., & Knutson, J. F. (2000). Maltreatment and disabilities: A population-based epidemiological study. *Child Abuse & Neglect, 24*(10), 1257–1273.

Waszyk-Nowaczyk, M., & Simon, M. (2009). Pharmaceutical care as an area of pharmacist–physician collaboration. *Farmacja Polska, 65*(10), 713–716.

Ylinen, S., Hämeen-Anttila, K., Sepponen, K., Lindblad, A. K., & Ahonen, R. (2010). The use of prescription medicines and self-medication among children – A population-based study in Finland. *Pharmacoepidemiology and Drug Safety, 19*(10), 1000–1008. doi:10.1002/pds.1963. Retrieved from https://www.ncbi.nlm.nih.gov/pubmed/20712023

Chapter 16

The Transferability of Primary Child Healthcare Systems

Paul Kocken, Eline Vlasblom, Gaby de Lijster, Helen Wells, Nicole van Kesteren, Renate van Zoonen, Kinga Zdunek, Sijmen A. Reijneveld, Mitch Blair and Denise Alexander

Abstract

There is considerable heterogeneity between primary care systems that have evolved in individual national cultural environments. Models of Child Health Appraised (MOCHA) studied how the transfer of models or their individual components can be achieved across nations, using examples of combinations of settings, functions, target groups and tracer conditions. There are many factors that determine the feasibility of successful transfer of these from one setting to another, which must be recognised and taken into account. These include the environment of the care system, national policy-making and contextual means of directing population behaviour — in the form of penalties and incentives, which cannot be assessed or expected to work by means of rational actions alone. MOCHA developed a list of criteria to assess transferability, summarised in a population characteristics, intervention content, environment and transfer (PIET-T) process. To explore the process and means of transferability, we obtained consensus statements from the researchers on optimum model scenarios and conducted a survey of stakeholders, professionals and users of children's primary care services that involved three specific health topics: vaccination coverage in infants, monitoring of a chronic or complex condition and early recognition of mental health problems. The results give insight into features of transferability — such as the availability and the use of guidelines and formal procedures; the barriers and facilitators of implementation and similarities and differences between model practices and the existing model of child primary care in the country. We found that successful transfer of an optimal model is impossible without tailoring the model to a specific country setting. It is vital to be aware of the sensitivity of the population and environmental characteristics of a country before starting to change the system of primary care.

Keywords: Transferability; implementation; model health services; health systems; child health; incentives

Introduction

The goal of the Models of Child Health Appraised (MOCHA) project is to define optimal models of primary child health care that have the potential of transfer to European Union (EU) countries. As we have seen, a model is only a simplified representation of a complex reality; however, the design of models of primary child health care is not a simple task because of the comprehensiveness of the componentry of healthcare systems (see Chapter 1). In this chapter, we study how the transfer of models of primary child health care can be achieved across nations, using examples of combinations of settings, functions and target groups. Tracer conditions we use to illustrate the options for transfer are preventive services for immunisation, treatment and monitoring of a chronic (asthma) or complex condition (traumatic brain injury), assessment of mental health problems of psychosocial and assessment of mental health problems ,and psychosocial assessment of adolescents for use of contraceptive services. These topics will be dealt with, using the framework developed by MOCHA to analyse the complex primary care systems and assess criteria for transferability.

To understand the structure, processes and outcome of care delivery, a usable set of primary care systems' components was distinguished by Kringos, Boerma, Hutchinson, Van der Zee, and Groenewegen (2010), including governance, economic conditions, workforce, access, comprehensiveness, continuity and coordination, quality, efficacy and equity. MOCHA chose the components access and workforce to categorise the primary child healthcare systems according to roughly two system structure components: the primary care lead practitioner, being a general practitioner (GP) or paediatrician, and referral processes to secondary or other care (gatekeeping or not) (Blair, Rigby, & Alexander, 2017). Combining the two components led to the following classification of primary care in EU countries:

- open access countries: countries with an open access referral process and any lead practitioner;
- gatekeeper and mixed-led countries: countries with a partial or usual gatekeeper and either a paediatrician-led primary care, or a mix of paediatrician-led and GP-led primary care; and
- gatekeeper and GP-led countries: countries with a partial or usual gatekeeper and primary care led by a GP.

The feasibility of the transfer of models from one setting to another is determined by many factors related to the population of a country, the characteristics of the model to be transferred and factors in the environment of the care system, including national policy-making and contextual means of directing population behaviour, such as penalties and rewards, called 'levers'. Keeping in mind the differences in care systems, the transfer of a model from one country to another requires tailoring to the specific country-setting. MOCHA has developed a long list of criteria for assessing transferability, summarised in a population characteristics, intervention content, environment and transfer (PIET-T) process model as shown in Figure 16.1 (Schloemer & Schröder-Bäck, 2018). The criteria match with models on intervention implementation (Damschroder et al., 2009; Fleuren, Wiefferink, & Paulussen, 2004). This is also discussed in detail in Chapter 18.

Understanding the significance of the PIET-T criteria is essential to successfully assess whether components of a model can be transferred to a different system. The next sections will assess feasibility of scenarios for improvement of primary care according to professional stakeholders from EU countries, expert views on implementation of good practices and legitimacy of levers – penalties and rewards – to achieve behaviour change.

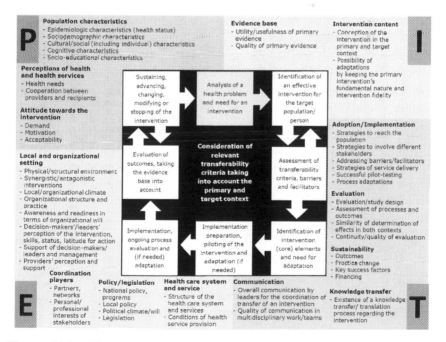

Figure 16.1. The PIET-T model with systematised criteria to determine transferability.

Listening to Professional Stakeholders

We undertook a study to obtain consensus statements from stakeholders in children's primary health care on what needs to change to optimise primary care health systems for children. They were asked about the acceptability and feasibility of changes towards potentially optimal ways to deliver primary care to children and how these potential changes might be achieved. Testimonials and opinions from experts in the fields of policy-making, practice, science and knowledge, and end-user advocacy were gathered via a survey and online focus groups. As a stimulus for discussion, we created imaginary scenarios on future provision of child health care (Kocken, Vlasblom, De Lijster, & Reijneveld, 2018).

The survey contained three health topics, accompanied by scenarios related to functions of primary child health care, the tracer conditions and children's age-groups. These topics were designed to reflect the comprehensiveness of a primary healthcare system for children:

- vaccination coverage in infants: prevention/ immunisation against measles/ 0−4 years old;
- treatment and monitoring of a chronic or complex condition: chronic care and complex care/asthma or traumatic brain injury/4−12 years old; and
- early recognition of mental health problems: school and adolescent health services/mental health/12−18 years old.

Vaccination Coverage in Infants

The stakeholder respondents considered a change of the care system's component 'public access to trustworthy information' as important. They called for more public information about vaccinations, to reduce vaccination hesitancy and thereby improving vaccination coverage in the population. Although the majority of stakeholders were positive about a scenario describing a specialised preventive child health service to improve vaccination coverage, a change from the current model in their country to any other was not given as a priority. A higher priority was given to combat vaccination hesitancy using public information. The stakeholders suggested the use of social media and opinion leaders to influence public opinion, even though literature suggests that combatting vaccination hesitancy through public information is less effective than providing information on vaccinations within an ongoing relationship between a specialised preventive child health professional and parents (Schollin Ask et al., 2017).

Treatment and Monitoring of a Chronic or Complex Condition

Almost all of the respondents were in favour of working in multidisciplinary teams to improve care for children with a chronic condition or complex needs (see Chapter 10). The added value of professionals with different skills working closely together was rated as important (see Chapter 13). However, our survey showed a large variability in opinions on the feasibility of changing towards multidisciplinary teams. Some stakeholders thought their country was too far away from the model and believed working in teams costly and in some cases, unnecessary. Stakeholders advocated the importance of understanding the families' perspective and providing clear information to them about how and where to address their healthcare needs. We know that special attention should be given to vulnerable families with complex needs, particularly those who do not have the capacity to organise their help in a sufficient way (Chapters 5 and 15; Keilthy, Warters, Brenner, & McHugh, 2017). It was generally agreed that facilitating the different professionals working together would be a challenge and that training in multidisciplinary working would be beneficial (see Chapter 13) (Brenner, O'Shea, & Larkin, 2017).

Early Recognition of Mental Health Problems in Adolescents

The stakeholders supported collaboration and communication between healthcare providers as components of health care that should be optimised in order to improve early recognition of mental health problems in adolescents. The majority of stakeholders also replied that they were positive about confidential access to adolescent health service; however, we received a variety of opinions on the subject. Some stakeholders thought guaranteeing confidentiality to adolescents when consulting primary care improves early recognition of mental health problems, through lowering the barrier to approach care and increasing the willingness of adolescents to discuss sensitive topics. Other stakeholders expressed their doubts or were against confidential access. They thought this hampers the inclusion of the family in the treatment process, which is considered key to optimal service delivery to adolescents with mental health problems. The stakeholders were clear at what stage of the patient consultation confidentiality can be given: namely in preventive activities, all kinds of psychological support and training or courses that are available for all children. However, for treatment of complex problems, medical treatment and prescription of medicines, consent of parents is needed and confidentiality cannot be given.

Feasibility, Barriers and Facilitators: Criteria for Transferability

The stakeholders of open-access countries seemed to answer most frequently to have a need for a change of the system. They were relatively more often in favour of a change than the two gatekeeper system countries across all three scenarios. The stakeholders from gatekeeper and mixed-led countries asked the least for a change towards confidential access. The primary care systems for children in countries with a gatekeeper function by GPs seemed to need the least amount of change (this applies to specialised preventive health services and multidisciplinary teams). The stakeholders from these countries indicated most often that the suggested scenario was already in place in their country.

The differences between care systems make clear that transferring an optimal model requires tailoring to the specific country-setting. The following criteria from the PIET-T process model seemed important (Schloemer & Schröder-Bäck, 2018).

Population Characteristics

Public attitude towards a health topic seemed to be important for change to be effective and for equitable service delivery (see Chapter 17). This is particularly relevant for issues such as vaccination, the way of accessing services and the age in which a young person can make use of a service without parental consent. MOCHA's research into public preferences for primary care for children showed large differences between countries in terms of respondents' agreement on the statement whether the child has the right to a confidential consultation with a primary care provider (Van Til, Groothuis-Oudshoorn, & Boere-Boonekamp, 2018). Samples from populations from Spain and Poland (gatekeeper and mixed-led country, respectively) agreed the least with this right for children, which corresponded with the views of the experts in study. As the public attitudes on, for instance, family involvement in the care of a child vary between countries, transferability of a healthcare system from one country to another very much depends on these opinions being embedded in the countries' culture (Zdunek, Schröder-Bäck, Blair, & Rigby, 2017).

Environment

In all scenarios, the current healthcare system and service provision in the country was regarded as a major barrier for moving towards the proposed changes in the systems' components. Relatively, the least challenging change was towards multidisciplinary working, although the issue of financing multidisciplinary teams, the slow process of changing the policy and legislation and the general need for more workforce was nevertheless mentioned as barriers. A well-functioning and accessible healthcare system was also seen as a facilitator in the sense that well-equipped school health services add to the early recognition of mental health problems in adolescents. The MOCHA project has demonstrated the value of extensive national policies, sometimes as shared responsibility with regional authorities, with regard to school and adolescent health services as an indicator for countries to have potentially good quality services for children and adolescents (see Chapter 11) (Jansen et al., 2018). National policies to ensure geographical and financial access were also identified by the PHAMEU project, as indicators for the presence of strong primary care in a country (Kringos et al., 2013).

Intervention Content

A facilitating factor mentioned several times by the stakeholders was the evidence base with regard to the targeted changes of improved communication on vaccination and confidential access to adolescent health services. With regard to the importance of interdisciplinary working for an effective primary healthcare system, the evidence base was already there according to the stakeholders. The importance of good e-health systems, such as patient record systems for coordination of care and reminder systems for vaccinating children, was also mentioned several times as a facilitator. A lack of evidence on the influence of such systems on the effectiveness, efficiency and quality of primary care hinders further development of the care system. Conducting research to find the evidence will facilitate changes in components of primary care.

Transfer

Favourable economic conditions, supportive policy-making and a good political climate will facilitate the sustainability of transfer of optimum components of primary care from one country to another (Schloemer & Schröder-Bäck, 2018). The barriers found in our study, such as lack of funding and a lack of qualified professionals need to be addressed in clear strategies and policies.

Expert Views on Implementation of Good Practices

This study went in more in depth what factors influence the implementation of good practices in primary child health care. Knowledge of these factors from the PIET-T model informs us whether transferability of optimal component to a specific healthcare system or country may be possible (Van Kesteren, Van Zoonen, Kocken, 2018). The study aimed to:

- obtain insight into the availability and use of good practices of measles immunisation, information provision on contraceptive advice for adolescents, assessment of mental health problems and asthma care in six European countries; and
- achieve a better understanding of the facilitators and barriers of implementation of suggested good practices within the context of various models of primary child care in Europe.

A cross-case research design was used to compare implementation conditions between good practices and countries. The experts were asked to fill out an online questionnaire to get insight into their views with regard to the use of good practices, barriers and facilitators. Experts from six European countries were included in this study: Germany, Cyprus, Sweden, The Netherlands, Italy and Poland. Countries were selected in such a way that they were more or less exemplary of the broad features of the types of primary care models in the EU (see Chapter 1). They varied in terms of lead practitioner (GP, primary care paediatrician, mixed) and open or gatekeeping systems of provision of health services. For this study, we added a third governance characteristic, namely whether the health care is state regulated or professionals have more or less autonomy in providing services, respectively, hierarchical or non-hierarchical systems (Bourgueil, Marek, & Mousquès, 2009).

The results give insight into the availability and use of guidelines and formal procedures, barriers and facilitators of implementation of the good practices studied and similarities and differences between good practices and models of child primary care.

Availability and Use of Guidelines and Formal Procedures

The influence of the type of primary care model on the availability of guidelines or formal procedures was studied. In general experts from Sweden, the Netherlands and Poland, with a hierarchical gatekeeping system seemed to be positive about the availability of guidelines. Non-hierarchical led countries seemed to have guidelines to a lesser extent. In Cyprus, a country with open access and where paediatricians deliver primary care for children, guidelines were the least available. Germany as a country with similar system characteristics was divergent in this respect and had guidelines available. It appeared that all countries have guidelines or formal procedures available for asthma, but that in spite of their availability, the use of these guidelines or formal procedures was limited. In contrast, guidelines or formal procedures for immunisation were generally used for nearly all children and the best implemented.

Barriers and Facilitators of Implementation of the Good Practices Studied

We examined barriers and facilitators of the implementation process of good practices related to a framework representing the implementation process and related categories of determinants, namely characteristics of the good practice itself (intervention content), the primary care professional, the organisational setting and the socio-political context (environment) (Fleuren et al., 2004; Schloemer & Schröder-Bäck, 2018).

The results showed that experts from most countries identified mostly facilitators with regard to communicating with vaccine-hesitant parents; barriers were notably found with regard to the conduct of spirometry for asthma and for conducting a psychosocial assessment for contraceptive services for sexually active adolescents.

Important facilitators at the level of the intervention were that the good practice is not too difficult to perform and fits well within routine practice such as with vaccination. Facilitators from the environment were the perception of the primary care professional that it is important to use good practice and that the good practice is supported by healthcare policy-makers. This was also especially the case with vaccination.

Important barriers that were mentioned by experts from almost all countries were in the field of financial resources and time available, knowledge and adequate training for doctors and nurses. With regard to performing spirometry for asthma diagnosis and management, some experts saw barriers were on the socio-political level with regard to policy support and legislation and regulation. With regard to the implementation of the good practice of conducting a psychosocial assessment in order to provide contraceptive information and services for sexually active adolescents, the experts identified mainly barriers. For conducting a risk assessment of the mental health problems in young people, the majority of countries identified both facilitators and barriers.

Poland, Italy, Germany and Cyprus, all countries with a paediatrician- or mixed paediatrician-/GP-led child primary care, experienced facilitators and barriers in the implementation of the good practices. The experts from the Netherlands and Sweden, all countries with hierarchical professional GP-led systems, experienced facilitators to a greater extent, in Sweden particularly in terms of motivating parents to vaccinate their child and use of spirometry.

Immunisation, spirometry and screening for mental health are all are clinical procedures, which have varying levels of complexity. Barriers and facilitators to changes may be understood from the Cynefin model on complexity (IBM) (Snowden & Boone, 2007). For example, vaccination is a more or less simple practice that can be changed with relative ease. Use of the spirometer in asthma care may be more complicated and dependent on variables which can be managed reasonably well in care, such as resources and professional consensus on the acceptance of the good practice. Risk assessment for mental health and sexual and reproductive health is a more complex good practice, due to the influence of societal, genetic and care determinants. The assessment of these health problems is therefore difficult and can be managed to a lesser extent.

Penalties, Rewards and Behaviour Change

This strand of the MOCHA programme focussed on the use of levers, which is the term adopted for the use of incentives and penalties to encourage certain choices, in European child healthcare contexts. It is suggested that the use of levers is likely to increase under conditions of neo-liberalism which apply to greater and lesser degrees in all MOCHA countries (Wells, 2017a). Where individuals are encouraged to believe that they should seek out opportunities to choose their own treatment and care, but the state cannot actually allow its citizens to make free choices that are not in the best interests of the wider group (such as in the case of immunisation and herd immunity), levers nudge citizens in particular directions while maintaining the illusion of free choice.

Financial levers in particular are in relatively widespread use across Europe (for both providers of and recipients of health care), combined with an implicit assumption that they were part of a good model of delivery (for more details, see Wells, 2017a). However, the research found very limited evidence of evaluations of levers, with those identified general only adopting a financial 'effectiveness' perspective, and mainly focussed on their use in relation to healthcare providers rather than recipients (Wells, 2017a). We concluded that the use of levers is not sufficiently considered within their particular socio-cultural context (e.g. the different political histories of countries, or the variously constructed relationships between citizens and their respective states). Nor is it being considered as part of complex ecological systems involving triadic relationships between emotional humans (child, parent and healthcare provider) rather than rational *homo economicus*, potentially leading to unwanted and unintended consequences. Identities such as 'professional' (on the provider side) and 'parent' (on the recipient side) may be affronted by the implication that a sum of money may be sufficient to change how we behave (Wells, 2017b). The presence of the child as a third person in a 'deal' between the state and a parent is a particular complication in this context, with parents required to choose whether or not they wish to accept the deal on behalf of a child who the parents may believe will actually be the bearer of any perceived risk (Wells, 2017b). Efforts to encourage parents to vaccinate their children are a particularly salient example of this tension.

A further consideration particularly generated by the use of penalties is the introduction of an instrumental and disciplinary relationship into one that should be characterised by normative commitment and trust. 'Gaming' (Eijkenaar, Emmert, Scheppach, & Schoffski, 2013; Mannion, 2014) is a term that describes when individuals become focussed on the ends, at the expense of the means. This is more likely where the state is seen to have reframed the interaction between itself and the public, or itself and professional healthcare providers, as instrumental (about gains and losses) rather than as normative (about doing something because it is the right thing to do) (Wells, 2017b).

Our research also suggests that an excessive focus on securing the outcome of behavioural change at the expense of proper consideration of the means – the processes via which the outcomes are achieved – is counterproductive. Systems should not aim to secure discrete changes in behaviour at any cost but instead focus on ensuring that its processes and policies increase the perceived legitimacy of the system and authorities. Ensuring that levers are operating in ways that are seen to be procedurally just (offering opportunities for voice, consistent usage, communication of motivation, respect, fairness and so on) (Lind & Tyler, 1988; Tyler, 1994) is essential for securing longer-term compliance with the state's objectives via its perceived legitimacy in the eyes of the leverage targets and is also closely related to transferability. The basic antecedents of a procedurally just experience appear to be transferable across demographics and contexts, and the limited application of the concepts in healthcare settings does seem to suggest relevant transferability, though there are suggestions that different value structures between countries may mean that some terms (such as 'fairness' and 'respect' perhaps) may vary according to context and therefore need further consideration (Cohen & Avrahami, 2006). There is, furthermore, reason for viewing quality patient experiences as a central aspect of any healthcare model, not as an added luxury, given that increased satisfaction also leads to increased compliance with treatment recommendations. Satisfied patients appear, therefore, to be healthier patients, and this is achieved via procedurally just treatment within relationships characterised by trust, respect and lack of bias that, in many cases, can be achieved at little or no extra cost to the system. Conversely, the costs to health (in the short and long term) of accidentally designing systems that do not value procedural justice are likely to be significant. These procedural justice considerations should be a facet of all levering policies and not be overlooked in pursuit of short-term targets for compliance. There is no point securing short-term behavioural change if the means of doing so alienate the provider or recipient from (all) authority in future and make them less compliant in the longer term (Hughes & Larson, 1991). It is necessary to see attempts at leverage as conveying messages about value, worth and respect to their intended recipients, not just as methods of securing behavioural change. For example, behavioural change approaches may tell us that people are more likely to be amenable to making changes at key life points such as when they become parents, or experience bereavement, but we should look to procedural justice approaches of basic fairness and equity of provision (Lind & Tyler, 1988; Tyler, 1994) to guide a healthcare system in targeting potentially vulnerable people in ways that do not make them feel exploited.

The MOCHA research also highlights significant equity issues relating to financial and intellectual resources, given that within any population not everyone has the same capacity to (1) understand what is being offered or threatened and in relation to what activity and (2) freely choose whether or not they wish to accept the offer, or endure the threat, that the state is making (e.g. where less wealthy parents may have to factor in financial benefit or hardship, while more wealthy parents may not) (Wells, 2017a).

As such, it is vital that the future use of levers is not underpinned by an assumption that behavioural change can be achieved through the manipulation of rational actors (and hence a neglect of issues such as emotion, capacity, justice and socio-cultural context). There are ways in which the use of levers can be rendered more procedurally fair, and more likely to secure longer-term compliance, but equity issues are likely to remain wherever resources and access are offered or withheld as a method of securing compliance with state objectives.

Summary

The MOCHA research presented in this chapter assessed criteria for transferability of models of primary child health care from one setting or country to another. It showed that stakeholders expressed a need for improvements to the child primary care system and valued the importance of system components in the field of public access to information about vaccination, coordination and continuity of care and open access to services for adolescents and confidentiality until treatment is in place. Heterogeneity was found between countries with regard to the presence of these components and their demand for change. Primary care systems with open access seemed to have the highest demand for changing system components. GP-led gatekeeper systems, generally rated as strong primary care systems, felt the least urgency for transforming system components.

The study into factors affecting the implementation of good practices also showed that models of primary care to a certain extent are relevant. It was found that GP- or mixed-led hierarchical professional systems seemed to have a positive influence on the availability of guidelines of formal procedures for several good practices. It is likely that governance features are important to ascertain the needed levels of guideline use and adherence. Good practices in the field of immunisation, asthma care and screening for mental health or reproductive issues are all clinical procedures with varying levels of complexity, requiring appropriate resources, training and public information and cultural 'acceptance' from a public and professional perspective. Guideline adherence to optimise effectiveness may be more likely in hierarchical professional systems with a certain level of state regulation.

With regard to the PIET-T criteria, public attitudes towards a health topic are important for changes with regard to effective vaccination coverage or service use without parental consent. Also, the current healthcare system and service provision in a country is regarded as a major facilitator or barrier for moving towards changes in the systems' components. A facilitating factor in the field of intervention content mentioned is the evidence base with regard to the targeted change. The study of good practices showed that the implementation is influenced by a range of facilitating or hindering factors that fall in the broad PIET-T categories intervention content and environment, such as service organisation and socio-political factors. The perceived legitimacy of levers for behaviour change of countries' citizens is reflected in the socio-cultural context and people's perceptions of the PIET-T model. Healthcare systems should not aim at securing discrete changes in behaviour at any cost but instead focus on ensuring that its processes and policies increase the perceived legitimacy of the system and authorities.

This chapter makes clear that transfer of an optimal model requires tailoring to the specific country-setting. It is important to be aware of the sensitivity of the population and environmental characteristics of a country and monitor them before starting changes to the system of primary child health care.

References

Blair, M., Rigby, M., & Alexander, D. (2017). *Final report on current models of primary care for children.* Retrieved from www.childhealthservicemodels.eu/wp-content/uploads/2017/07/MOCHA-WP1-Deliverable-WP1-D6-Feb-2017-1.pdf

Bourgueil, Y., Marek, A., & Mousquès, J. (2009). *Three models of primary care organization in Europe, Canada, Australia and New-Zealand.* Institute for research and information in health outcomes, Issues in health economics, 141.

Brenner, M., O'Shea, M., & Larkin, P. (2017). *Final report on the current approach to managing the care of children with complex care needs in member states.* Retrieved from http://www.childhealthservicemodels.eu/wp-content/uploads/2015/09/20170725_Deliverable-D8-2.1-Final-report-on-the-current-approach-to-managing-the-care-of-children-with-complex-care-needs-in-Member-States.pdf

Cohen, A., & Avrahami, A. (2006). The relationship between individualism, collectivism, the perception of justice, demographic characteristics and organisational citizenship behaviour. *The Service Industries Journal, 26*(8), 889—901. doi:10.1080/02642060601011707

Damschroder, L. J., Aron, D. C., Keith, R. E., Kirsh, S. R., Alexander, J. A., & Lowery, J. C. (2009). Fostering implementation of health services research findings into practice: A consolidated framework for advancing implementation science. *Implementation Science, 4*, 50–65. doi:10.1186/1748-5908-4-50

Eijkenaar, F., Emmert, M., Scheppach, M., & Schoffski, O. (2013). Effects of pay for performance in health care: A systematic review of systematic reviews. *Health Policy, 110*, 115–130. doi:10.1016/j.healthpol.2013.01.008

Fleuren, M. A. H., Wiefferink, K., & Paulussen, T. (2004). Determinants of innovation within health care organizations: Literature review and Delphi study. *International Journal for Quality in Health Care, 16*, 107–123. doi:10.1093/intqhc/mzh030

Hughes, T., & Larson, L. (1991). Patient involvement in health care: A procedural justice viewpoint. *Medical Care, 29*(3), e159–e165.

Jansen, D. E. M. C., Visser, A., Vervoort, J. P. M., van der Pol, S., Kocken, P., Reijneveld, S. A., & Michaud. (2018). *School and adolescent health services in 30 European countries: A description of structure and functioning, and of health outcomes and costs.* Retrieved from http://www.childhealthservicemodels.eu/wp-content/uploads/Deliverable-173.1_Final-report-on-the-description-of-the-various-models-of-school-health-services-and-adolescent-health-services.pdf

Keilthy, P., Warters, A., Brenner, M., & McHugh, R. (2017). *Final report on models of children's social care support across the EU and the relationship with primary health care.* Retrieved from http://www.childhealthservicemodels.eu/wp-content/uploads/2017/07/20170728_Deliverable-D9-2.2-Final-report-on-models-of-children%E2%80%99s-social-care-support-across-the-EU-and-the-relationship-with-primary-health-care.pdf

Kocken, P., Vlasblom, E., De Lijster, G., & Reijneveld, M. (2018). *A report containing consensus statements on most optimal models with guidance on potential benefits and how these might be achieved.* Retrieved from http://www.childhealthservicemodels.eu/wp-content/uploads/Deliverable-D18-9.2-A-report-containing-consensus-statements-on-most-optimal-models-with-guidance-on-potential-benefits-and-how-these-might-be.pdf

Kringos, D. S., Boerma, W. G., Hutchinson, A., Van der Zee, J., & Groenewegen, P. P. (2010). The breadth of primary care: A systematic literature review of its core dimensions. *BMC Health Services Research, 10*(1), 65. doi:10.1186/1472-6963-10-65

Kringos, D., Boerma, W., Bourgueil, Y., Cartier, T., Dedeu, T., Hasvold, T. … Groenewegen, P. (2013). The strength of primary care in Europe: An international comparative study. *British Journal of General Practice, 63*(616), e742–50. doi:10.3399/bjgp13X674422

Lind, E., & Tyler, T. (1988). *The social psychology of procedural justice.* London: Plenum Press.

Mannion, R. (2014). Take the money and run: The challenges of designing and evaluating financial incentives in healthcare; Comment on "Paying for performance in healthcare organisations". *International Journal of Health Policy Management, 2*(2), 95–96.

Schloemer, T., & Schröder-Bäck, P. (2018). Criteria for evaluating transferability of health interventions: A systematic review and thematic synthesis. *Implementation Science, 13*(1), 88. doi:10.1186/s13012-018-0751-8

Schollin Ask, L., Hjern, A., Lindstrand, A., Olen, O., Sjogren, E., Blennow, M., Örtqvist, Å. (2017). Receiving early information and trusting Swedish child health centre nurses increased parents' willingness to vaccinate against rotavirus infections. *Acta Paediatrica, 106*(8), 1309–1316. doi:10.1111/apa.13872

Snowden, D. J., & Boone, M. E. (2007). A leader's framework for decision making. *Harvard Business Review, 85*(11), 68–76.

Tyler, T. (1994). Psychological models of the justice motive: Antecedents of distributive and procedural justice. *Journal of Personality and Social Psychology, 67*(5), 850–863.

Van Kesteren, N. M. C., Van Zoonen, R., & Kocken, P. L. (2018). *Validated optimal models of children's prevention orientated primary health care: An E-Book showcasing conditions for implementation of examples of good practices in primary child health care in European countries.* Retrieved from http://www.childhealthservicemodels.eu/wp-content/uploads/20180131_Deliverable-D15-9.1-An-e-book-showcasing-conditions-for-implementation-of-examples-of-best-practices-in-primary-child-health-care-in-Europe-v2.pdf

Van Til, J., Groothuis-Oudshoorn, K., & Boere-Boonekamp, M. M. (2018). *Public priorities for primary child health care for children.* MOCHA. Retrieved from http://www.childhealthservicemodels.eu/wp-content/uploads/member-files/Final-Report-POCHA_14-08-2018.pdf

Wells, H. (2017a). Contribution to Blair, M., Rigby, M., Alexander, D. (2017) *Final report on current models of primary care for children.* Part I. Chapter 8. Retrieved from www.childhealthservicemodels.eu/wp-content/uploads/2017/07/MOCHA-WP1-Deliverable-WP1-D6-Feb-2017-1.pdf

Wells, H. (2017b). Contribution to Contribution to Blair, M., Rigby, M., Alexander, D. (2017) *Final report on current models of primary care for children.* Part II. Chapter 8. Retrieved from www.childhealthservicemodels.eu/wp-content/uploads/2017/07/MOCHA-WP1-Deliverable-WP1-D6-Feb-2017-1.pdf

Zdunek, K., Schröder-Bäck, P., Blair, M., & Rigby, M. (2017). *Report on the contextual determinants of child health policy.* Retrieved from http://www.childhealthservicemodels.eu/wp-content/uploads/member-files/Context-Culture-Report-WP-1-task-7-a-12.03.2017.-PRE-FINALdocx.pdf

Chapter 17

National and Public Cultures as Determinants of Health Policy and Production

Kinga Zdunek, Mitch Blair and Denise Alexander

Abstract

The Models of Child Health Appraised (MOCHA) project recognises that child health policy is determined to a great extent by national culture; thus, exploring and understanding the cultural influences on national policies are essential to fully appraise the models of primary care. Cultures are created by the population who adopt national rituals, beliefs and code systems and are unique to each country. To understand the effects of culture on public policy, and the resulting primary care services, we explored the socio-cultural background of four components of policy-making: content, actors, contexts and processes. Responses from the MOCHA Country Agents about recent key national concerns and debates about child health and policy were analysed to identify the key factors as determinants of policy. These included awareness, contextual change, freedom, history, lifestyle, religion, societal activation and tolerance. To understand the influence of these factors on policy, we identified important internal and external structural determinants, which we grouped into those identified within the structure of health care policy (internal), and those which are only indirectly correlated with the policy environment (external). An important child-focused cultural determinant of policy is the national attitude to child abuse. We focused on the role of primary care in preventing and identifying abuse of children and young people, and treating its consequences, which can last a lifetime.

Keywords: Health policy; population; culture; transferability; child health; values; child abuse

Introduction

Child health policy is influenced and determined to a great extent by national culture. In order to fully understand and appraise models of child primary care, it is essential to explore the cultural influences upon the policies and actions that create the individual systems.

Culture is not abstract, but is created by individuals and organisations, who use material, organisational and political resources to develop their own systems of cultural codes which are made into rituals and passed on to others (Turner, 2012). The specificity and separateness of culture do not depend on the multiplicity and originality of elements but rather on the relationships between them (Dyczewski, 1993). Culture is characterised by a range of interacting influences: (1) it has individual character, as we create and are influenced by culture; (2) it has social character as it is created by interpersonal communication; (3) it simultaneously connects some people together, and separates others; and (4) it is dynamic and can evolve in some conditions and lessen in others (Dyczewski 1993, cited in Majchrowska, 2002). Culture remains in a relationship of interdependence with the social system therefore changes in one system entail changes in the other (Dyczewski, 1993).

To understand the effects of culture on public policy and on primary care services, we explored the socio-cultural background of four components of policy-making, namely, content, actors, contexts and processes (Buse, Mays, & Walt, 2005; Walt & Gilson, 1994). This work also formed an important background in the development of the Models of Child Health Appraised (MOCHA) conceptual child-centric framework (see Chapter 4). To investigate how culture influences child health policy, we interrogated the European Values Study (EVS) (2015a), alongside a MOCHA survey on child health-specific influences on policy. Finally, we look at how the primary care systems interact specifically with the very important topic of child abuse and neglect.

European Values Study

The most significant element of culture is values. They are the baseline for its existence and development (Dyczewski, 1993). The worldwide socio-cultural transformations across various aspects of life affect the system of values in terms of both declarations and actions (Bogusz, 2004). Therefore, our theoretical preposition is that the process of multi-level contextual changes over time, causes the shifts in normative systems (see Chapter 4), and influences attitudes towards child and childhood, child health and child health care and policy.

The European Values Study (EVS) is an international survey of the values held by a sample of Europeans and aids our understanding of the opinions of Europeans about such matters as family life, social issues and beliefs. In the MOCHA project, we looked at the EVS from the perspective of a value-based approach. Although it is a survey of adult attitudes, EVS contains several issues that are pertinent to children and also relevant to child health services and policy, such as family and marriage, a topic which contains questions about what constitutes a successful marriage, attitude towards child care, marriage, children and traditional family structures. The EVS (2015b) survey is conducted every 10 years, and the next results will be available in 2019; currently, the latest data are from 2008. Nevertheless, despite their age, there is likely to be an influence on policy from these values in the past nine years.

In most European countries, the family and children are extensively valued with between 95% and 100% of Europeans declaring that family is either very or quite important in their lives (EVS, 2011e) and 80% of the respondents in most countries (73% in Denmark) stating that children are very or rather important for a successful marriage (EVS, 2011a).

Generally, Europeans do not consider having a child as their societal duty. The majority of those surveyed in Bulgaria (71%) believe this to be the case; but elsewhere, the agreement with this statement varies from above 40% in Malta, Cyprus and Portugal and Czech Republic to 10% or less in the UK, Finland, the Netherlands and Sweden (EVS, 2011b)

The belief that a woman needs a child to be fulfilled increases in rates, the further south in Europe that the survey is conducted. The difference is noticeable in countries such as Great Britain, Ireland, Norway, Sweden and Finland where the indicators do not exceed 20%, compared to continental Europe, where most of the countries, except the Netherlands and Belgium, report quite positive attitudes towards this statement. (EVS, 2011c)

The percentage of people that agree or agree strongly with the statement that 'a job is alright but what most women really want is a home and children' is lower in northern Europe and the Scandinavian region and higher in the southern and eastern regions, ranging from 83% of Romanians to 11% of Danes (EVS, 2011d).

The EVS demonstrates that not only are children an important feature in people's lives and values, but that children are no longer an inevitability, but for most people a considered choice and as such, they are placed at a high value in many families. As the EVS states:

> Children requir[e] and deserv[e] high investments and intense emotional involvement from their parents. Where the father used to be the centre of the family, home has slowly transformed into a child-centred haven. (EVS, 2015a)

This is, in part, some explanation as to why issues involving children's health and well-being can be very potent influences on public attitudes and consequently child health policy.

Public Opinion and Drivers

The MOCHA project investigated the extent to which societal views on the content and quality of children's health care, influence how policy-makers respond.

To achieve this, we used a hybrid approach, which linked the constructionist data-driven inductive perspective (Charmaz, 2006), with the elements of deductive coding which was based on the classification of contextual determinants by Leichter (1979). In our study, the constructionist constant comparative method was supported by elements of deductive thematic analysis.

The MOCHA Country Agents (CAs) (Chapter 1) were asked to identify the three strongest public and professional discussions related to child health services in their countries in the past five years (2011−2016). As these are strongly embedded within national context and influenced by various external factors, we used the results to analyse the contextual determinants of subsequent child health policies in Europe.

Semi-structured questionnaires were developed in accordance with the following criteria designed by the researchers: identification of the object and area of public concern, characteristics of the broader context of the case and identification of the level of discussion, the characteristic of the vehicles of public expression and the outcomes of the case.

The research stages have been described in full in Blair, Rigby, and Alexander (2017), Zdunek, Schröder-Bäck, Blair, and Rigby (2017), but in summary, they were as follows:

- Data was collected from the MOCHA CAs (see Chapter 1).
- The data were reviewed by a MOCHA researcher and then incorporated into a qualitative analysis software programme (NVivo 11).
- The data were then coded, by analysing the phrases used to transform the text into codes.
- The data were then categorised in terms of their significance, common themes were extracted, and patterns were identified. This allowed us to define the properties of the extracted themes and analysis of the data.

The analytical phase of the work was based on the adapted classification of contextual determinants, as proposed by Leichter (1979), of four categories: cultural, structural, situational and international factors. We adapted them to our survey as socio-cultural, structural (external and internal), situational and international factors. Seventy-one cases resulted from the MOCHA exercise, the analysis of which revealed the contextual determinants. We grouped the inductively identified codes into categories, which were subsequently assigned into four groups, reflecting Leichter's determinants. A number of sub-elements which influence child health policy were further identified.

Socio-cultural Factors

Socio-cultural factors constitute everyday choices, behaviours and attitudes that affect the way the things are done. We identified several elements which affected child health policy in European countries. The CAs gave detailed examples of national issues, which are described in full in Zdunek et al. (2017). Although there was a huge range of national debates, many started by a single incident or awareness of a perceived injustice; it was possible to classify the socio-cultural factors that influenced subsequent policy developments into eight categories.

(1) Awareness: This includes individuals or institutions raising awareness of a problem, or awareness of its impact; it also involves information and misinformation.

(2) Contextual change: This can manifest as shifts in the proximal and/or distal child environment. It might be a phenomenon at the macro or micro level.

(3) Freedom: Discussion about the rights of the child and the family to medical treatment or provision.

(4) History: Tradition is usually strongly embedded in a country's culture; thus, history was extracted as a separate category from the data of the case studies. The impact of the past policies and solutions, as well as inherited traditions, may help or hinder an issue.

(5) Lifestyle: Digital media and its use in schools is a component of modern lifestyle interpreted as a set of behaviours which directly or indirectly may positively or negatively affect child health status. Lifestyle is also the component which should be taken into consideration while defining child health policy priorities.

(6) Religion: Attitudes and religious beliefs affect national debates as well as individual lifestyle choices.

(7) Societal activation: The level of societal activation in the country determines what is initiated within child health policy as well as care and often is driven by public sensitivity for child-related issues. Activation can be twofold: either in terms of public involvement in the policy modifications or as a lack of involvement.

(8) Tolerance: Among the issues analysed and discussed in Europe, we observed that they reflected contemporary socio-cultural dilemmas. Migration and the changes to the traditional family pattern brought about the emergence of discourse in terms of tolerance.

What was interesting in our analysis was the similar nature of many of the discussions that emerged in the different countries that were surveyed. Many debates could also be classified under different headings to the ones that were given; it was only subtle differences that differentiated them from each other. Vaccination was a common source of debate, lifestyle factors and fears about changes in lifestyle that lead to sedentary behaviour, childhood obesity and the influence of the digital revolution, including artificial intelligence are seen in many countries. Religion influences debates about changes in society, for example in Malta, changes in the influence of religion have been discussed as a possible contributor to the rise in single-parent families and subsequent child poverty. The full list of characteristics is described in Blair et al. (2017).

Structural Determinants

Among the many determinants of child health care and policy, we identified some as structural in character, meaning that it is proximal and distal elements of the child health care system itself that influence the way services are provided. In particular, the relationships of primary care services with other models of care are crucial (see Chapters 10 and 15). We divided the structural determinants into two groups and defined them as internal and external determinants. The internal determinants are those identified within the structure of health care and policy, whereas the external determinants relate to the elements indirectly correlated with health care and policy.

Internal Structural Determinants

Our data identified interdependent processes such as access to care and provision of care, which are often very closely related to access issues. Other internal structural determinants of policy change or for demand for change include the issues of organisational culture, workforce and organisational functionality of the system. The examples of internal structural determinants that were subject to debate and policy change, as a result of contextual and societal action, are described in full in Blair et al. (2017) and Zdunek et al. (2017).

- Access to care: This includes the provision of services that allow access, particularly in rural or remote regions of Europe; protests at the cessation or centralisation of services which means fewer local services; access to specific forms of care, such as mental health care available locally. National debates emerged between the need for quality as a justification for centralisation of services; and the need for locally accessible services.
- Provision of care: These issues closely interrelate to access issues and continue debates about centralisation of care, for example paediatric services only available in large national hospitals, and the restructuring of eligibility criteria to access services for free.
- Workforce: Issues identified here include proposed changes in medical training to work with children in primary care, the ageing of the primary care medical workforce, workforce shortages which were correlated with adverse events and outcomes for child patients and a lack of interest in the medical or nursing professions among young people.
- Organisational issues: Identified here were exposures of a lack of procedures in emergencies, poor capacity of the health system to deal with emergency situations, inefficiency in the health care system, out-dated methods of caring for children and lack of capacity for long-term care of children in need of child protection or needing complex care.

External Structural Determinants

Child health policy is not created in isolation. When discussing determinants, it is essential to take into account factors which directly and indirectly affect the way health policy is formulated or provided. These external factors may influence the hierarchy of priorities and the position of child health among other values. External structural determinants are interpreted as factors on a macro-level which influence the way problems are solved and issues are negotiated in child health care. Our data reveal a strong influence of politics, policy, the economy and finance. Many of these determinants are closely connected, for example, the level of political awareness is expressed by the initiatives undertaken at the policy level. This is expressed, among others, by the implementation of legal solutions.

- Politics: Many child health policies were formed or discussed as a result of pre-election promises – about, for example, changes to medical training or to combat public health issues such as childhood obesity. Other politically-sensitive topics included the treatment of migrant and asylum-seeking populations, particularly that of unaccompanied child migrants. A lack of political awareness or action about issues such as the rights of disabled children to equal access to health and other services was also subject to national debate.
- Policy: National debates around issues such as exposure of children to passive smoking, childhood obesity and the rights of disabled children were reflected in policy decisions, such as amendments to national law or changes in public health policy. In some cases, policy decisions prompted protests, such as those supporting disabled children who, it was felt, were disadvantaged due to recent policy changes, or the further marginalisation of families already at risk of poverty or social exclusion as a consequence of policy decisions that limit services or access to services.
- Economy: A major influence on public action and child health policy decisions was the economic downturn in Europe and subsequent austerity measures that were adopted by a number of countries. These were seen to increase hardship for populations already experiencing social problems or poverty. Public service cuts were seen to directly increase child poverty, child mental health issues, education and family security. Homelessness was seen as a particular concern. Cuts to services were also seen to affect the quality and workforce of health services, which in turn affected access and child health outcomes.

International Determinants

Membership of regional and global organisations facilitates information exchange and also obligates a country to respect shared values and adapt to commonly agreed rules. Globally published evidence may not always be available nationally and illuminates the existence of a problem. International comparison drives discussions that aim to solve the problem. The MOCHA project identified three categories of international determinants from our data. These are as follows:

- Global evidence: Global reports and comparison studies were cited by many countries as an important source of information that provoked or supported national discussions about an issue. Many cited sources of such evidence in Europe were the Health Behaviour in School-Aged Children (HBSC) Study (2018), the World Health Organization (WHO) (2018) and the Organisation for Economic Co-operation and Development (OECD) (2018). Other less authoritative global evidence was also used, as can be seen in the countries where there was considerable debate about vaccine safety, despite using questionable research as sources.

- Cross-nationality: The surge in global and national reports is correlated with the cross-nationality of many child health policy and care issues. The issues of obesity, vaccination, child abuse or care for migrant children are not contained within the border of one country but connected to global changes of lifestyle, increased awareness of personal health due to ease of communication and increased awareness of children's rights. This has been linked to issues such as the institutionalisation of child care and shifts in European normative systems. Often, such cross-national comparison has resulted in exchange of views, ideas and learning from experiences of other countries. Examples of such cross-national debates are the proposed changes in medical education in the Czech Republic, international evidence to support changes in laws on tobacco smoking in Latvia and the outcry at discrimination against disabled children in Croatia, which contravened children's rights as set out by the United Nations.

- Global processes and movements: Global influences affect many national discussions. One of the most influential was the global economic crisis, which influenced the functioning of child health care and policy in most European countries. Spain, Portugal, Greece, Malta and Ireland, in particular, struggled with child poverty and homelessness. The global humanitarian crisis and the plight of unaccompanied asylum-seekers were items of discussion in the UK and Finland. The combination of migrant status in countries affected by the economic crisis was particularly potent, because these families were already vulnerable to poverty and hardship. Globalisation also contributed to diagnosis and treatment decisions in primary care and health services in general, in particular, medication. Specific examples of these global movements becoming issues debated within a country and leading to policy change include that of the effect of increasing digital media on children's mental health in Germany, and the use of medication in high numbers of children with ADHD in Iceland, leading to claims of over-medicalising normal behaviour.

Situational Aspects

The particular situations which contributed to the intensification of the debate were correlated with the socio-cultural, systemic and international factors mentioned above. The scope of those is reflected by behavioural episodes, procedural and institutional episodes and the global situation. Examples of such phenomena have been classified into three categories:

(1) Behavioural episodes: Situations identified as key national discussions ranged from the exposure of historical child sexual abuse by schools or other institutions in a country and health system actions as a result of current child abuse claims, to discussions about the safety of vaccinations, vaccination hesitancy and the ability of the health service to effectively refute poor research evidence. Related to these situations is a lack of trust in governmental decisions and evidence.

(2) Procedural and institutional events: These included changes in the law such as the recognition of same-sex marriages in certain countries which gave rise to discussions about emergency contraception and the content of sex education curricula. Other such events included the introduction or cessation of compulsory vaccination before certain benefits or rights to state education could be accessed (see also Chapter 16); governmental dysfunctionality or potential corruption that compromises safety for the population, economic decisions that increase child poverty and decisions that were publicly understood to have an effect on children's health — such as the cessation of physical activity in schools and a rise in childhood obesity levels.

(3) Global situation: The main global issues that influenced Europe in recent years were the wave of migrants entering Europe and the economic crisis. Other global issues that were of concern among European nations were the growth in childhood obesity and the pro/anti vaccination movements.

Full descriptions of these events have been reported previously in Zdunek et al. (2017).

Attitudes to Abuse from the Perspective of Contextual Determinants

MOCHA did not specifically address the issue of child abuse as part of its remit, but in the process of research into children's use of primary care and into the services primary care provides for children in the European Union and European Economic Area, the issue of child protection, maltreatment and safety are essential topics that warrant discussion, particularly in the light of the contextual determinants identified by the MOCHA project. Primary child health care has an important role to play in the prevention and identification of child abuse at both an individual and a population levels. This involves identifying abuse, helping to prevent abuse and treating the consequences of abuse (which can continue for a lifetime). The training of the primary care workforce to recognise, and as importantly, to report and deal with cases of abuse is vital, and one which the lack of child focus in training curricula suggests that might not be optimal (see Chapter 13). Existing research seems to suggest that although primary care services are able to identify potential abuse, it is the subsequent effective collaborative working to report and act on suspicion that is lacking (Cossar, Brandon, & Jordan, 2011; Rees et al., 2010; Richardson-Foster, Stanley, Miller, & Thomson, 2012; Stanley, Miller, & Richardson Foster, 2012).

School and adolescent health services are particularly important in this respect, because most children of all socio-economic classes and almost all social groups will attend school. School nurses and teachers often work together to help identify families at risk and may be the first point of contact for children in need. School is also an important venue for protection interventions, as stated by Sethi et al. (2018). They are an ideal setting where children can be empowered and learn to avoid and report instances of abuse (including the various forms of bullying), without increasing stigma. The WHO report, however, found that less than half the countries in the WHO European region provide primary school programmes about recognition of abuse and harm and how to disclose worries to trusted adults. In MOCHA, mental health (with the exception of Greece, Malta and Poland) and behavioural problems (with the exception of Denmark, Greece, Hungary, Lithuania, Norway and Portugal) are also main priority needs of pupils. Coping with stress, anxiety and learning disorders, bullying, depression, social and emotional learning and self-esteem are all mentioned as examples of mental health topics for pupils covered by SHS. In terms of behavioural problems, the main topic is aggression and abuse.

As part of the national and public cultural context of policy, an extremely potent element in the subject of abuse is the *societal attitudes* towards it. For instance, a recent report by the WHO Regional Office for Europe has reiterated the need for a reduction in corporal punishment:

> Societal attitudes need to be shifted to discourage the use of violent discipline and reinforce the benefits of nonviolent approaches. Universal campaigns can positively shift population attitudes away from physical punishment and other risk factors for child maltreatment. (Sethi et al., 2018)

Awareness of child abuse, and the stimulation of national debates about child protection issues, including what constitutes abuse, and what actions are best for prevention and treatment has featured in the MOCHA project. In our research into contextual determinants, we found that issues involving vulnerable children or that compromise the safety of children are particularly emotive and provoke intense discussion. Certain situation-specific 'trigger' events were identified in our research that prompted changes or calls for changes in national primary care systems. For example, reports of child abuse in boarding schools in Iceland; and reports of abuse that occurred in a nursery school in the Czech Republic. These trigger events are analysed further in Zdunek et al. (2017).

Awareness is also raised by increased visibility of the issues as a result of the use and publication of results of international standardized survey tools such as the Health Behaviour of School Children (HBSC) involving 11-, 13- and 15-year-olds. It was this survey that highlighted the issue of the extent of bullying in schools (described above) for Latvian policy-makers when compared to other countries (Zdunek et al., 2017). This underlines the need for informative and robust data, as well as highlighting some of the difficulties in collecting data about children (see Chapter 7).

A greater awareness of the risk factors for child abuse has led to the sensitisation of national and public cultures to the issue. The risk to children's health by living with certain risk factors has been identified in the MOCHA project, migrant children, children in the care system (see Chapter 5) and children with disability (see Chapter 15). In addition, public recognition of risk factors and potential adverse consequences of this has also been identified in the project. Examples of this include the advocacy work carried out by NGOs, health and social protection groups in Spain, on behalf of children who were subject to increasing levels of poverty and unemployment. The Centre for Legal Resources in Romania, suspecting child abuse, compiled a list of issues in relation to possible inappropriate medication use in residential facilities for vulnerable disabled children, and the police investigative procedures uncovered widespread sexual abuse among missing children in Northern Ireland (the UK) (Zdunek et al., 2017).

In MOCHA's investigation into the interface between primary health and social care, we found that the legal framework for protection varies immensely between countries. All countries report the presence of a child protection framework; the Fundamental Rights Agency reports that a main law for child protection is present in only 18 EU countries. A specific legal framework for protection of children with disabilities is present in 15 of 26 (58%) of countries with further variation for federal countries such as Spain or Austria (Kielthy, Warters, Brenner, & McHugh, 2017) (Chapter 15). In MOCHA's investigation into the care of children with complex needs, the system's ability to coordinate the work of several agencies to the benefit of a vulnerable child and family was described. At the service level, the degrees of collaborative and integrated work between agencies also vary with half of responding countries having a specific care coordinator. The presence of such a system certainly is known to reduce stress of families and also may lessen the emotional environment in a household that may lead to maltreatment or abuse.

Migrant children and those in the care system are especially vulnerable and MOCHA has demonstrated a wide variation in legal entitlement to primary child health care as well as discover some innovative service models which place the child as the centre of a holistic multiagency collaborative endeavour in the best case scenario where the service follows the child – an important aspect especially for highly mobile populations likely to fall through the service safety nets (Hjern & Østergaard, 2016; Chapter 5).

Summary

The importance of context in the process of child health care and policy-making is more significant than ever. The changes within the last two decades, such as proliferation of actors, reconfiguration of their power and the new context of health, has provoked the shift from health governance to governance for health.

It also sheds new light on the factors which influence the style of child health care and policy-making. The determinants characterised in this chapter, including attitudes to abuse, play a regulatory function towards child health care and policy. They affect public activity which often is the reaction to public discontent. The reactions of society to events, and subsequent policy changes results in the implementation and/or introduction of new procedures, action plans and guidelines. This has then influenced the level of awareness, intensified the scrutiny, increased the access and availability of services, provoked the introduction of structural changes or withdrawn unfavourable changes.

References

Blair, M., Rigby, M., & Alexander, D. (2017). *Final report on current models of primary care for children.* Retrieved from www.childhealthservicemodels.eu/wp-content/uploads/2017/07/MOCHA-WP1-Deliverable-WP1-D6-Feb-2017-1.pdf

Bogusz, R. (2004). Zdrowie jako wartość realizowana i deklarowana. In W. Piątkowski (Ed.), Zdrowie, choroba, społeczeństw. Studia z socjologii medycyny. Wydawnictwo Uniwersytetu Marii Curie-Skłodowskiej, Lublin.

Buse, K., Mays, N., & Walt, G. (2005). *Making health policy.* Maidenhead: Open University Press.

Charmaz, K. (2006). *Constructing grounded theory. A practical Guide through Qualitative Analysis.* London: Sage.

Cossar, J., Brandon, M., & Jordan, P. (2011). *'Don't make assumptions': Children's and young people's views of the child protection system and messages for change.* London: Office of the Children's Commissioner.

Dyczewski, L. (1993). Trwałość kultury polskiej. In Wartości w kulturze polskiej, L. Dyczewski (Ed.), Fundacja pomocy szkołom polskim na wschodzie im. Tadeusza Goniewicza, Lublin.

European Values Study. (2011a). *Percentage of people that think children are very or rather important for a successful marriage.* Retrieved from http://www.atlasofeuropeanvalues.eu/new/europa.php?ids=145&year=2008

European Values Study. (2011b). *Percentage of people that agree or agree strongly with the statement that it is a duty towards society to have children.* Retrieved from http://www.atlasofeuropeanvalues.eu/new/europa.php?ids=156&year=2008

European Values Study. (2011c). *Percentage of people that think a woman has to have children in order to be fulfilled.* Retrieved from http://www.atlasofeuropeanvalues.eu/new/europa.php?ids=149&year=2008

European Values Study. (2011d). *Percentage of people that agree or agree strongly with the statement that a job is alright but what most women really want is a home and children.* Retrieved from http://www.atlasofeuropeanvalues.eu/new/europa.php?ids=161&year=2008&country=

European Values Study. (2011e). *Percentage of people that say family is very or quite important in their lives.* Retrieved from http://www.atlasofeuropeanvalues.eu/new/europa.php?ids=2&year=2008

European Values Study. (2015a). *About EVS.* Retrieved from www.europeanvaluesstudy.eu/page/about-evs.html

European Values Study. (2015b). *Family: Marriage – Children – Unconditional love – Role of women – Transmission of values.* Retrieved from http://www.europeanvaluesstudy.eu/page/family.html

Health Behaviour in School-Aged Children. (2018). *HBSC.* Retrieved from http://www.hbsc.org/

Hjern, A., & Østergaard, L. S. (2016). *Migrant Children in Europe: Entitlements to Health Care.* Retrieved from http://www.childhealthservicemodels.eu/wp-content/uploads/2015/09/20160831_Deliverable-D3-D7.1_Migrant-children-in-Europe.pdf

Kielthy, P., Warters, A., Brenner, M., & McHugh, R. (2017). *Final report on models of children's social care support across the EU and the relationship with primary health care.* Retrieved from http://www.childhealthservicemodels.eu/publications/deliverables/

Leichter, H. (1979). *A comparative approach to policy analysis: Health care policy in four nations.* Cambridge: Cambridge University Press.

Majchrowska, A. (2003). cited Dyczewski L. (1993) Kulturowe podstawy życia społecznego, (in:) Wybrane elementy socjologii: Podręcznik dla studentów i absolwentów wydziałów pielęgniarstwa i nauk o zdrowiu akademii medycznych, (red) A. Majchrowska, Czelej, Lublin.

Organisation for Economic Co-operation and Development. (OECD). (2018). Retrieved from http://www.oecd.org/

Rees, G., Gorin, S., Jobe, A., Stein, M., Medforth, R., & Goswami, H. (2010). *Safeguarding young people: Responding to young people 11 to 17 who are maltreated.* London: The Children's Society. Retrieved from https://www.childrenssociety.org.uk/sites/default/files/tcs/research_docs/Safeguarding%20Young%20People%20-%20Responding%20to%20Young%20People%20aged%2011%20to%202017%20who%20are%20maltreated_0.pdf

Richardson-Foster, H., Stanley, N., Miller, P., & Thomson, G. (2012). Police intervention in domestic violence incidents where children are present: Police and children's perspectives. *Policing & Society, 22,* 220–234. doi:10.1080/10439463.2011.636815

Sethi, D., Yon, Y., Parekh, N., Anderson, T., Huber, J., Rakovac, I., & Meinck, F. (2018). *European status report on preventing child maltreatment.* Copenhagen: World Health Organization Regional Office for Europe. Retrieved from http://www.euro.who.int/__data/assets/pdf_file/0017/381140/wh12-ecm-rep-eng.pdf?ua=1

Stanley, N., Miller, P., & Richardson Foster, H. (2012). Engaging with children's and parents' perspectives on domestic violence. *Child and Family Social Work, 17,* 192–201. doi:10.1111/j.1365-2206.2012.00832.x

Turner, J. (2012). *Struktura teorii socjologicznej.* Warszawa: PWN.

Walt, G., & Gilson, L. (1994). Reforming the health sector in developing countries. The central role of policy analysis. *Health Policy and Planning, 9*(4), 353–370.

World Health Organization. (2018). *Maternal, newborn, child and adolescent health: Child Health.* Retrieved from https://www.who.int/maternal_child_adolescent/child/en/

Zdunek, K., Schröder-Bäck, P., Blair, M., & Rigby, M. (2017). *Report on the contextual determinants of child health policy.* Retrieved from http://www.childhealthservicemodels.eu/wp-content/uploads/member-files/Context-Culture-Report-WP-1-task-7-a-12.03.2017.-PRE-FINALdocx.pdf

Chapter 18

Bringing MOCHA Lessons to Your Service

*Magda Boere-Boonekamp, Karin Groothuis-Oudshoorn,
Tamara Schloemer, Peter Schröder-Bäck, Janine van Til,
Kinga Zdunek and Paul Kocken*

Abstract

Identifying the qualities of primary care that have the potential to produce optimal health outcomes is only half the story. The Models of
Child Health Appraised (MOCHA) project has not only explored how
to transfer these to other national contexts, but also which successful
components should be transferred. It is important to assess the population criteria of the identified sociodemographic, cultural and social
characteristics and the population perspectives on a care system's components. The project analysed public experiences and perceptions of the
quality of primary care for children from a representative sample of the
general public in five European Union member states. The public perception of children's primary care services, in particular the perceived
quality of care and expectations with regard to care for children, is
important to understand before MOCHA lessons can be effectively
adopted in a country. We found that the socio-cultural characteristics
of a country inform the population perceptions and preferences with
regard to the care system. In the five countries surveyed, there was
agreement about aspects of quality of care – such as accessible opening
hours, confidential consultations for children and timeliness of consultation for an illness, but there was a difference in opinion about giving
priority to items such as making an appointment without a referral, or a
child's right to a confidential consultation. The cultural context of
transferability and the means of addressing this such as defining the target audience and the different means of disseminating important

messages to the wider community to address contextual factors can act as barriers or facilitators to the introduction of new components of primary care models.

Keywords: Health policy; transferability; culture; values; child health; quality of care

Introduction

The Models of Child Health Appraised (MOCHA) project has identified the qualities of primary care health systems that have the potential to produce optimal health outcomes for children in European Union (EU) countries. The question can then be asked what successful components of a care system should be transferred from one country to another. For instance, to reach accessible services with child friendly opening hours (see Chapter 11), or continuous professional–client relationships responsive for a child's changing needs. MOCHA developed a long list of criteria for assessing this transferability. The criteria have been summarised in a population characteristics, intervention content, environment and transfer – transferability (PIET-T) process model (see Chapter 16) (Figure 18.1) (Schloemer & Schröder-Bäck, 2018). This chapter focuses on the population criteria for transferability, including sociodemographic, cultural and social characteristics, the population's perceptions of health and health services and the population's attitude towards the care system's components.

The public perceptions and preferences included in the PIET-T model are vital. MOCHA conducted a client preference study among EU citizens of five countries to obtain insight into the public's perceptions and attitudes of the care systems in a selection of EU countries (Van Til, Groothuis-Oudshoorn, & Boere-Boonekamp, 2018). The perceptions of primary health care services imply that the public builds preferences on the basis of the experiences with the system (see the P section of Figure 18.1). Public perceptions have been shown to be important for transferring new methods of primary care delivery.

Principles of Transferability with Special Attention to Influences from the Perspective of the Public

In order to bring MOCHA lessons to your service, it is essential to identify, discuss and – ultimately – apply evidence-based good practice and implement these in new contexts. This idea of good or best practice exchange in health care is a main principle of EU Public Health. With limited directive power, the European Commission has the potential to facilitate such good or best practice exchange and stimulate in such a way the improvement of health care across the EU. The identification of good and best practices – a lead task for DG SANTE but also for research projects within the Horizon 2020 scheme such as

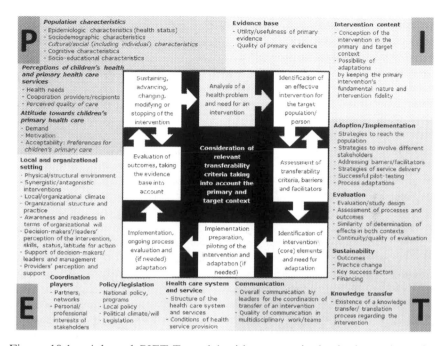

Figure 18.1. Adapted PIET-T model with systematised criteria to determine transferability with 'P' concretised for children's primary health care *Source*: Adapted from Schloemer & Schröder-Bäck, 2018.

MOCHA – is thus of great importance. In addition to research, Commission activities exist to support the identification and exchange of good and best health practices research. However, to identify a good or best practice in one context (e.g. in one EU member state) does not mean that this practice will also be effective if implemented in another context (e.g. in another EU member state). To give a concrete example, compulsory measles immunisation might be effective and a best practice in some countries (as is the case in Czech Republic and Hungary) and might be introduced in other EU member states but it remains to be seen if it is effective in that country and may well be an unacceptable option for other EU countries.

The concept of transferability is crucial to any good and best practice exchange, yet, relatively little research exists that supports the understanding of transferability of health interventions in European public health and offers tools to facilitate this. The MOCHA project has aimed to identify validated criteria to inform transferability of good and best practices.

An explorative analysis of facilitators and barriers in setting effective policies, considering good and best practice exchange, and a systematic review resulted in the creation of two models of transferability (Schloemer & Schröder-Bäck, 2018). Firstly, the conceptual PIET-T describes, from the perspective of decision and policy-makers, the primary context (in which evidence of good and best practices were gained) and the target context, to which these practices shall be transferred and in which they could be implemented. Contexts in this regard could be different EU countries, but also smaller-scale contexts, such as cultural, administrative region, provinces or municipalities.

A second model created was the Process Model for the Assessment of Transferability. This model presents – in accordance with the conceptual model – the criteria of transferability grouped under four headings:

(1) population characteristics;
(2) intervention characteristics;
(3) environmental characteristics; and
(4) aspects of transfer.

These criteria help determine which information is relevant for the target context and allow a comparison with existing information on the primary context. By assessing these criteria, we can identify facilitators and barriers. However, transferability cannot be measured using existing information from this phase, but can only be anticipated. To make these criteria operational, a detailed overview of descriptive themes, criteria and subcriteria is essential. To this end, we have created a checklist tool (Schloemer & Schröder-Bäck, 2018). This model reflects themes related to population that play a role in the (non)implementation of good and best practices, because they can facilitate or inhibit transferability. The term population here mainly refers to the potential recipients of child primary health care and related persons in a country. We therefore underline the population themes with a focus on the public's perceptions of children's primary healthcare services, in particular perceived quality of care. Furthermore, acceptability is an important criterion, and so, we emphasise public preferences with regard to child primary health care. Our third focus is on cultural population characteristics as these may vary greatly depending on the specific context and might influence transferability of services. These aspects of the population are highlighted in italics in Figure 18.1.

Public Experiences and Priorities in Primary Care for Children

In order to create optimal primary care for children, the views of all stakeholders on which changes are necessary and are achievable in policies are of utmost importance. This includes the opinions of citizens. Data on citizens' experiences and preferences are described in the Population part of the PIET-T process model of Schloemer and Schröder-Bäck (2018) (Figure 18.1) and can be used to estimate whether strengths in one country can be transferred to another country.

We elicited public experiences and perceptions of the quality of primary care for children using a cross-sectional study and a representative sample of the general public (Van Til et al., 2018) (see Chapter 3). We also asked about priorities of primary care in respect of children. These tasks are shown in Figure 18.1, in the section entitled Preferences. The following countries were chosen for this study:

- the United Kingdom and the Netherlands (both GP-led system with GP gate-keeper to other healthcare services);
- Germany and Spain (both primary care paediatrician-led, respectively, open access to secondary care and gatekeeper); and
- Poland (mixed system and gatekeeper).

The questions in the Preferences For Child Health Care Assessed (POCHA)-questionnaire were related to nine potential quality attributes of a primary care system from child-, youth- and carer-centred perspectives: accessible, affordable, appropriate, confidential, continuous, coordinated, empowering, equable and transparent (Van Til et al., 2018).

In total, 2,403 respondents filled out the questionnaire: 469 from Germany, 469 from the Netherlands, 478 from Poland, 491 from Spain and 496 from the United Kingdom. Of all respondents, 36.3% had one or more children below 18 years of age, 23.3% had older children, and 40.4% did not have children.

Experiences

Based on their experiences or perceptions, respondents indicated to what extent they were satisfied with the quality of primary care for children in their country, on a scale of 1 (very dissatisfied) to 10 (perfectly satisfied). Mean satisfaction scores differed significantly between countries, ranging from 5.5 (Poland) to 7.2 (Spain).

Each respondent rated the quality of the primary care system on ten out of 40 quality aspects (five-point Likert agree-disagree scale). The average agreement over all 40 items was highest in the Netherlands (70%), followed by the United Kingdom (68%), Germany (64%), Spain (62%) and Poland (56%). The item that was judged highest was the setting of the services being clean and appealing (range 73–84%). The item judged lowest was whether the child has the possibility to limit his parents' access to his medical records (range 12–36%). For some items, the respondents' perceived quality was comparable across countries, for instance that primary care facilities have ample opening hours (range 52–59%). For other items, there were large differences between countries, for example for a child's right to have a confidential consultation with a primary care provider. Agreement scores for these items were consistently lower in Poland and Spain.

Priorities

For priority setting, we used a best–worst scaling case 1 methodology, with eight different sets of combinations of ten statements on quality items. Two random sets of ten statements were presented to each respondent.

Universal priorities for primary care for children according to respondents in this study are as follows: timeliness related to severity, adequate skills and competencies of practitioners; efficacy. Items which were consistently prioritised as low in all countries were as follows: convenient appointment system, the child's possibility to limit their parents' access to the child's medical records and to express his opinions about his health management independently from his parents.

Each country also showed its very specific priorities, probably related to the country's history and culture. For instance, very important to respondents in Poland was that children and/or their parents can make an appointment with other healthcare providers without a referral. In the top ten priorities in the Netherlands, there was the child's right to a confidential consultation with the primary care provider. Finally, that a child's health is not influenced by the parents' background characteristics was very important to respondents from Germany, but less important in other countries.

Experiences versus Priorities

There were national differences in the public's experiences and priorities. To account for this, we combined priority scores with experience scores for each country separately. This allowed the identification of areas of potential improvement based on the importance given to them by the respondents from that country. In Spain, for example, the potential for improvement was highest with regard to opening hours of primary care services and availability of specialised care (Table 18.1).

A major strength of this approach was that by combining priority scores with an evaluation of perceived quality, the most important areas of potential improvement in each country can be identified.

Cultural Aspects

Closely related to the PIET-T model criteria, research carried out by MOCHA explored the phenomenon of the culture of 'evidence-based practice' (Zdunek, Schröder-Bäck, Rigby, & Blair, 2018) and that the wider health policy is not only directed to the population, but that the population also drives the content of health policy. The work concluded that an awareness, acknowledgement and addressing of the contextual factors are essential for successful transfer of knowledge to another country or region. The importance of socio-cultural factors has been described in Chapter 17; here, we address their effect on policy-making and the most likely methods of transition across borders.

The MOCHA project conducted a survey of the project Country Agents (see Chapter 1) and also surveyed stakeholders in primary care services for children across the EU and EEA countries. For further details of the methodology, see Zdunek et al. (2018). What became evident in this research was that the content of policy varies from country to country, and, together with the analysis of contextual factors, forms a baseline for developing a map of the current status of child health care in Europe. Public awareness of child issues can be measured by

Table 18.1. Overview of the quality aspects with a high potential for improvement, presented for each of the five countries.

Country	Attribute	Quality Aspect
Germany	Continuous	All healthcare providers involved in the care of a child know about each other's involvement, trust each other and work well together
	Accessible	Primary care services for children have ample opening hours, the after-hour care arrangements are good enough, and home-visits are planned if needed
	Coordinated	If the main primary care provider of a child is not able to meet the needs of that child, that care can be given by other health professionals within the primary care practice
	Coordinated	If a child needs specialised and long-term care, hospitals and primary care providers collaborate to offer care close to the child's home
	Affordable	The effort needed to get coverage and/or repayment for any out-of-pocket cost of primary care for a child is reasonable and feasible
Netherlands	Appropriate	Primary care providers are able to dedicate enough time to working with a child
	Accessible	Children and/or their parents know about the range of services available in primary care and how they can access them
Poland	Continuous	All healthcare providers involved in the care of a child know about each other's involvement, trust each other and work well together
	Appropriate	In primary care, the facilities and equipment are available to deliver the services that are needed for children
	Accessible	Children and/or their parents can make an appointment with other primary care providers without a referral from the main primary care provider
	Coordinated	Specialised care (e.g. physiotherapy, dental health care, psychological care, specialised

Table 18.1. (*Continued*)

Country	Attribute	Quality Aspect
		chronic care nurses) is available to a child within the primary care provider's practice
	Accessible	Primary care providers provide care within a reasonable amount of time, given the severity of the health issue
Spain	Accessible	Primary care services for children have ample opening hours, the after-hour care arrangements are good enough, and home-visits are planned if needed
	Coordinated	Specialised care (e.g. physiotherapy, dental health care, psychological care, specialised chronic care nurses) is available to a child within the primary care provider's practice
United Kingdom	Continuous	All health care providers involved in the care of a child know about each other's involvement, trust each other and work well together
	Accessible	Primary care services for children have ample opening hours, the after-hour care arrangements are good enough, and home-visits are planned if needed
	Appropriate	Primary care providers are able to dedicate enough time to working with a child

the level of activity of actors who play the main role in the theatre of child health care (see Chapter 3). Two trends of approaching the contextual environment are the scientific approach and the institutional approach (see Figure 18.2).

This evidence is not valuable for transfer of knowledge to different service environments without considering its context. As our respondents commented in the survey:

> it is also not always possible to meet all criteria of the evidence-based medicine to one hundred percent. In some subjects, this is also difficult - for example, in paediatrics. (Austrian CA)

We found that contextual factors, particularly the media in each country, were powerful factors in forming barriers or facilitating policy change. The Greek Country Agent, for example, stated that: 'results and suggestions by the report [into problems in the primary care health system and suggestions for

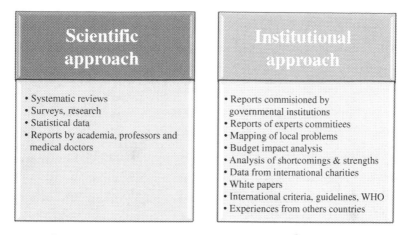

Figure 18.2.   Evidence usage in child health policy-making.

change] were used mainly through news media (TV and printed press), in facilitated discussions between representatives of the political parties, health professionals and administrative staff of the health system' (Zdunek et al., 2018). The media in Romania played a significant role in national debates about vaccination – at the beginning of a phenomenon of vaccine refusal by many parents, the media were said to have a lack of neutrality, giving a prime-time voice to a number of anti-vaccination voices alone on media outlets, without giving opportunity for a pro-vaccination voice to facilitate debate through the plurality of opinions. The most challenged vaccinations were against measles and polio. However, after a measles epidemic occurred, a shift in risk perceptions was observed in the Romanian media, which became an important actor advocating in favour of vaccination. Journalistic campaigns began to report illness and death and pressured the government to take concrete measures to limit the epidemics.

The media not only promotes awareness of existing evidence, but also about awareness of context. For example, the Bulgarian CA stressed that:

> the obvious truth is that the outcome of treatment of many chronic diseases depends on the effect of the medical measures, but depends also on the social environment in which these measures are undertaken. If these social factors are not taken into account, there is a high risk that the medical measures are not implemented. (Bulgarian CA)

In the MOCHA Stakeholder survey, we asked about the most influential stakeholders, who can play a strategic role in circulating recommendations about optimal models of child health care in Europe. The respondents concluded that the most respected and influential were medical and professional associations, as well as health professionals and patient organisations. These stakeholders not only are important in the circulation of the information, but also play a role in implementing the newly proposed solutions.

The stakeholders also concluded that transferability of knowledge was also achieved by a range of recommendations. A combination of new formal policies, guidelines and recommendations together with personal contact was seen as important. Seminars, conferences and workshops are significant facilitators of exchange of information, not only between countries but also between competent authorities. The experts highlighted the strategic role of media, including social media in the circulation of information about innovative solutions in terms of child primary health care. This facilitates the process of active implementation of proposed solutions.

What is important is to identify the most appropriate recipients for the new policy or idea in developing a new model. These take into account the agents of the child in the proximal and distal (wider) environment (see Chapter 4). What was found to be important was to match the format of recommendations to the audience profile, as one respondent commented, the format of advice 'should be suited to the target audience's profile, either individual or priority groups, that is peer-reviewed journal and/or seminar for stakeholders and professionals', and another concluded that 'implementation work must adapt to the relevant audience. Mostly reports, scientific publications, seminars and news items are either useless or make a temporary change. The format must appear useful for the person receiving it, and it must be followed up regularly to ensure actual implementation' (see Zdunek et al., 2018).

The MOCHA data suggest there are several types of the most effective format for communicating scientific results. The scientific approach is relevant, popular and expected, accompanied by administrative and formal reports, strategies and recommendations. However, for successful transferability, as described in the PIET-T model above, data must be presented in an appropriate manner to the general population and those who are aware of the emerging possibilities of improvement in the quality of health care and health services. Thus, the media of television, radio, social media and other electronic media are also vital. Additionally, there is a need of public involvement in the discussion of newly proposed solutions. This is correlated with health education activities at the primary care level (see Chapter 11), health personnel (see Chapter 13), meetings with parents, young people and other citizens (see Chapter 3), decision-makers and public discussions. These different means of dissemination of knowledge and awareness of contextual and cultural factors is illustrated in Figure 18.3.

This proposed classification helps to adapt the format of the recommendations to the appropriate audience population, as shown in Figure 18.1. In the case of the audience in the proximal environment, a popular and personal format may be the most relevant. The audience in the distal environment would probably benefit more from the scientific and administrative format of data.

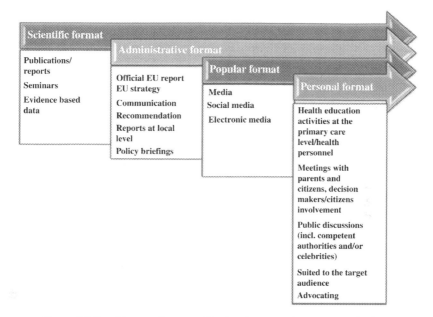

Figure 18.3.   Types of most effective format of recommendations.

Summary

The implementation of a good or best practice from one country to another depends on many factors, which are described in the PIET-T process model of Schloemer and Schröder-Bäck (2018). The MOCHA project designed this model to compare the countries' receptivity for inclusion of optimal features of care systems that have demonstrated improvement of quality of primary health care for children. This chapter focused on the Population section of the model. Public's perceptions of children's primary healthcare services, particularly perceived quality of care, and preferences with regard to child care services, will influence the transferability of services, depending also on socio-cultural characteristics of the population.

A study into the preferences of a representative sample from the general public of five EU countries showed that there was a difference between countries and also within countries in agreement about experiences with quality aspects of the primary care system, such as accessible opening hours or confidential consultations for children. Items such as timeliness related to severity of an illness were prioritised highly by all countries while countries differed in terms of giving priority to items such as making an appointment without a referral or a child's right to a confidential consultation. The socio-cultural characteristics of a country seem important for these population's perceptions and preferences with regard to the care system. The citizen's experiences and priorities, which are described in the Population part of the PIET-T process model, are relevant for estimating whether care systems' strengths in one country can be transferred to another. This can be done by comparing the PIET-T data of combinations of countries, as important differences might influence transferability. In this way, facilitators and barriers for transferability can be determined by analysing context-relevant criteria shown in Figure 18.1. Finally, we looked at the importance of the cultural context of transferability, and means of addressing this, defining a target audience and the different means of disseminating important messages to the wider community, and so addressing the contextual factors that can act as barriers or facilitators to knowledge transfer.

References

Schloemer, T., & Schröder-Bäck, P. (2018). Criteria for evaluating transferability of health interventions: A systematic review and thematic synthesis. *Implementation Science, 13*(1), 88. doi:10.1186/s13012-018-0751-8

Van Til, J., Groothuis-Oudshoorn, K., & Boere-Boonekamp, M. M. (2018). *Public priorities for primary child health care for children. A report on public preferences for patient-centred and prevention oriented primary child health care models for children.* Retrieved from http://www.childhealthservicemodels.eu/publications/technical-reports/

Zdunek, K., Schröder-Bäck, P., Rigby, M., & Blair, M. (2018). *The culture of evidence-based practice in child health policy — A report.* Retrieved from http://www.childhealthservicemodels.eu/publications/technical-reports/

Chapter 19

Evidence to Achieve an Optimal Model for Children's Health in Europe

Mitch Blair, Michael Rigby and Denise Alexander

Abstract

Models of Child Health Appraised (MOCHA) was a wide-ranging, multi-disciplinary and multi-method study that aimed to identify the best models of provision of primary care for the children of the European Union. The research has identified two main conclusions: (1) The depth of interdependency of health, economy and society. Primary care needs to be an active partner in public debate about current child health concerns. It should orientate more effectively in addressing wider societal influences on child health through advocacy and collaborative intersectoral public health approaches with those agencies responsible for public and community health if it is to address effectively issues such as childhood obesity, mental health and vaccine hesitancy. As part of this, it needs to address its workforce composition and skills, not least in two-way communication. (2) The European Community has many visions and commitments to children and child health policies, but their effectiveness is largely unfulfilled. The Commission can strengthen its impact on children's health and healthcare services within current remits and resources by focusing on a number of key fields: planned and structured research, providing insight into optimal human resources and skills in child primary care, developing and using ethical means of listening to children's views, remedying the invisibility of children in data, measuring the quality of primary care from a child-centric perspective, understanding the economics of investing in children's health, developing e-health standards and evaluation, collaborative and harmonised use of downloaded research databases, understanding and respecting children's rights and equity, and appreciating and allowing for children's evolving autonomy as they grow up. An optimal model of primary care for children is proactive, inclusive, corporately linked, based on and providing robust evidence, and respects the wider determinants of health and children's involvement in their health trajectory.

Keywords: Child; primary care health services; optimum models; health outcomes; intersectoral; interdependency; autonomy

Introduction

As indicated in the opening chapter of the Models of Child Health Appraised (MOCHA) report (Chapter 1), this large-scale comprehensive project was established to use research to identify the best models for provision of effective primary care for the children of Europe. In a wide-ranging multi-disciplinary and multi-method study, it achieved many scientific results but was not able to deliver the holy grail of an optimum model, or choice of validated models. In this respect we agree with the findings of the European Commission Expert Group on Health Systems Performance (2016), which recently noted:

> While highlighting variations between countries, it is often diffi-
> cult for practitioners and policy makers to interpret what a coun-
> try positioning means in terms of performance, and what policy
> action should be taken in order to improve performance.

But what MOCHA has established, as described in detail in its deliverables, and in summary in the 19 chapters of this volume of integrated results, is two things:

(1) the depth of interdependency of health, economy and society; and
(2) the European Community has many visions and commitments to chil-
    dren, and child and health-related policies, but the effectiveness is
    largely unfulfilled because there is no Model for European commitment
    to children.

While these may have been understood as truisms by many, an achievement of MOCHA has been to use scientific scrutiny to assess the many aspects of health and health care for children that make these two conclusions stand out so strongly.

Meanwhile, one of the founding questions that led to creation of the MOCHA project proposal — 'Which type of primary care doctor is better for delivering effective primary care for children?' — has been shown to be marginal on two grounds: the modest (though clearly important) role of doctors and indeed health care on children's health compared to the greater influence of the wider determinants (Chapter 9) and the demographic dynamic within the medical workforce which itself is changing the pattern of primary care practice for children (Chapter 13).

Intertwining of Health, Economy and Society

Economic Context

All citizens, and particularly children, are deeply influenced by their social and physical environments. The preconditions for good parenting and provision of a safe and learning rich home environment is highly dependent on adult security which is considerably influenced by the economy of the country and on the services available to support the family. And in turn those providing services, not least health services, are dependent on the national economy to fund those services, either directly through taxation of though a vibrant insurance system.

Thus, the well-being of the economy has major effects on the health of children in profound ways. In an attempt to look at overall effects, and also the progress of countries in improving the health of their children, in the absence of meaningful comparable illness or morbidity rates (see Chapter 7), the MOCHA study examined trends in mortality in young adults, after the end of the complete period of childhood. Hypothesising that deaths of young adults other than in accidents were in great part likely to be the outcome of the health services and determinants received throughout their childhood, we extracted data for the 30 study countries, showing numbers and rates, absolute change and rate of change in the past decade, and these are presented in Table 19.1.

Economic data for these countries are shown in Chapter 9 and confirm the effect, but what Table 19.1 shows is the strong gradient from the poorer New Member States countries to the more affluent countries, and also the progress being made by these countries in improving the standards of primary medical care. For example, increasing use of guidelines and evidence-based medicine, primary care staffing and e-health together with improved social and economic policies to support poor nutrition and housing and other upstream determinants of child health appear to be yielding strong gains.

In this setting, the type of doctor, and the skill mix, is less important than their knowledge and use of latest relevant evidence and their optimal utilisation of the available resources. We return to this theme in the context of harmonisation later, while details of workforce and education are the subject of Chapter 13.

Societal Context

We looked at the societal context of the delivery of primary care in five ways. First, Chapter 3 reports on how we undertook direct interviewing of children and parents in five very different European countries and found some strong threads. Health services need to be sensitive to needs, delivered in a non-patronising way and accessible in physical, economic and social meanings of accessibility. Secondly, as also reported in that chapter, we undertook societal studies on expectations of and attitudes to primary healthcare services for children. Thirdly, we undertook detailed study of the evolution of current societal attitudes to children, and the importance in the twenty-first century of taking a

Table 19.1. Total non-accidental deaths and Rate of Change in 20–24-year-olds (2006–2016) (GBD Study).

Total Non–accidental Deaths 2006–2016, 20–24 Year Olds, GBD Study

Country	Rate of Mortality (Per 100k), Both Genders				Rate of Mortality (Per 100k), Males				Rate of Mortality (Per 100k), Females			
	2006	2016	Absolute Change	% Change	2006	2016	Absolute Change	% Change	2006	2016	Absolute Change	% Change
Austria	20.54	15.63	4.91	-23.90	26.48	19.48	7.00	-26.44	14.48	11.61	2.87	-19.82
Belgium	14.33	11.85	2.48	-17.31	18.03	14.15	3.88	-21.52	10.60	9.47	1.13	-10.66
Bulgaria	33.41	28.26	5.15	-15.41	41.69	35.82	5.87	-14.08	24.56	20.34	4.22	-17.18
Croatia	21.20	17.36	3.84	-18.11	27.10	21.90	5.20	-19.19	15.07	12.60	2.47	-16.39
Cyprus	21.12	16.89	4.23	-20.03	26.77	22.82	3.95	-14.76	15.27	10.74	4.53	-29.67
Czech Rep.	17.32	14.53	2.79	-16.11	21.80	17.61	4.19	-19.22	12.59	11.28	1.31	-10.41
Denmark	17.59	13.88	3.71	-21.09	23.55	16.49	7.06	-29.98	11.45	11.15	0.30	-2.62
Estonia	47.09	31.23	15.85	-33.65	65.03	43.92	21.11	-32.46	28.24	17.52	10.72	-37.96
Finland	23.34	17.86	5.48	-23.48	32.01	25.12	6.89	-21.52	14.27	10.27	4.00	-28.03
France	14.94	12.15	2.79	-18.67	17.78	14.65	3.13	-17.60	12.09	9.59	2.50	-20.68
Germany	15.43	12.64	2.79	-18.08	18.80	15.03	3.77	-20.05	11.98	10.12	1.86	-15.53
Greece	23.24	19.41	3.83	-16.48	32.65	25.48	7.17	-21.96	13.12	13.00	0.12	-0.91%
Hungary	18.83	15.92	2.91	-15.45	22.95	19.43	3.52	-15.34	14.56	12.20	2.36	-16.21
Iceland	19.00	16.36	2.64	-13.89	23.22	17.27	5.95	-25.62	14.65	15.38	-0.73	4.98
Ireland	22.36	20.24	2.12	-9.48%	29.76	28.01	1.75	-5.88	14.82	11.92	2.90	-19.57
Italy	14.50	12.53	1.97	-13.59	18.16	15.49	2.67	-14.70	10.71	9.42	1.29	-12.04
Latvia	31.80	22.49	9.31	-29.28	43.00	27.40	15.60	-36.28	20.04	17.22	2.82	-14.07
Lithuania	32.45	23.71	8.74	-26.93	44.96	32.51	12.45	-27.69	19.59	14.43	5.16	-26.34
Luxembourg	19.20	14.45	4.75	-24.74	24.99	16.61	8.38	-33.53	13.13	12.17	0.96	-7.31%
Malta	21.61	17.02	4.59	-21.24	26.28	22.34	3.94	-14.99	15.94	12.22	3.72	-23.34
Netherlands	13.31	11.16	2.15	-16.15	15.23	13.39	1.84	-12.08	11.36	8.88	2.48	-21.83
Norway	24.95	18.14	6.81	-27.29	32.84	24.29	8.55	-26.04	16.78	11.59	5.19	-30.93
Poland	18.38	16.27	2.11	-11.48	23.91	21.27	2.64	-11.04	12.67	11.04	1.63	-12.87
Portugal	19.31	15.78	3.53	-18.28	22.20	18.67	3.53	-15.90	16.34	13.84	2.50	-15.30
Romania	28.46	28.89	-0.43	1.51%	34.01	34.48	-0.47	1.38%	22.59	22.93	-0.34	1.51%
Slovakia	19.93	16.85	3.08	-15.45	25.33	20.70	4.63	-18.28	14.27	12.83	1.44	-10.09
Slovenia	16.58	12.25	4.33	-26.12	20.89	15.16	5.73	-27.43	12.05	9.22	2.83	-23.49
Spain	14.92	11.12	3.8	-25.47	18.60	13.31	5.29	-28.44	11.05	8.84	2.21	-20.00
Sweden	17.55	16.95	0.6	-3.42%	23.00	23.58	-0.58	2.52%	11.86	9.97	1.89	-15.94
UK	22.58	18.57	4.01	-17.76	28.76	23.10	5.66	-19.68	16.36	13.88	2.48	-15.16

Table 19.1. (*Continued*)

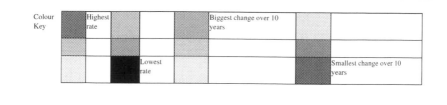

Notes: *Rate per 100k population of 20–24-year-olds.
**Accidents (excluded) include transport injuries, road injuries, unintentional injuries, exposure to mechanical forces, animal contact, foreign body, self-harm and interpersonal violence, forces of nature, conflict and terrorism, and executions and police conflict.
Data extracted from the results tool from the Global Burden of Disease study. Presentation: S. Deshpande

child-centric view throughout, reported in Chapter 4. Fourthly, we ascertained from all countries the child health-related issues that had hit the headlines or in other ways attracted strong societal interest, looking particularly at triggers and expectations (Chapter 17). Fifthly, we took three approaches to researching what changes to services would be acceptable and indeed hoped for. One was a sample public attitude study on attitudes to health services for children (van Til, Groothuis-Oudshoorn, & Boere-Boonekamp, 2018). The second asked a number of stakeholders in a range of countries their attitudes to a number of child primary care policy issues (Kocken, Vlasblom, de Lijster, & Reijneveld, 2018). And as a collation of all these issues in a policy change context, we looked at theories and practice on transferability of policy and evidence to new settings, and the societal environment featured in this (Schloemer, & Schröder-Bäck, 2018; Zdunek, Schroder-Back, Rigby, & Blair, 2018).

All these studies initiated by MOCHA in public consultation were inevitably small, and not statistically significant in quantitative science terms, but our mixed and varied methods and sources should be enough to show the importance of society as the operational context of primary care services. And in a different way, Chapter 14 raised the use of social media and health, being not only a potential threat and risk, but also a new modality for delivering knowledge and care.

So from this brief summary, but more so from the variety of society-related studies in the detailed MOCHA work and reported on the website www.child-healthservicemodels.eu, it is clear that society is strong, complex and has its own dynamics. Primary care for children cannot operate effectively in defiance of society (vaccine resistance and increasing child obesity are immediate examples of this), but also good primary care services are expected by society, and indeed, health services should be the servant of the people and not a meritocracy operating in isolation. Health service leaders must contribute to societal debate and influences, but, in a way, which is acceptable to society in a wider sense.

So for this reason too, it is not possible to define a single optimal model of child primary care provision. Instead, health systems need to be in harmony in the context of the society within which it operates, while also being evidence-based.

Health Policy and Provision in the European Community Context

A complexity in undertaking any research on health policy in EU countries is that that policy and operation of health services, and also social care and welfare services, are the prerogative and competency of individual member states. The European Commission itself has no competency in health care and cannot intervene in states' policies. However, in addition to the European endeavour of boosting member states' economies through free trade and development of social standards and thus benefiting health and health care, the Commission has three core functions which directly can enable primary healthcare systems across Europe: Research, Information and Communication Technologies (including e-health) and Public Health.

Additionally, there are activities related to harmonising Education and Training and addressing Social Inclusion. Finally, there are support and monitoring functions. Eurostat is the most relevant example of a support function, as reliable comparative data are an important tool in assisting policy-makers and service providers, while the Fundamental Rights Agency defines rights including those of children. Monitoring includes the function of DG Justice for monitoring implementation of the United Nations Convention on the Rights of the Child by member states.

However, there is no clear mechanism whereby this significant set of functions, and respective Directorates General, harmonises their work either on a topic basis or more generally on either health issues or children's interests. From our findings, we assess that there is considerable scope for the Commission to strengthen its impact on children's health and healthcare services, within current remits and resources, and based on its vision of a knowledge-based economy enabling European solidarity though robust collaborative member states.

Of course, the European Commission works within the wider geographical compass to the European Regional Office of the World Health Organization, and in June 2018, the Health Ministers for the whole of Europe met in Tallinn and confirmed a shared vision on Health Systems for Prosperity and Solidarity: leaving no one behind (World Health Organization Regional Office for Europe, 2018). That vision featured, additional to investment, Inclusion and Innovation. The meeting committed to Solidarity. We see these intentions as exactly what is needed within Europe to progress the strengths of the Commission to support better primary care for Europe's children. We share this vision in the next section, based on our findings and our frustrations.

Potential for the EU to Boost Primary Care for Children within Existing Actions

The MOCHA project has identified a number of potential areas for more focused research, and policy and service development described in the next sections.

Optimal Human Resources in Child Primary Care

The workforce is the biggest resource in any health system and the more so in primary care. We have identified in Chapter 13, the unsatisfactory situation in which there is no knowledge or evidence about optimal professional mix, or the most needed and productive skills within professions and how to assure these. There is a clear requirement for research in this area, not only because of the urgency now becoming apparent with the rapidly shifting demography of primary care providers but also to ensure appropriate training of the workforce to optimally meet the needs of children and young people now and in the future. In Chapter 13, we identify significant differences in basic education patterns for medical doctors, and even more so for nurses. There is also a European risk here, in that, these are mutually recognised qualifications between European Member States, yet there is not a matching of skills and competencies.

DG Employment, Social Affairs and Inclusion (2018) is responsible for the European Skills/Competences, Qualifications and Occupations (ESCO) initiative which has a section for Health Professionals. However, this seems to stop at a high level. Meanwhile DG Education and Culture have responsibility for harmonisation of third-level education across Europe, but there is limited harmonisation of contents even when related to professional competencies leading to mutually accepted profession recognition.

From the totality of the findings in Chapter 13, we can identify the potential significant benefit if research could be addressed to identify optimal medical and nursing knowledge and competencies, which in turn could lead to strengthening of the ECSO reference skill sets. European children would benefit from better, more effective and safer services.

Ethical means of Listening to Children

We were able, within the scope of MOCHA, to interview 81 children in five countries, reported in Chapter 3. The value to the project in terms of clarifying patient and parent perceptions about how the health system works for the individual was enormous and helped to inform development of standards and give insight onto some of the important issues such as coordination and communication skills with professionals. A recommendation would be the development of the tools we used successfully, to create a more systematic and representative survey across Europe about experiences. This could also build on the experience of the country agent reports on participation of children and young people in such surveys.

Europe has successfully developed the European Health Interview Survey and the European Health Examination Survey, which enable compilation of comparative data, and there is a European Health Interview & Health Examination Surveys Database website (https://hishes.wiv-isp.be/index.php?hishes=home). When these survey tools were designed more than a decade ago, children were excluded for reasons of methodology. However, with the development of techniques such as those applied by MOCHA, the exclusion of the voices of children is no longer defensible. Work is needed to create for children the tools and knowledge bases now in existence for adult citizens.

Improving the visibility of children in data

A large part of the project has required the hunting down of key clinical, epidemiological, workforce and economic data related to children and their services – Chapter 7 details this. In fact, often the analyses are not available, but at field capture level, the data are there. Adding appropriate coding and analysis is not a large job in the total system of data assembly, but is not done, and children are the victims. This is not a new problem. For example, the Child Health Indicators of Life and Development project was co-funded in 2000–2002 by the European Commission to give visibility to children through a planned balanced indicator set (Rigby, Köhler, Blair, & Mechtler, 2003), but has never been actioned. Our scientific understanding of the importance of life course development and its importance for human potential has grown since then. There is increased recognition that both vertical and horizontal integration of services is a necessity to tackle the latest forms of morbidity and enhance well-being. We cannot afford to wait another 18 years to agree and actively use an appropriate set of shared measures and outcomes in the whole child health system which reflects these two dimensions.

However, there are good examples of such harmonisation in the area of perinatal health (http://www.europeristat.com/) and also neonatal intensive care, which has an extensive network across Europe. Many disease registers also have European harmonisation requirement and those that are linked to clinical networks of health professionals, including public health, have higher quality information on which to base policy and practice. However, the full age range of children and the full range of health and health-related conditions are still excluded from virtually all European data systems. In effect, European statistical systems do not honour the United Nations Convention on the Rights of the Child.

There are also good examples of the use of e-health in the more recent EU countries, for example Estonia and Slovenia, where they have been able to leapfrog technology and provide national scale data on linked primary and specialist care data allowing the possibility of assessing the contribution of different parts of the health system to health outcomes.

The European Child Public Health Observatory network could provide a data infrastructure which would allow for the monitoring of child health trends over time in different countries and potentially give an early warning to systems about emerging issues and provide information to help plan services in member states. It would also enhance the monitoring of child health against the Region's WHO strategy for child and adolescent health.

Improving the Measurement of Child Primary Care Quality

Most techniques for measuring the quality of primary care tend to have little focus on children's care. MOCHA has found the PHAMEU initiative to measure the quality of primary care (Kringos, Boerma, van der Zee, & Groenewegen, 2013) has been widely used but this initiative is set for all ages. However, our own surveys of stakeholders indicates the desirability of developing a framework which takes into account both the development of the child and young person over time and the necessity to consider the different domains of structure process and outcome in relation to children and young people more carefully, for example when considering access, continuity and advocacy for this age group.

Investing in Child Health

It is incredibly difficult to identify the spend on and the activity of health services for children, as elaborated in Chapters 7 and 9. In order for spend to be optimised, innovative means of identifying financial spend on children and return on investment need to be developed. An actuarial approach across the life course would help policy-makers to exercise some choice in policy options. The Commission has an Expert Panel on Innovative Ways of Investing in Health (https://ec.europa.eu/health/expert_panel/home_en), and we would see merit in linkage with other activities so as to give evidence-based guidance on cost-effective and actuarially based investments which would benefit children's health (such possibly as professional education, evaluated prevention programmes and e-health).

Improving Child Centric e-Health Standards and Evaluation

DG CONNECT leads an active e-health research and development programme. However, our work on e-health found little focus on children despite their health service needs and also their being eager users of social media and health technologies – including exposure to un-validated ones with potential risks (see Chapter 14). There is opportunity here for focused research on development of appropriate standards and evaluation of effectiveness of these technologies.

MOCHA itself has managed in a modest way to kick-start linkage with the Trillium II project (https://trillium2.eu/) on Patient Summaries led by the European office of the HL7 Foundation and created a strong interest within that project in focusing on children's record summaries (see Chapter 14). However, this work is unfunded. The wish and potential opportunity are to commence with immunisation (involving also the European Centre for Disease Control (ECDC)), then move on to other child record aspects and possibly to interact with WHO in the optimisation and standardisation of data contained in national schemes for Home-based Records (see Deshpande, Rigby, Alexander, & Blair, 2018).

MOCHA has also identified the need for focussed research on the optimal data items in Electronic Health Records and for functionalities including algorithms for disease detection and other child EHR decision support applications. Indeed, as reported in Chapter 14, this need has been identified globally but is not being addressed. It could be a valuable field in which Europe could show leadership through its active e-health programme.

Collaborative and Harmonised Use of Downloaded Research Databases

In Chapter 7, we described the initiative within MOCHA to identify the many research databases in Europe compiled from operational record systems. We identified 147 of these relevant to evaluation of primary care for children, but in the event, very few could be used within the resources and timescale of the project, despite the willingness of each one to be registered with the project and to complete a metadata collation. Barriers included variation in data models and data representation, lack of resource at the individual database management level, setting of prohibitive fees and also the need to seek ethical approval for each enquiry for each database.

Exploitation within an ethical framework of very large databases is a much advocated new dimension to health research. Europe could set a lead on this – not least from the degree of opportunity we have identified. And given the paucity of data on children's health care, there is a very large need waiting to be met. We also recommend that there should be developed a common large database research governance framework which is operationalised across the EU. Ethical guidelines and a high-level ethical process could be defined collaboratively at EU level with the intention of establishing key ethical principles and codes of conduct and above all mutual recognition. Existence of this during our work could have led to much more robust evidence for our findings.

Promoting Child Rights and Equity

Europe is rightly strong on the principle of supporting Children's Rights, and indeed, DG Justice leads on monitoring this. However, many rights are focussed in high-level terms and are difficult to make meaningful at child level. The MOCHA project has sought to be innovative in selecting a number of rights statements and framing service delivery principles for child primary care as a means of delivering on those rights – see Chapter 4. Not only is further work needed to find parallel underpinning healthcare evidence, but also this initiative could be developed into a more proactive rights-achieving initiative.

Further means of monitoring equity are also needed. Chapters 5 and 8 show the current paucity of effective measurement in this field, due to a considerable degree to the lack of child-centric published data.

Recognising Children's Evolving Autonomy

Throughout this report, we have demonstrated the need for health practitioners and services to adapt to the evolving autonomy of the child and young person, whether through improved communications skills or decision making regarding treatment or developing salutogenic behaviours. Yet, technically in most countries, the law considers children to be dependents until their 18th birthday (or in some respects, until 16 years). In our work on human papilloma virus immunisation, we found countries where parents could veto the child having the protection, or conversely compulsorily injecting the child at the parent's request.

However, children are not dependent infants for 17 years – they are increasingly enquiring, active and responsible human beings seeking to set their own course in life, adjusted to their own characteristics. Europe has recognised that this simple 'incompetent unless fully competent' attitude is inappropriate for older citizens, whose drive and whose cognitive ability may gradually reduce, but who do not want a sudden and irreversible progression from legal competence to legal dependence. Hence, Europe has initiated opportunities and frameworks for assisted decision-making, whereby the citizen can delegate (or be relieved of) some responsibilities, while still being able to express basic preferences and choices. We believe that there is an urgent need to initiate similar innovation for children, so that as their comprehension, decision-making and actions progressively increase, so they can formally express and have recorded their preferences and wishes. This was well demonstrated in Chapters 11 and 12. We see the scope for further work on this, with a view to developing a European set of principles matching at the early stage of life of the assisted decision-making principles for the late stages of life.

Conclusion

MOCHA set out with the goal of identifying through research the optimal models of primary care for children. For the reasons cited, this is an impossible challenge as environment and society so dominate citizen health, and acceptable means of delivering health care, that no one model will fit all. But we have seen the importance of evidence-based approaches and have been increasingly frustrated and saddened at the inability to marshal strong evidence, or undertake local comparisons, due to avoidable barriers. One barrier is the lack of focus on applied research to enhance children's healthcare systems – such as by being able to research relative importance of different professional skills or e-health optimisation. The second is failure to marshal existing raw data into accessible information systems yielding data that matter about children.

Yet despite these avoidable gaps, Europe has most if not all of the skills and organisations to enable better evidence to be created by applied research, and linked across European institutions and directorates, to lead to an improvement both in evidence-informed policy and in care delivery. Healthcare provision remains a national competence, but if Europe through further collaborative research could produce strong and convincing evidence on optimum components of models and design principles, thus enabling member states and populations to make evidence-informed informed decisions, this should have as much beneficial influence as European solidarity has had on, for example, environment, workplace safety or sustainability.

So in conclusion, our Optimal Model for Children's Primary Health Care in Europe is one where the European Commission is proactive, in a joined up corporate way, to enable and provide robust evidence on which member states and their populations and institutions can make informed policy decisions on intersectoral intervention on the wider determinants of child health, service structure, professional competencies, investment levels and child co-involvement in their health trajectory.

References

Deshpande, S., Rigby, M., Alexander, D., & Blair, M. (2018). *Home based records.* Retrieved from www.childhealthservicemodels.eu/wp-content/uploads/R15-Home-Based-Records-Report.pdf

DG Employment, Social Affairs and Inclusion. (2018). *European skills/competencies, qualifications and occupations.* Retrieved from https://ec.europa.eu/esco/portal/home

European Commission. (2016). *So what? Strategies across Europe to assess quality of care — Report by the expert groups on health systems performance assessment.* Retrieved from https://ec.europa.eu/health/sites/health/files/systems_performance_assessment/docs/sowhat_en.pdf

Kocken, P., Vlasblom, E., de Lijster, G., & Reijneveld, M. (2018*). Consensus statements of stakeholders on most optimal models of child primary healthcare with guidance on potential benefits and how these might be achieved.* Retrieved from http://www.childhealthservicemodels.eu/wp-content/uploads/Deliverable-D18-9.2-A-report-containing-consensus-statements-on-most-optimal-models-with-guidance-on-potential-benefits-and-how-these-might-be.pdf

Kringos, D. S., Boerma, W., van der Zee, J., & Groenewegen, P. (2013). Europe's strong primary care systems are linked to better population health but also to higher health spending. *Health Affairs, 32*(4), doi:10.1377/hlthaff.2012.1242

Rigby, M. J., Köhler, L. I., Blair, M. E., & Mechtler, R. (2003). Child health indicators for Europe — A priority for a caring society. *European Journal of Public Health, 13*(3 Supplement), 38–46.

Schloemer, T., & Schröder-Bäck, P. (2018). Criteria for evaluating transferability of health interventions: A systematic review and thematic synthesis. *Implementation Science, 13*(1), 88. doi:10.1186/s13012-018-0751-8

van Til, J., Groothuis-Oudshoorn, K., & Boere-Boonekamp, M., (2018). *Public priorities for primary care for children.* Retrieved from http://www.childhealthservicemodels.eu/publications/technical-reports/

World Health Organization Regional Office for Europe. (2018, June 13−14). *Health systems for prosperity and solidarity: Leaving no-one behind.* Tallinn, Estonia. Retrieved from http://www.euro.who.int/__data/assets/pdf_file/0008/373688/tallinn-outcome-statement-eng.pdf?ua=1

Zdunek, K., Schroder-Back, P., Rigby, M., & Blair, M. (2018). *The culture of evidence-based practice in child health policy − A report.* Retrieved from http://www.childhealthservicemodels.eu/publications/technical-reports/

Appendix 1: List of MOCHA Scientists

Work Package 1: Identification of Models of Children's Primary Health Care

Mitch Blair	**Imperial College, London, UK**
Barbara Corso	CNR Institute of Neuroscience (CNR-IN), Padua, Italy
Ingrid Wolfe	King's College, London, UK
Daniela Luzi	CNR Institute of Research on Population and Health Policy (IRPPS), Rome, Italy, Rome, Italy
Denise Alexander	Imperial College, London, UK
Fabrizio Pecoraro	CNR Institute of Research on Population and Health Policy (IRPPS), Rome, Italy, Rome, Italy
Filipa Ferreira	University of Surrey, UK
Harshana Liyanage	University of Surrey, UK
Helen Wells	Keele University, UK
Ilaria Rocco	CNR Institute of Neuroscience (CNR-IN), Padua, Italy
Kinga Zdunek	Medical University of Lublin, Poland
Manna Alma	University Medical Center Groningen, Netherlands
Michael Rigby	Imperial College, London, UK
Nadia Minicuci	CNR Institute of Neuroscience (CNR-IN), Padua, Italy
Oscar Tamburis	CNR Institute of Research on Population and Health Policy (IRPPS), Rome, Italy
Peter Schröder-Bäck	Maastricht University, Netherlands
Rosie Satherley	King's College, London, UK
Sapfo Lignou	King's College, London, UK
Simon de Lusignan	University of Surrey, UK
Tamara Schloemer	Maastricht University, Netherlands
Uy Hoang	University of Surrey, UK

Work Package 2: Interfaces of Models of Primary Health Care with Secondary, Social and Complex Care

Maria Brenner	**Trinity College Dublin, Ireland**
Anne Clancy	University of Tromsø, Norway
Austin Warters	Trinity College Dublin, Ireland
Colman Noctor	Trinity College Dublin, Ireland
Daniela Luzi	CNR Institute of Research on Population and Health Policy (IRPPS), Rome, Italy
Eleanor Hollywood	Trinity College Dublin, Ireland
Elena Montañana Olaso	Trinity College Dublin, Ireland
Fabrizio Pecoraro	CNR Institute of Research on Population and Health Policy (IRPPS), Rome, Italy
Harriet Hiscock	Murdoch Children's Research Institute, Australia
Ingrid Wolfe	King's College, London, UK
Jay Berry	Boston Children's Hospital
Keishia Taylor	Trinity College Dublin, Ireland
Miriam O'Shea	Trinity College Dublin, Ireland
Oscar Tamburis	Trinity College Dublin, Ireland
Phil Larkin	University College Dublin, Ireland
Rebecca McHugh	University College Dublin, Ireland
Stine Lundstroem Kamionka	University of Southern Denmark, Denmark
Tricia Keilthy	Trinity College Dublin, Ireland

Work Package 3: Effective Models of School Health Services and Adolescent Health Services

Danielle Jansen	**University Medical Center Groningen, Netherlands**
Annemieke Visser	University Medical Center Groningen, Netherlands
Eline Vlasbom	TNO (Netherlands Organisation for Applied Scientific Research), Netherlands

(*Continued*)

Johanna P. M. Vervoort	University Medical Center Groningen, Netherlands
Magda Boere-Boonekamp	University of Twente, Netherlands
Sijmen A. Reijneveld	University Medical Center Groningen, Netherlands
Paul Kocken	TNO (Netherlands Organisation for Applied Scientific Research), Netherlands
Pierre-André Michaud	University Hospital of Lausanne, Switzerland
Simon van der Pol	University Medical Center Groningen, Netherlands

Work Package 4: Identification and Application of Innovative Measures of Quality and Outcome

Nadia Minicuci	**CNR Institute of Neuroscience (CNR-IN), Padua, Italy**
Barbara Corso	CNR Institute of Neuroscience (CNR-IN), Padua, Italy
Daniela Luzi	CNR Institute of Research on Population and Health Policy (IRPPS), Rome, Italy
Fabrizio Pecoraro	CNR Institute of Research on Population and Health Policy (IRPPS), Rome, Italy
Gary Freed	Murdoch Children's Research Institute, Australia
Ilaria Rocco	CNR Institute of Neuroscience (CNR-IN), Padua, Italy
Oscar Tamburis	CNR Institute of Research on Population and Health Policy (IRPPS), Rome, Italy

Work Package 5: Identification and Use of Derivatives of Large Data Sets and Systems to Measure Quality

Simon de Lusignan	**University of Surrey, UK**
Filipa Ferreira	University of Surrey, UK
Harshana Liyanage	University of Surrey, UK
Uy Hoang	University of Surrey, UK

Work Package 6: Economic and Skill Set Evaluation and Analysis of Models

Heather Gage	**University of Surrey, UK**
Anne Clancy	University of Tromso, Norway
Daniela Luzi	CNR Institute of Research on Population and Health Policy (IRPPS), Rome, Italy
Ekelechi MacPepple	University of Surrey, UK
Fabrizio Pecoraro	CNR Institute of Research on Population and Health Policy (IRPPS), Rome, Italy
Filipa Ferreira	University of Surrey, UK
Graham Cookson	University of Surrey, UK
Nadia Minicuci	CNR Institute of Neuroscience (CNR-IN), Padua, Italy

Work Package 7: Ensuring Equity for All Children in all Models

Anders Hjern	**Karolinska Institute, Sweden**
Arzu Arat	Karolinska Institute, Sweden
Sharon Goldfeld	Murdoch Children's Research Institute, Australia

Work Package 8: The Role of Electronic Records and Data to Support Safe and Efficient Models

Michael Rigby	**Imperial College London, UK**
Adamos Hadjipanayis	European University of Cyprus, Cyprus
Fabrizio Pecoraro	CNR Institute of Neuroscience (CNR-IN), Padua, Italy
Filipa Ferreira	University of Surrey, UK
Geir Gunnlaugsson	University of Iceland, Iceland
Grit Kühne	Imperial College London, UK
Shalmali Deshpande	Imperial College London, UK
Simon de Lusignan	University of Surrey, UK

Work Package 9: Validated Optimal Models of Children's Prevention-orientated Primary Health Care

Paul Kocken	**TNO (Netherlands Organisation for Applied Scientific Research), Netherlands**
Eline Vlasbom	TNO (Netherlands Organisation for Applied Scientific Research), Netherlands
Gaby de Lijster	TNO (Netherlands Organisation for Applied Scientific Research), Netherlands
Janine van Til	University of Twente, Netherlands
Kinga Zdunek	Medical University of Lublin, Poland
Kyriakos Martakis	Maastricht University, Netherlands
Magda Boere-Boonekamp	University of Twente, Netherlands
Mitch Blair	Imperial College London, UK
Michael Rigby	Imperial College London, UK
Nicole van Kesteren	TNO (Netherlands Organisation for Applied Scientific Research), Netherlands
Peter Schröder-Bäck	Maastricht University, Netherlands
Renate van Zoonen	TNO (Netherlands Organisation for Applied Scientific Research), Netherlannds
Tamara Schloemer	Maastricht University, Netherlands

Work Package 10: Dissemination

Michael Rigby	**Imperial College London, UK**
Adamos Hadjipanayis	European University of Cyprus, Cyprus
Christine Chow	Imperial College London, UK
Danielle Jansen	University Medical Center Groningen, Netherlands
Denise Alexander	Imperial College London, UK
Kinga Zdunek	Medical University of Lublin, Poland
Maria Brenner	Trinity College Dublin, Ireland
Mitch Blair	Imperial College London, UK
Peter Schröder-Bäck	Maastricht University, Netherlands

Work Package 11: Project Management

Mitch Blair	**Imperial College London, UK**
Bernardo Hourmat	Imperial College London, UK
Christine Chow	Imperial College London, UK
Denise Alexander	Imperial College London, UK
Michael Rigby	Imperial College London, UK

MOCHA External Advisory Board

Richard Parish CBE	**Chair of External Advisory Board**
Aagje Ieven	Eurochild
Agata D'Addato	Eurochild
Aneela Ahmed	European Patients' Forum
Christopher Clouder	Alliance for Childhood
Jeni Bremner	European Health Management Association
Johan Hansen	Independent expert
Johanna Pacevicius	Assembly of European Regions
Katrin Fjeldsted	Standing Committee of European Doctors (CPME)
Lembe Kullamaa	European Patients' Forum
Neal Halfon	Independent expert
Ragnheiður Ósk Erlendsdóttir	Independent expert
Stefano del Torso	European Academy of Paediatrics
Valentina Strammiello	European Patients' Forum
Vivian Barnekow	Independent expert

Appendix 2: List of MOCHA Country Agents

http://www.childhealthservicemodels.eu/partnerlisting/country-agents/

Austria	Dr Reli Mechtler, Lilly Damm
Belgium	Dr Sophie Alexander, Dr Liesebeth Borgermans
Bulgaria	Prof Vladimir Pilossoff, Dr Georgi Christov
Croatia	Dr Ivan Pristas, Dr Marko Brkic
Cyprus	Dr Adamos Hadjipanayis
Czech Republic	Dr Ales Bourek
Denmark	Prof Carsten Obel, Niklas Munksgaard Berg
Estonia	Dr Toomas Veidebaum, Eha Nurk, Lagle Suurorg
Finland	Prof Mika Gissler
France	Dr Christine Edan
Germany	Prof Ulrike Ravens-Sieberer, Ann-Katrin Meyrose
Greece	Dr Dina Zota
Hungary	Dr Péter Altorjai
Iceland	Dr Geir Gunnlaugsson
Ireland	Carol Hilliard
Italy	Dr Roberto Buzzetti
Latvia	Prof Anita Villerusa, Irisa Zile
Lithuania	Dr Indrė Būtienė
Luxembourg	Dr Yolande Wagener
Malta	Dr Natasha Azzopardi-Muscat
Netherlands	A. Prof Danielle Jansen
Norway	Prof Anne Karin Lindhal, Dr Ingrid Sperre Saunes
Poland	Dr Kinga Zdunek
Portugal	Prof Margarida Gaspar de Matos
Romania	Dr Maria Roth

(*Continued*)

Slovakia	Prof Jozef Suvada
Slovenia	Dr Polonca Truden, Dr Jernej Zavrsnik
Spain	Prof Luis Martin Alvarez
Sweden	Dr Anders Hjern
United Kingdom	Prof Mitch Blair, Marcia Philbin, Lisa Cummins

Index

Printed in the United States
By Bookmasters